Library
Education Centre
Royal Liverpool University Hospital
Prescot Street
Liverpool
L7 8XP

D1389574

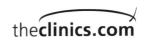

GASTROENTEROLOGY CLINICS OF NORTH AMERICA

Dysplasia and Cancer in Inflammatory Bowel Disease

GUEST EDITOR
Francis A. Farraye, MD, MSc

September 2006 • Volume 35 • Number 3

SAUNDERS

An Imprint of Elsevier, Inc.
PHILADELPHIA   LONDON   TORONTO   MONTREAL   SYDNEY   TOKYO

W.B. SAUNDERS COMPANY
A Division of Elsevier Inc.

Elsevier Inc. • 1600 John F. Kennedy Blvd., Suite 1800 • Philadelphia, Pennsylvania 19103-2899

http://www.theclinics.com

**GASTROENTEROLOGY CLINICS
OF NORTH AMERICA**
September 2006
Editor: Kerry Holland

Volume 35, Number 3
ISSN 0889-8553
ISBN 1-4160-4015-3

Copyright © 2006 Elsevier Inc. All rights reserved. No part of this publication may be reproduced or transmitted in any form or by any means, electronic or mechanical, including photocopy, recording, or any information retrieval system, without written permission from the publisher.

Single photocopies of single articles may be made for personal use as allowed by national copyright laws. Permission of the publisher and payment of a fee is required for all other photocopying, including multiple or systematic copying, copying for advertising or promotional purposes, resale, and all forms of document delivery. Special rates are available for educational institutions that wish to make photocopies for non-profit educational classroom use. Permissions may be sought directly from Elsevier's Rights Department in Philadelphia, PA, USA; phone: (+1) 215 239 3804, fax: (+1) 215 239 3805, e-mail: healthpermissions@elsevier.com. Requests may also be completed on-line via the Elsevier homepage (http://www.elsevier.com/locate/permissions). You may also contact Rights & Permissions directly through Elsevier's home page (http://www.elsevier.com), selecting first 'Customer Support', then 'General Information', then 'Permissions Query Form'. In the USA, users may clear permissions and make payments through the Copyright Clearance Center, Inc., 222 Rosewood Drive, Danvers, MA 01923, USA; phone: (978) 750-8400, fax: (978) 750-4744, and in the UK through the Copyright Licensing Agency Rapid Clearance Service (CLARCS), 90 Tottenham Court Road, London WIP 0LP, UK; phone: (+44) 171 436 5931; fax: (+44) 171 436 3986. Other countries may have a local reprographic rights agency for payments.

Reprints. For copies of 100 or more, of articles in this publication, please contact the Commercial Reprints Department, Elsevier Inc., 360 Part Avenue South, New York, New York 10010-1710. Tel. (212) 633-3813 Fax: (212) 462-1935 e-mail: reprints@elsevier.com.

The ideas and opinions expressed in *Gastroenterology Clinics of North America* do not necessarily reflect those of the Publisher. The Publisher does not assume any responsibility for any injury and/or damage to persons or property arising out of or related to any use of the material contained in this periodical. The reader is advised to check the appropriate medical literature and the product information currently provided by the manufacturer of each drug to be administered to verify the dosage, the method and duration of administration, or contraindications. It is the responsibility of the treating physician or other health care professional, relying on independent experience and knowledge of the patient, to determine drug dosages and the best treatment for the patient. Mention of any product in this issue should not be construed as endorsement by the contributors, editors, or the Publisher of the product or manufacturers' claims.

Gastroenterology Clinics of North America (ISSN 0889-8553) is published quarterly by Elsevier Inc., 360 Park Avenue South, New York, NY 10010-1710. Months of issue are March, June, September, and December. Business and Editorial Offices: 1600 John F. Kennedy Blvd., Suite 1800, Philadelphia, PA 19103-2899. Customer Service Office: 6277 Sea Harbor Drive, Orlando, FL 32887-4800. Periodicals postage paid at New York, NY and additional mailing offices. Subscription prices are $195.00 per year (US individuals), $100.00 per year (US students), $290.00 per year (US institutions), $206.00 per year (Canadian individuals), $345.00 per year (Canadian institutions), $255.00 per year (international individuals), $130.00 per year (international students), and $345.00 per year (international institutions). Foreign air speed delivery is included in all *Clinics* subscription prices. All prices are subject to change without notice. POSTMASTER: Send address changes to *Gastroenterology Clinics of North America*, Elsevier Periodicals Customer Service 6277 Sea Harbor Drive, Orlando, FL 32887-4800. **Customer Service: 1-800-654-2452 (US). From outside of the US, call 1-407-345-4000. E-mail: hhspcs@harcourt.com**

Gastroenterology Clinics of North America is also published in Italian by Il Pensiero Scientifico Editore, Rome, Italy; and in Portuguese by Interlivros Edicoes Ltda., Rua Commandante Coelho 1085, 21250 Cordovil, Rio de Janeiro, Brazil.

Gastroenterology Clinics of North America is covered in *Index Medicus, Excerpta Medica, Current Contents/Clinical Medicine, Science Citation Index, ISI/BIOMED*, and *BIOSIS*.

Printed in the United States of America.

Dysplasia and Cancer in Inflammatory Bowel Disease

GUEST EDITOR

FRANCIS A. FARRAYE, MD, MSc, Clinical Director, Section of Gastroenterology; and Professor of Medicine, Boston University Medical Center, Boston, Massachusetts

CONTRIBUTORS

CARY B. AARONS, MD, Surgical Research Fellow, Department of Surgery, Boston University School of Medicine, Boston, Massachusetts

JAMES M. BECKER, MD, FACS, James Utley Professor of Surgery; Chairman; and Surgeon-in-Chief, Department of Surgery, Boston University Medical Center, Boston, Massachusetts

CHARLES N. BERNSTEIN, MD, Department of Internal Medicine, University of Manitoba and the University of Manitoba Inflammatory Bowel Disease Clinical and Research Centre, Winnipeg, Manitoba, Canada

ERICK P. CHAN, MD, Fellow, Division of Gastroenterology, University of Pennsylvania School of Medicine, Philadelphia, Pennsylvania

SONIA FRIEDMAN, MD, Assistant Professor, Department of Medicine, Harvard Medical School; and Associate Physician, Division of Gastroenterology, Brigham and Women's Hospital, Boston, Massachusetts

WOLFRAM GOESSLING, MD, PhD, Instructor in Medicine, Harvard Medical School; Department of Medical Oncology, Dana-Farber Cancer Institute; Department of Medicine, Brigham and Women's Hospital; and Gastrointestinal Unit, Department of Medicine, Massachusetts General Hospital, Stem Cell Program and Division of Hematology/Oncology, Children's Hospital, Boston, Massachusetts

STEVEN H. ITZKOWITZ, MD, FACP, FACG, The Dr. Burrill B. Crohn Professor of Medicine, and Associate Director, The Dr. Henry D. Janowitz Division of Gastroenterology, Mount Sinai School of Medicine, New York, New York

ROBERT T. KAVITT, MD, Resident Department of Medicine, University of Chicago, Chicago, Illinois

RALF KIESSLICH, MD, PhD, I. Med. Klinik und Poliklinik Johannes Gutenberg Universität Mainz, Mainz, Germany

GARY R. LICHTENSTEIN, MD, Professor of Medicine; and Director, Center for Inflammatory Bowel Disease, Division of Gastroenterology, University of Pennsylvania School of Medicine, Philadelphia, Pennsylvania

EDWARD V. LOFTUS, JR, MD, Associate Professor of Medicine, Division of Gastroenterology and Hepatology, Mayo Clinic College of Medicine, Rochester, Minnesota

ROBERT J. MAYER, MD, Professor of Medicine, Harvard Medical School; Director, Center for Gastrointestinal Affairs; Department of Medical Oncology, Dana-Farber Cancer Institute; and Department of Medicine, Brigham and Women's Hospital, Boston, Massachusetts

MARKUS F. NEURATH, MD, PhD, I. Med. Klinik und Poliklinik Johannes Gutenberg Universität Mainz, Mainz, Germany

ROBERT D. ODZE, MD, FRCPC, Chief, Gastrointestinal Pathology Service; and Associate Professor, Department of Pathology, Brigham and Women's Hospital, Harvard Medical School, Boston, Massachusetts

DAVID T. RUBIN, MD, Assistant Professor of Medicine, Section of Gastroenterology, The MacLean Center for Clinical Medical Ethics, and, The Reva and David Logan Center for Research in Gastroenterology, University of Chicago, Chicago, Illinois

ARTHUR F. STUCCHI, PhD, Associate Research Professor, Departments of Surgery, Pathology, and Laboratory Medicine, Boston University School, Boston, Massachusetts

GASTROENTEROLOGY CLINICS
OF NORTH AMERICA

Dysplasia and Cancer in Inflammatory Bowel Disease

CONTENTS　　　　　　　VOLUME 35 • NUMBER 3 • SEPTEMBER 2006

> Patients with ulcerative colitis (UC) are at increased risk of colorectal cancer (CRC), but a series of population-based studies published within the past 5 years suggest that this risk has decreased over time. The crude annual incidence rate of CRC in UC ranges from approximately 1 in 500 to 1 in 1600. In some cohorts, an elevated risk of CRC relative to the general population can no longer be demonstrated. The exact mechanism for this decrease in risk remains unclear but may be attributable to a combination of more widespread use of maintenance therapy and surveillance colonoscopy as well as more judicious reliance on colectomy. In addition to the classic risk factors of increased extent and duration of UC, it seems that primary sclerosing cholangitis, a family history of sporadic CRC, severity of histologic bowel inflammation, and young age at colitis onset are independent risk factors for cancer.

> Morphologic identification of dysplasia in mucosal biopsies is the best and most reliable marker of an increased risk for malignancy in patients who have inflammatory bowel disease, and it forms the basis of the recommended endoscopic surveillance strategies that are in practice for patients who have this illness. In ulcerative colitis (UC) and Crohn's disease (CD), dysplasia is defined as unequivocal neoplastic epithelium that is confined to the basement membrane, without invasion into the lamina propria. Unfortunately, unlike in UC, only a few studies have evaluated the pathologic features and biologic characteristics of dysplasia and carcinoma in CD specifically. As a result, this article focuses mainly on the pathologic features, adjunctive diagnostic methods, and differential diagnosis of dysplasia in UC.

Colorectal cancer (CRC) develops from a dysplastic precursor lesion, regardless of whether it arises sporadically, in the setting of high-risk hereditary conditions, or in the context of chronic inflammation like inflammatory bowel disease (IBD). This review focuses on the molecular alterations associated with CRC pathogenesis in IBD. Although none of the molecular alterations to be discussed have yet been integrated into clinical practice, there is potential for molecular diagnostics to enhance the management of patients with long-standing IBD.

Dysplasia can be a marker that cancer is already present or is coming in the near future. Hence, physicians should not be cavalier in approach to finding it or in approach once it is found, whether it is in flat mucosa or raised mucosa. Low-grade dysplasia should garner similar respect to high-grade dysplasia, if for no other reason than the difficulty that expert pathologists have in distinguishing it with certainty from high-grade dysplasia. There is no sure way to reduce the likelihood that dysplasia will arise in ulcerative colitis. Some investigators have promoted the use of 5-ASA; however, there is no definitive evidence that 5-ASA can reduce cancer incidence.

Colorectal cancer (CRC) remains a significant cause of mortality in patients with inflammatory bowel disease (IBD). Although most of the studies on the risk of CRC in IBD have been performed in patients with ulcerative colitis (UC), there is convincing evidence that patients with Crohn's disease (CD) have a similar risk of developing neoplasia. Although the risk of cancer in IBD remains rare, the fact that it occurs in the setting of known risk factors and at a younger age than non–IBD-related colon cancer therefore warrants prevention strategies. Current guidelines for prevention of cancer in IBD recommend routine surveillance colonoscopies with random biopsies and consideration of proctocolectomy if precancerous dysplasia is identified and confirmed. Although this approach remains of good clinical rationale, the evidence for its benefit is minimal or lacking. This article reviews the rationale and evidence for such a practice and compares current guidelines.

The newly developed high-resolution and magnification endoscopes offer features that allow more and new mucosal details to be seen. They are commonly used in conjunction with chromoendoscopy. The analysis of mucosal surface details is beginning to resemble histologic examination. More accurate recognition of small flat and depressed neoplastic lesions is possible. Endoscopic prediction of neoplastic and nonneoplastic tissue is possible by analysis of surface architecture of the mucosa, which influences the endoscopic management. For the diagnosis of flat adenomas, chromoendoscopy should be a part of the endoscopist's armamentarium. In inflammatory bowel disease, chromoendoscopy can be used for patients with long-standing UC to unmask flat intraepithelial neoplasia and is likely to become the new standard method for surveillance colonoscopy in the near future. The new detailed images seen with magnifying chromoendoscopy are the beginning of a new era in which advances in optical development, such as confocal endomicroscopy, allow a unique look at detailed cellular structures.

There has been a multitude of case reports, population studies, and studies from inflammatory bowel disease referral centers that links Crohn's disease to intestinal and extraintestinal cancers. There is good evidence to support an increased risk for colorectal cancer and small bowel adenocarcinoma. There is less evidence to support a link between Crohn's disease and lymphomas, leukemias, and carcinoids. For the cancers of the colon, small intestine, and of chronic perianal fistulas, vigilance on the part of the physician is required. For lymphomas, leukemias, and carcinoids, more studies are needed to better define an association, if any, with Crohn's disease.

Inflammatory bowel disease (IBD) clearly increases the risk for gastrointestinal (GI) malignancies, especially colorectal cancer (CRC). Surgery remains the only effective treatment for IBD-related CRC. Although the surgical options for GI cancers can vary, the indications for surgical intervention are similar for all patients who have IBD. When the appropriate surgical technique is used in IBD-related small bowel, colon, or rectal cancer, along with neoadjuvant or adjuvant chemotherapy when necessary, prognosis, function, and long-term outcomes generally are good. Although the prognosis following surgical treatment for patients who have IBD-related CRC is no worse than for those whose cancers arise sporadically, the outcomes remain poor for patients who have both Crohn's disease and small bowel adenocarcinomas, primarily because of their advanced stage at detection.

One of the most promising and important approaches to decrease the risk of colorectal carcinoma in patients with long-standing inflammatory bowel disease is chemoprevention. This strategy focuses on the primary prevention of dysplasia and carcinoma through the regular administration of medications. Although multiple agents have been investigated for such a beneficial effect, the data remain mixed, and additional studies are needed. This article reviews the current evidence supporting or refuting a chemoprotective effect of existing and emerging therapies.

Inflammatory bowel disease (IBD) is an acknowledged predisposing factor for the development of intestinal and extraintestinal cancers. In general, an increased risk for colorectal cancer exists for patients who have both ulcerative colitis (UC) and Crohn's disease (CD). Small bowel tumors are extremely rare in the general population, but their incidence is enhanced 40-fold in patients who have CD. UC confers a marginally increased risk for myeloid leukemia, whereas patients who have CD may have a trend toward a higher incidence of lymphoma. This article reviews the therapeutic options for the most common malignant complication, colorectal carcinoma, as well as specific recommendations regarding the impact of the underlying disease upon the tolerance and efficacy of chemotherapy in these patients.

ELSEVIER
SAUNDERS

GASTROENTEROLOGY CLINICS
OF NORTH AMERICA

THE CLINICS ARE NOW AVAILABLE ONLINE!

Access your subscription at:
http://www.theclinics.com

Gastroenterol Clin N Am 35 (2006) xi–xiii

GASTROENTEROLOGY CLINICS
OF NORTH AMERICA

Preface

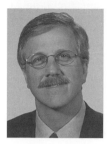

Francis A. Farraye, MD, MSc

Guest Editor

P atients with long-standing ulcerative colitis and extensive Crohn's colitis are at an increased risk for developing dysplasia and colorectal carcinoma (CRC). In addition, patients with Crohn's disease of the small intestine are at an increased risk for developing small bowel adenocarcinoma. Cancer is one of the most feared complications of inflammatory bowel disease (IBD). At present, despite a lack of evidence from randomized controlled trials, surveillance colonoscopy is the best and most widely used method to detect dysplasia and CRC in IBD patients. In this issue of the *Gastroenterology Clinics of North America*, nationally and internationally known experts review all aspects of the diagnosis and management of dysplasia and cancer in IBD. The practical information presented in this issue can be immediately incorporated into your practice to help in the management of patients with IBD at risk for developing dysplasia and CRC.

It has been appreciated for some time that an increased extent and duration of IBD are risk factors for developing CRC. Several novel risk factors have been elucidated over the past 10 to 15 years, including primary sclerosing cholangitis, family history of colorectal cancer, and endoscopic and histologic severity of inflammation. Dr. Edward Loftus from the Mayo Clinic reviews the epidemiology and risk factors for the development of dysplasia and cancer in patients with IBD. Recent studies suggest that the risk of IBD patients developing CRC may be decreasing. Although the explanation for this is not certain, Dr. Loftus suggests that several factors, including widespread introduction of maintenance therapy and surveillance colonoscopy, along with the judicious use of colectomy, may be playing a beneficial role.

At present, the morphologic identification of dysplasia in mucosal biopsies is the best and most reliable marker of an increased risk of malignancy in patients

0889-8553/06/$ – see front matter
doi:10.1016/j.gtc.2006.08.001
© 2006 Elsevier Inc. All rights reserved.
gastro.theclinics.com

with IBD and forms the basis of the currently recommended endoscopic surveillance strategies. Dr. Robert Odze from the Brigham and Women's Hospital reviews the pathology of flat and polypoid dysplasia as well as cancer in patients with IBD. The difficulties facing pathologists in the interpretation of dysplasia are highlighted, and possible adjunctive histochemical measures are discussed.

Colon carcinogenesis in IBD is a consequence of sequential episodes of somatic genetic mutation and clonal expansion. Dr. Steven Itzkowitz from the Mount Sinai Hospital discusses the molecular alterations associated with the pathogenesis of CRC in IBD. There is potential for molecular diagnostics to one day enhance the management of patients with long-standing IBD, although these advances are not yet ready for immediate clinical application.

Dysplasia in IBD may occur in flat mucosa (endoscopically invisible) or as an elevated lesion on endoscopy. Although the finding of flat high-grade dysplasia in endoscopic biopsy samples, when confirmed by at least two expert gastrointestinal pathologists, is usually considered an indication for colectomy, the indications for colectomy for low-grade dysplasia are controversial. Additionally, recent data suggest that polypoid dysplasia, if entirely resected endoscopically and unassociated with flat dysplasia elsewhere in the colon, can be managed with continued surveillance colonoscopy. Dr. Charles Bernstein from the University of Manitoba, Canada reviews the incidence, natural history, and controversies in the management of flat and polypoid dysplasia.

The performance of surveillance colonoscopy (number of biopsies, intervals, etc.) is quite variable across gastroenterology clinical practices. Drs. David Rubin and Robert Kavitt from the University of Chicago discuss the rationale and evidence for the benefit of surveillance colonoscopy to detect dysplasia and CRC in patients with IBD. Present recommendations for the performance of surveillance colonoscopy and differences between the guidelines are reviewed. In addition, surveillance for patients with ileal pouch anal anastomosis is discussed.

Newer techniques are needed to facilitate the identification of dysplastic and neoplastic lesions in patients with IBD. Chromoendoscopy may be the technique most readily applicable in clinical practice today. Drs. Ralf Kiesslich and M.F. Neurath from the University of Mainz, Germany review the technique, benefits, and limitations of chromoendoscopy. They also discuss possible future imaging modalities, including narrow-band imaging, optical coherence tomography, fluorescence endoscopy, and confocal laser endomicroscopy.

There is good evidence to support an increased risk of small and large bowel cancer as well as both squamous and adenocarcinoma associated with perianal fistulizing disease in patients with Crohn's disease. There is less evidence to support a link between Crohn's disease and lymphomas, leukemias, and carcinoids. Dr. Sonia Friedman from the Brigham and Women's Hospital critically evaluates the literature on neoplasia and Crohn's disease of the small and large bowel.

Surgery remains the only effective treatment for patients with IBD-related CRC. Surgical therapy for cancer or dysplasia in IBD is based not only on general oncologic principles but also on the procedure appropriate for the IBD diagnosis. Drs. Arthur Stucchi, Cary Aarons, and James Becker from the Boston University Medical Center review the surgical approach to colorectal and small bowel cancer in patients with IBD. Preoperative evaluation, staging, surgical options, controversies regarding ileal pouch anal procedures, and postoperative surveillance are all clearly reviewed.

Given the inherent problems associated with colonoscopic surveillance for dysplasia and cancer in patients with IBD, it has been suggested that chemoprevention be explored as a potential method to lower the risk of developing dysplasia and CRC in IBD. Chemoprevention refers to the primary prevention of dysplasia and carcinoma through the regular administration of medications. Drs. Erik Chan and Gary Lichtenstein from the University of Pennsylvania review the current evidence supporting or refuting a chemoprotective effect of the 5-ASA compounds, corticosteroids, immune modulators, ursodeoxycholic acid, folate, calcium, and statins.

Unique problems face oncologists in managing IBD patients with advanced CRC. Drs. Wolfram Goessling and Robert Mayer from the Dana Farber Cancer Institute focus on the role of the oncologist in the treatment of CRC in the setting of IBD. The authors review specific recommendations regarding the impact of the underlying IBD upon the tolerance for and efficacy of chemotherapy. Specific chemotherapy regimens are discussed.

The risk of dysplasia and colorectal cancer is a concern for both patients and their physicians. I would like to thank the authors, who did a superb job in reviewing the literature, presenting the data in a clinically useful fashion, and making this issue of the *Gastroenterology Clinics of North America* immediately applicable for readers as they manage their patients with inflammatory bowel disease.

Francis A. Farraye, MD, MSc
Section of Gastroenterology
Boston University Medical Center
85 East Concord Street
Boston, MA 02118, USA

E-mail address: francis.farraye@bmc.org

Gastroenterol Clin N Am 35 (2006) 517–531

GASTROENTEROLOGY CLINICS
OF NORTH AMERICA

Epidemiology and Risk Factors for Colorectal Dysplasia and Cancer in Ulcerative Colitis

Edward V. Loftus, Jr, MD

Division of Gastroenterology and Hepatology, Mayo Clinic College of Medicine, 200 First Street SW, Rochester, MN 55905, USA

Crohn and Rosenberg [1] of Mount Sinai Hospital in New York are credited with the first case report of colorectal cancer (CRC) occurring in the setting of ulcerative colitis (UC) in 1925. Shortly thereafter, Bargen [2] of the Mayo Clinic published a case series of 20 patients with UC with malignant disease of the colon. A series of reports over the next several decades firmly established the link between UC and CRC [3–5], and by the 1970s, some reports described a cumulative probability of developing CRC as high as 60% after a duration of UC of at least 40 years [6]. It became recognized that extensive involvement of the colon by UC and increased duration of the condition were risk factors for CRC. By this point in time, many surgeons advocated the consideration of prophylactic colectomy for patients with UC with extensive involvement and duration of at least 10 years. Indeed, the increased risk of CRC, coupled with the finding of decreased overall survival of patients with UC compared with the general population, led to difficulties for some patients with UC in securing life insurance and health insurance policies at a reasonable cost or at all.

Recently performed studies hint at a changing picture, however. Not only do patients with UC in many cohorts not seem to have a significantly increased risk of CRC [7–9], but overall survival in some of these cohorts is equal to or better than what would have been expected in the general population [10,11]. Furthermore, over the past 15 years, a number of intriguing risk factors for CRC in UC, beyond disease extent and duration, have been identified. It therefore seems timely to review the descriptive epidemiology of colorectal neoplasia in inflammatory bowel disease (IBD), with a focus on UC. Risk factors for colorectal neoplasia in UC are also reviewed. The relation between Crohn's

Dr. Loftus has received research support in the past 12 months from Procter and Gamble, Abbott, and Schering-Plough. He has served as a consultant in the past 12 months for Abbott, UCB, Elan, Shire, and Prometheus Laboratories.

E-mail address: loftus.edward@mayo.edu

0889-8553/06/$ – see front matter © 2006 Elsevier Inc. All rights reserved.
doi:10.1016/j.gtc.2006.07.005

disease and CRC is beyond the scope of this article and is reviewed elsewhere in this issue. Intriguing protective factors for colorectal neoplasia have recently been proposed and studied, most notably medical therapy for IBD (eg, 5-aminosalicylic [5-ASA]) and surveillance colonoscopy, but each of these topics is reviewed elsewhere in this issue.

RISK OF COLORECTAL CANCER IN ULCERATIVE COLITIS
The reported "risk" of CRC in UC has varied considerably, and these differences can be attributed to numerous factors, including marked differences in study design, geographic differences in CRC risk, secular changes in CRC risk over time, and even differences in the definition of "incidence" [12,13]. As one might expect, studies based on patients evaluated at tertiary care facilities or hospitals tend to demonstrate a higher cancer risk and worse prognosis than those based on population-based cohorts from a defined geographic region. Some studies exclude CRC diagnosed within a certain time period of UC diagnosis, whereas others do not. The completeness of follow-up varies considerably across studies.

Absolute Risk (Prevalence, Incidence, and Cumulative Probability)
Eaden and colleagues [14] attempted to pool the results of 116 studies involving 54,478 patients with UC, in whom 1698 CRCs were detected, in a meta-analysis published in 2001 (Table 1). This was a mixture of referral center–based, hospital-based, and population-based studies of variable methodologic quality and level of detail. The overall "prevalence" of CRC in UC (ie, cases of CRC divided by cases of UC) was 3.7% [14]. The clinical significance of prevalence in this context is debatable, however, because this value is derived from cross-sectional studies and studies of quite variable degrees of longitudinal follow-up. A more appropriate measure of absolute risk is incidence (ie, cases of CRC divided by person-years of follow-up among all UC cases). In the meta-analysis by Eaden and colleagues [14], the overall incidence of CRC in the 41 studies that reported duration of UC was three cases of CRC per 1000 person-years of UC follow-up (see Table 1). Stated another way, the annual risk of CRC in UC was 0.3%, or 1 in 333. This figure does not take into account varying degrees of annual risk based on duration of UC, however. In a qualitative review of CRC risk in UC published the year before, the same authors [15] noted annual CRC incidence rates of 1 in 100 to 1 in 200 based on studies from Sweden [16] and the early St. Mark's Hospital experience [17].

Based on 19 studies that reported CRC incidence at 10-year intervals of UC duration, Eaden and colleagues [14] were able to estimate the cumulative probability of CRC (see Table 1). After 20 years' duration of UC, the cumulative risk of CRC was 8.3% (95% confidence interval [CI], 4.8–11.7), and this figure rose to 18.4% (95% CI, 15.3–21.5) after 30 years of disease. In other words, one would expect to diagnose CRC in almost one in five individuals with UC and intact colons after 3 decades of the condition.

Table 1
Findings from the meta-analysis of colorectal cancer risk in ulcerative colitis conducted by Eaden and Colleagues

Parameter	Value (95% CI)
CRC prevalence, %[a]	3.7 (3.2–4.2)
Overall annual CRC incidence, %[b]	0.3 (0.2–0.4)
Annual CRC incidence in first decade of UC, %[c]	0.2 (0.1–0.2)
Annual CRC incidence in second decade of UC, %[c]	0.7 (0.4–1.2)
Annual CRC incidence in third decade of UC, %[c]	1.2 (0.7–1.9)
Cumulative CRC incidence after 10 years, %[c]	1.6 (1.2–2.0)
Cumulative CRC incidence after 20 years, %[c]	8.3 (4.8–11.7)
Cumulative CRC incidence after 30 years, %[c]	18.4 (15.3–21.5)

Abbreviations: CI, confidence interval; CRC, colorectal cancer; UC, ulcerative colitis.
[a]Includes results from all 116 studies.
[b]Includes results from 41 studies reporting duration of UC.
[c]Includes results from 19 studies reporting results at 10-year intervals of UC duration.
Data from Eaden JA, Abrams KR, Mayberry JF. The risk of colorectal cancer in ulcerative colitis: a meta-analysis. Gut 2001;48:526–35.

Several population-based estimates of the incidence of CRC in UC have been reported since publication of this meta-analysis (Table 2), and the results of these studies suggest a lower incidence [7,9,18–20]. Palli and coworkers [7] reported cancer incidence in a population of patients with IBD diagnosed in Florence, Italy between 1978 and 1992. They identified 10 CRCs among 689 patients with UC followed for 7877 person-years, equating to an annual incidence rate of 0.13% or approximately 1 in 700. Bernstein and colleagues [18] identified 36 colon cancers and 13 rectal cancers among 2672 patients with UC who were diagnosed between 1984 and 1997 and were followed for 19,665 person-years in the Canadian province of Manitoba. The annual risks of colon and rectal cancer were 0.16% and 0.06%, respectively, for a combined annual risk of approximately 0.2%, or 1 in 500. In an inception cohort from Copenhagen County, Denmark diagnosed between 1962 and 1987, 13 CRCs were reported among 1160 patients with UC followed for 22,290 person-years, yielding an annual risk of 0.06% or 1 in 1600 [19]. The 30-year cumulative probability of CRC was only 2.1%. In the Hungarian province of Veszprem, 723 patients with UC diagnosed over a 30-year period were followed for 8564 person-years [20]. Thirteen CRCs were detected, yielding an annual crude incidence of 0.15%, or approximately 1 in 650. The 30-year probability of CRC was 7.5% [20]. Finally, a much smaller cohort of 378 patients with UC diagnosed between 1940 and 2001 in Olmsted County, Minnesota were followed for 5567 person-years, and 6 CRCs were detected [9]. The crude annual risk of CRC in this UC cohort was approximately 0.1%, or 1 in 1000. The 30-year cumulative risk of CRC was only 2.0% [9]. It is interesting to note that no Olmsted County resident diagnosed with UC after 1980 developed CRC.

These five population-based studies [7,9,18–20] would suggest that the con temporary incidence rate of CRC in UC, ranging from 1 in 500 to 1 in 16(

Table 2

Recent population-based studies of colorectal cancer risk in ulcerative colitis

Study (reference)	Location	Dates	UC cohort size (n)	Person-years follow-up	Colorectal cancers (n)	Annual crude incidence rate (%)	Cumulative incidence at 30 years (%)	Relative risk (95% CI)[a]
Palli, et al [7]	Florence, Italy	1978–1992	689	7877	10	0.12%	NR	1.79 (0.9–3.3)
Bernstein, et al [18]	Manitoba, Canada	1984–1997	2672	19,665	36 colon	0.16%	NR	2.75 (1.9–4.0)
Bernstein, et al [18]	Manitoba, Canada	1984–1997	2672	19,665	13 rectal	0.06%	NR	1.90 (1.0–3.4)
Winther, et al [19]	Copenhagen County, Denmark	1962–1987	1160	22,290	13	0.06%	2.1%	1.05 (0.6–1.8)
Lakatos, et al [20]	Veszprem, Hungary	1974–2004	723	8564	13	0.15%	7.5%	NR
Jess, et al [9]	Olmsted County, Minnesota	1940–2001	378	5567	6	0.1%	2.0%	1.1 (0.4–2.4)

Abbreviations: CI, confidence interval; NR, not reported; UC, ulcerative colitis.

[a]Reported as incidence rate ratio in study by Bernstein and colleagues [18] and as standardized morbidity ratio in the other studies [7,9,19].

annually, may be considerably lower than the pooled estimate of 1 in 300 in the 2001 meta-analysis [14]. The reasons for this apparent decline in incidence remain unclear, but possibilities include more widespread institution of surveillance colonoscopy, a higher prevalence of patients on maintenance therapy (which, in turn, could lead to a lower prevalence of chronic bowel inflammation or to another mechanism of chemoprevention), and a fairly aggressive surgical approach in the case of the Copenhagen County and Olmsted County cohorts [9,19], with 30-year colectomy rates of between 20% and 30%. There also remains the possibility that factors completely unrelated to IBD are playing a role in the declining incidence (eg, changes in diet, differences in water supply).

The findings of these recently published population-based estimates of CRC incidence are further corroborated by data arising from the large colonoscopic surveillance program at St. Mark's Hospital between 1970 and 2001 [21]. Six hundred patients with UC with extensive involvement were followed for 5932 person-years, and 30 CRCs were detected (annual risk of 0.5%). The cumulative probability of CRC in patients with UC undergoing surveillance was only 7.6% after 30 years of disease [21]. Linear regression suggested that CRC incidence declined over the course of the study. Furthermore, a study of pathology records at the Karolinska Institute in Stockholm, Sweden revealed a 15-fold decrease in the frequency of UC-related CRC between the 1950s and 1990s, despite a steady incidence rate of UC and a growing population in Stockholm County [22].

Relative Risk

The risk of CRC can also be expressed in relative terms, as a standardized morbidity ratio (SMR; observed cancers in a UC cohort divided by expected cancers, with expected rates derived from the general population) or an incidence rate ratio (IRR; observed incidence of cancers in a UC cohort divided by observed incidence of cancers in a control cohort of the general population). Population-based studies from Sweden have demonstrated a fourfold to sixfold increased risk of CRC relative to what would have been expected in the general population [16,23]. Population-based estimates elsewhere do not suggest a relative risk this high, however. Bernstein and colleagues [18] were able to compare the incidence rate of CRC in a cohort of patients with UC and a non-IBD patient cohort. The IRR for colon cancer in UC was 2.75 (95% CI, 1.91–3.97), and for rectal cancer, it was 1.90 (95% CI, 1.05–3.43) (see Table 2). This elevation in risk was statistically significant but considerably lower than what had been described in Sweden.

Studies of population-based cohorts from Florence [7], Copenhagen County [19], and Olmsted County [9] would suggest an even lower relative risk of CRC (see Table 2). In the Florence study, 689 patients with UC diagnosed between 1978 and 1992 were followed for a total of 7877 person-years, and 10 CRCs were diagnosed [7]. Based on cancer rates in Tuscany over the same time period, 5.6 CRCs would have been expected, suggesting that the risk was 80% higher than expected (SMR = 1.79; 95% CI, 0.9–3.3) [7]. The SMR for CRC in patients with UC from Copenhagen County was estimated to be only 1.05 (95% CI, 0.56–1.79) [19]. In Olmsted County, the SMR for CRC in patients with UC was 1.1 (95% CI, 0.4–2.4) [9]. In other words, none of these studies could demonstrate an elevated risk of CRC relative to the general population.

Although these studies suggest that the relative risk of CRC is considerably lower than previously described and perhaps no longer "statistically significant," clinicians treating patients with UC should not relax their vigilance in detecting colorectal neoplasia. Some would argue quite the opposite–that the low rates of CRC observed in these studies are the successful result of timely and appropriate access to good health care, including maintenance therapies, surveillance colonoscopy, and surgery [24].

INCIDENCE OF COLORECTAL DYSPLASIA

The incidence of colorectal dysplasia in UC is more difficult to determine than the incidence of CRC. First of all, unlike the "hard end point" of CRC, there is considerable interobserver variability in the diagnosis of dysplasia, especially low-grade dysplasia (LGD) [25]. More importantly, because dysplasia is generally asymptomatic, its detection depends on the frequency and intensity of colonoscopic surveillance. Thus, reports arising from surveillance programs with high compliance rates may indicate higher rates of dysplasia than those from "real-world" practice. Finally, varying treatment practices with respect to maintenance therapies and colectomy may have an impact on the incidence of dysplasia.

Two population-based studies have examined the incidence of colorectal dysplasia in UC [26,27]. In Örnsköldsvik, Sweden, 204 patients with UC (66% with pancolitis) were followed for 3664 person-years (median of 16.5 years per person), and compliance with colonoscopic surveillance was high [26]. Fifty-two patients (24%) developed dysplasia at some point in their disease course, and a total of 88 lesions were identified. The cumulative risk of dysplasia was not calculated. A crude incidence rate can be calculated based on the number of dysplastic lesions and person-years of follow-up and is approximately 2.4% annually. Dysplastic lesions included polypoid dysplasia (n = 17), high-grade dysplasia (HGD; n = 9), and LGD (n > 41). In Olmsted County, Minnesota, where surveillance colonoscopy was recommended but not performed under a rigid protocol, 22 dysplastic lesions were identified among 378 patients with UC, including 8 flat or polypoid lesions, 12 adenomas or adenoma-like lesions within an area of active colitis, and 2 adenomas proximal to the area of active colitis [27]. The cumulative incidence of dysplasia in this cohort was 9.2% after 25 years of disease.

Another recent estimate of colorectal neoplasia incidence comes from the St. Mark's Hospital program, where 600 patients underwent a total of 2627 colonoscopies (median of 3 per patient) over 5080 person-years (mean follow-up of 8.5 years) [21]. Forty-seven patients (7.8%) developed 78 episodes of LGD, and

19 patients (3.2%) developed 30 episodes of HGD. Polypoid dysplasia was identified in 20 patients, and 32 patients were noted to have sporadic adenomas. All told, the cumulative probability of developing dysplasia or CRC was 7.7% at 20 years and 15.8% at 30 years [21].

DEMOGRAPHICS OF PATIENTS WITH ULCERATIVE COLITIS WITH COLORECTAL CANCER

What are the typical demographic characteristics of patients with UC who develop CRC? In the meta-analysis by Eaden and colleagues [14], the mean age at CRC diagnosis was 43.2 years (95% CI, 40.5–45.9) and the mean duration of UC at CRC diagnosis was 16.3 years (95% CI, 15.0–17.6). In a study of 241 patients with UC with CRC evaluated at the Mayo Clinic in Rochester, Minnesota between 1976 and 1996, these values were remarkably similar—the median age at UC diagnosis was 27 years (range: 6–76 years), the median duration of UC at CRC diagnosis was 16 years (range: 0–64 years), and the median age at CRC diagnosis was 46 years (range: 17–85 years) [28]. Thus, the typical patient with UC-CRC seems to have been diagnosed with UC at an age slightly younger than usual and has had the condition for a decade and a half before CRC diagnosis. The role of younger age at onset of IBD is further explored as a putative risk factor for UC-CRC elsewhere in this article.

Surprisingly little has been written about gender distribution of UC-CRC. Some studies hint that men may be at greater risk, but the data are conflicting. In the Manitoba study, the increased risk of colon cancer was higher among men than women (IRR: 3.2 versus 2.2) [18]. In the Mayo Clinic study of 241 patients with UC-CRC, 67% were male [28]. Furthermore, in Olmsted County, two thirds of the cases of CRC detected in the UC cohort occurred in men [9]. Finally, a preliminary report of a case-control study from an IBD endoscopy database at the University of Chicago on the role of inflammation in dysplasia and CRC risk in UC suggested that male gender was an independent risk factor for colorectal neoplasia even after controlling for other important variables, such as duration and extent of disease [29]. Conversely, male gender did not seem to influence cancer risk in Uppsala, Sweden [16], Copenhagen County [19], or Veszprem [20] or in the surveillance program at St. Mark's Hospital [21].

RISK FACTORS FOR COLORECTAL DYSPLASIA AND CANCER
Duration of Inflammatory Bowel Disease

The mechanisms by which UC leads to CRC are beyond the scope of this article and are presented elsewhere in this issue; nevertheless, it stands to reason that the mechanisms are related to chronic inflammation and that the longer the chronic bowel inflammation is ongoing, the higher is the risk for colorectal dysplasia and CRC. In the landmark study by Ekbom and colleagues [16] from Uppsala, Sweden, an analysis stratified by duration of UC showed that the relative risk of CRC, as measured by SMR, rose from approximately threefold in years 5 through 9 to approximately 17-fold in years 25 though 29. (The absolute risk, as measured by crude annual CRC incidence, rose from 0.1% to 1.3% over the same duration intervals.) Eaden and colleagues [14] were able to quantify the relation between duration of UC and CRC risk in their meta-analysis (see Table 1). When the results of the 19 studies reporting CRC risk in 10-year increments were pooled, the annual incidence of CRC in the first decade of disease was 0.2%, rising to an annual risk of 0.7% in the second decade of UC and to 1.2% annually in the third decade. In some studies, this annual risk rises exponentially with duration beyond 30 years and has led some societies to call for surveillance colonoscopy every 1 to 3 years between years 8 and 20 and then every 1 to 2 years after year 20 [30]. Conversely, some of the recently published population-based studies could not demonstrate a clear-cut relation between UC duration and cancer risk [9]. Furthermore, in the large St. Mark's Hospital surveillance colonoscopy program, the slope of the actuarial cumulative incidence curve of CRC remained constant over time, suggesting that the frequency of surveillance did not have to be increased over time [21]. This particular point remains controversial.

Extent of Inflammatory Bowel Disease

The other "classic" risk factor for UC-related CRC is increased extent of colitis. The Uppsala study demonstrated this in stark fashion: patients with proctitis alone had a CRC risk that was only 70% higher (and not significantly different) than expected, those with left-sided colitis had a risk 2.8 times higher than expected, and patients with pancolitis had a cancer risk greater than 14 times higher than expected [16]. This observation was further quantified in the meta-analysis by Eaden and colleagues [14]. The overall prevalence of CRC among patients with UC in all 116 studies was 3.7%, but when restricted to the 35 studies that stratified their analyses by extent of UC, the prevalence of CRC among patients with extensive involvement rose to 5.4%. Even in the Olmsted County study, where the overall risk was not significantly elevated compared with the general population, a subgroup analysis by extent showed a risk gradient, with the SMR rising from 0 in patients with proctitis to 0.8 in patients with left-sided UC and to 2.4 in patients with extensive or pancolonic involvement [9]. It seems reasonable to continue to risk-stratify patients with UC based on the extent of their disease.

Primary Sclerosing Cholangitis

In 1992, Broome and colleagues [31] noted in a case-control study that the prevalence of primary sclerosing cholangitis (PSC) was 28% in their 17 patients with UC with colorectal dysplasia or DNA aneuploidy versus 0% in their 55 patients without precancerous abnormalities, raising the possibility that PSC, which normally has a prevalence in UC of approximately 5%, might be a risk factor for colorectal neoplasia. Numerous studies conducted since then have for the most part demonstrated that patients with PSC and UC are at particularly increased risk for CRC and colorectal dysplasia [32–42]. The strongest evidence comes from studies from Sweden. In a small referral-based cohort from Huddinge University Hospital, the cumulative probability of dysplasia or cancer in 40 patients with PSC-IBD was much higher (31% after 20 years of UC) than in a control group of patients with UC without PSC who were matched for age, onset of UC, and extent (5% after 20 years) [33]. In one study, a cohort of 125 patients with cholangiographically documented PSC was followed by linkage to the Swedish National Cancer Registry [38]. Among the 104 patients with PSC with intact colons at the time of PSC diagnosis, the cumulative risk of CRC was 16% at 10 years after PSC diagnosis. When assessed from the date of UC diagnosis, the cumulative CRC risk was 33% at 20 years and 40% at 30 years after UC diagnosis [38]. Several years later, Bergquist and colleagues [41], through a network of Swedish hepatologists, assembled a cohort of 604 patients with PSC diagnosed in Sweden between 1970 and 1998 and followed them through 1998 by linkage to the Swedish National Cancer Registry. Twelve CRCs developed over 4123 person-years of follow-up (crude annual risk of 0.3%), with only 1.2 cancers expected, yielding an SMR of 10.3 (95% CI, 5.3–18.1). Neither study had a comparison group of patients with UC without PSC.

There has been some debate as to the mechanism of this association. Is PSC a marker for subclinical long-standing pancolitis, or is there something intrinsically different about PSC-related IBD, such that PSC is a risk factor independent of duration and extent? It is difficult, if not impossible, to design studies to answer these questions, especially because PSC is relatively rare, both diseases can be insidious in onset, and the outcome variable itself, at least in the case of dysplasia, is subject to interobserver variability.

Evidence to support the concept that PSC is strongly associated with a quiescent to mild pancolitis can be gleaned from a variety of sources. In one study, 9 patients with PSC without clinical symptoms to suggest IBD underwent a colonoscopy with biopsies [43]. Endoscopic findings were subtle and variable, but 7 patients (77%) had histologic evidence of IBD, 1 already had LGD, and 1 had indefinite dysplasia, suggesting that the subclinical colitis may have been long-standing. The same group of investigators compared colonic disease activity in 29 patients with PSC-IBD and in 58 patients with extensive UC but no PSC and found that patients with PSC were twice as likely to have never required corticosteroid treatment for their IBD (52% versus 24%; $P < .05$) and three times as likely to have never required hospitalization for treatment of IBD (55% versus 19%; $P < .02$) [44]. In a Mayo Clinic comparison of 71 patients with PSC-IBD and 142 patients with extensive UC without PSC, proctocolectomy was significantly less likely in patients with PSC [42].

Other evidence, however, suggests that long-standing subclinical extensive colitis alone cannot explain the increased risk in patients with PSC-IBD. A case-control study and a post-hoc secondary analysis of a randomized clinical trial suggest that ursodeoxycholic acid (UDCA) may reduce the risk of colorectal dysplasia and CRC in patients with PSC-IBD [45,46]. The case-control study of 59 patients with PSC-IBD found a 50% prevalence of UDCA use among the patients with dysplasia and an 85% prevalence of UDCA use in those without dysplasia, yielding an odds ratio (OR) for dysplasia of 0.18 (95% CI, 0.05–0.61) [45]. Among 105 patients with PSC enrolled into a randomized, double-blind, placebo-controlled trial of UDCA in the treatment of PSC, 85 had PSC-IBD and 52 were eligible for the post-hoc analysis [46]. (The others were excluded for a previous proctocolectomy or a recent or concurrent diagnosis of dysplasia or CRC.) The median duration of treatment was between 40 and 42 months. Colorectal dysplasia or CRC developed in 3 patients initially assigned to UDCA (10%) and in 8 patients initially assigned to placebo (35%), yielding a relative risk of dysplasia or CRC of 0.26 in the UDCA group (95% CI, 0.1–0.9) [46]. There is no reason to suspect that UDCA would reduce CRC risk in PSC-IBD unless PSC somehow exerted a carcinogenic effect through alteration in the colonic bile acid milieu.

Regardless of the exact mechanism of the association, it is clear that patients with PSC-IBD are at especially high risk for colorectal dysplasia or CRC. In a Mayo Clinic study of 71 patients with PSC-IBD with intact colons, the cumulative probability of dysplasia or cancer at 10 years after the latest of three dates (first Mayo visit, diagnosis of PSC, or diagnosis of IBD) was greater than 50% [42]. For this reason, patients with UC who are diagnosed with PSC should be enrolled immediately in a colonoscopic surveillance program regardless of UC duration, and patients with PSC without IBD, even those who are asymptomatic, should undergo a full colonoscopy with extensive biopsies even if no endoscopic abnormalities are present.

Family History of Colorectal Cancer

Nuako and colleagues [47] performed a case-control study of risk factors for CRC in UC and found that a family history of sporadic CRC (first-degree relatives only), irrespective of a family history of IBD, was independently associated with a twofold risk of CRC in patients with UC. Eaden and coworkers [48] also identified a family history of sporadic UC as an independent risk factor (OR = 5.0, 95% CI, 1.1–23), although this was more broadly defined as CRC in any relative. When using the more stringent definition of a first-degree relative, the association remained positive but no longer statistically significant (OR = 3.5, 95% CI, 0.7–17). Askling and colleagues [49] used four population-based cohorts from Sweden to identify 10,649 patients with UC and found that a family history of sporadic UC was independently associated with a twofold increase in CRC risk. In a more recent case-control study from the Mayo Clinic, a family history of CRC remained independently associated with CRC risk in patients with UC even after controlling for other important variables, such as PSC, surveillance colonoscopy, presence of pseudopolyps, 5-ASA therapy, and use of nonsteroidal anti-inflammatory drugs or aspirin (OR = 3.7, 95% CI, 1.0–13.2) [50]. The weight of evidence does seem to support the observation that a family history of CRC is an additional risk factor for cancer in patients with UC.

Severity of Chronic Bowel Inflammation

Despite the long-standing belief of many that the risk of CRC in UC must be related to chronic bowel inflammation, until recently, no clinical study could link the severity of colonic inflammation with CRC risk, with the exception of a single study in 1964 [51]. A number of detailed case-control studies found no significant association with the severity of colitis, as measured by hospitalization, frequency of diagnostic testing, and frequency of symptomatic exacerbations [48,52]. These studies relied on markers that were primarily based on symptoms and not on the degree of endoscopic or histologic inflammation. Rutter and colleagues [53] at St. Mark's Hospital took this a step further by reviewing in detail the endoscopy reports and pathology reports of 68 patients with UC with CRC or dysplasia and 136 patients with UC without colorectal neoplasia and assigning a severity score (0–4 on a 5-point scale) to each segment of the colon for each colonoscopy based on retrospective review of the reports. Univariate analysis suggested a strong link between endoscopic (OR = 2.5, 95% CI, 1.4–4.4) or histologic (OR = 5.1, 95% CI, 2.4–11.1) score and colorectal neoplasia. After controlling for other important risk factors, the association between neoplasia and histologic score remained significant (OR = 4.7, 95% CI, 2.1–10.5) [53]. This association was recently confirmed in a preliminary report from the University of Chicago [29]. The corollary to this is that certain endoscopic findings, generally those indicative of long-standing and perhaps severe inflammation, may also be associated with neoplasia [54]. In the same group of cases and controls from St. Mark's Hospital, Rutter and coworkers [54] demonstrated that CRC or dysplasia risk was linked to postinflammatory polyps (OR = 2.3) and strictures (OR = 4.6) but that a macroscopically normal-appearing colon may be inversely associated with neoplastic risk (OR = 0.4).

Age at Ulcerative Colitis Diagnosis

Whether young age at onset of UC is a risk factor for CRC, independent of duration of UC, is unsettled. In the meta-analysis by Eaden and colleagues [14], the overall crude annual incidence rate of 0.6% in studies restricted to pediatric-onset UC was numerically higher than that calculated for adults (0.3%). Individual population-based studies from Sweden seem to indicate that young age at onset of IBD is indeed a risk factor for cancer [16,23]. For example, in the Uppsala cohort, even after controlling for other factors (eg, extent, duration), patients with UC diagnosed before the age of 15 years were four times more likely than those diagnosed with UC between the ages of 15 and 29 years to develop CRC, whereas older age groups were significantly less likely to develop CRC [16]. When the Stockholm County cohort was divided into three strata by age at diagnosis, the significantly elevated CRC risk was observed only in the youngest onset stratum (less than 30 years old at UC diagnosis) [23]. In Manitoba, the highest IRR of CRC observed was in those patients with IBD diagnosed when they were younger than 40 years of age [18]. Similar numeric trends, not statistically significant, have been observed in Copenhagen and Olmsted Counties [9,19]. The weight of evidence would suggest that younger age at colitis onset is an independent risk factor for CRC.

Backwash Ileitis

The term *backwash ileitis* was first used by Crohn and Rosenak [55] in 1936 to describe mild mucosal inflammation of the extremely distal terminal ileum in patients with UC with pancolonic involvement. The colon resection specimens of 590 patients with UC who underwent a proctocolectomy with ileal pouch–anal anastomosis at a single German referral center were examined for histologic evidence of backwash ileitis, pancolitis, CRC, and colorectal dysplasia [56]. The prevalence of CRC in those with backwash ileitis was 29% compared with a CRC prevalence of only 9% in patients with pancolitis without backwash ileitis and 1.8% in those with left-sided colitis ($P < .001$). In multivariate analysis, using CRC as the dependent variable and adjusting for other factors, such as dysplasia, increased duration, and PSC, pancolitis with backwash ileitis remained a significant risk factor (OR = 19.4, 95% CI, 4.6–136), and this was higher than the OR observed with pancolitis without ileitis (OR = 9.6, 95% CI, 2.4–66) [56]. Selection bias may have influenced the results (ie, only those undergoing a colectomy were included), however, and other studies have not been able to reproduce these findings [42,54]. A detailed pathologic study of 200 patients with UC, including 34 with histologically confirmed backwash ileitis, found no difference in the frequency of dysplasia or CRC in those patients with or without backwash ileitis [57].

Geography?

The meta-analysis by Eaden and coworkers [48] found that the highest crude annual incidence rates were higher in the United Kingdom and the United States (0.4% and 0.5%, respectively), whereas rates were lower in Scandinavia and elsewhere (0.2% annually). The recent publication from Olmsted County indicates that, at least in this small region of the United States, the crude incidence rate of UC has dropped considerably, however [9]. Whether geographic differences in CRC risk still exist is unclear.

SUMMARY

Patients with UC are at increased risk of CRC, but a series of population-based studies published within the past 5 years suggest that this risk has decreased over time. The crude annual incidence rate of CRC in UC ranges from approximately 1 in 500 to 1 in 1600. In some cohorts, an elevated risk of CRC relative to the general population can no longer be demonstrated. The exact mechanism for this decrease in risk remains unclear but may be attributable to a combination of more widespread use of maintenance therapy and surveillance colonoscopy as well as more judicious reliance on colectomy. In addition to the classic risk factors of increased extent and duration of UC, it seems that PSC, a family history of sporadic CRC, severity of histologic bowel inflammation, and young age at colitis onset are independent risk factors for cancer.

References
  [1] Crohn BB, Rosenberg H. The sigmoidoscopic picture of chronic ulcerative colitis (nonspecific). Am J Med Sci 1925;170:220–7.

[2] Bargen JA. Chronic ulcerative colitis associated with malignant disease. Arch Surg 1928;17:561–76.
[3] Svartz N, Ernberg T. Cancer coli in cases of colitis ulcerosa. Acta Med Scand 1949;135: 444.
[4] Dukes CE, Lockhart-Mummery HE. Practical points in the pathology and surgical treatment of ulcerative colitis. Br J Surg 1957;45:25–36.
[5] Rosenqvist H, Ohrling H, Lagercrantz R, et al. Ulcerative colitis and carcinoma coli. Lancet 1950;1:906–8.
[6] Devroede GJ, Taylor WF, Sauer WG, et al. Cancer risk and life expectancy of children with ulcerative colitis. N Engl J Med 1971;285:17–21.
[7] Palli D, Trallori G, Bagnoli S, et al. Hodgkin's disease risk is increased in patients with ulcerative colitis. Gastroenterology 2000;119:647–53.
[8] Winther KV, Jess T, Langholz E, et al. Survival and cause-specific mortality in ulcerative colitis: follow-up of a population-based cohort in Copenhagen County. Gastroenterology 2003;125:1576–82.
[9] Jess T, Loftus EV, Velayos FS, et al. Risk of intestinal cancer in inflammatory bowel disease: a population-based study from Olmsted County, Minnesota. Gastroenterology 2006;130: 1039–46.
[10] Masala G, Bagnoli S, Ceroti M, et al. Divergent patterns of total and cancer mortality in ulcerative colitis and Crohn's disease patients: the Florence IBD study 1978–2001. Gut 2004;53:1309–13.
[11] Jess T, Loftus EV, Harmsen WS, et al. Survival and cause-specific mortality in patients with inflammatory bowel disease: a long-term outcome study in Olmsted County, Minnesota, 1940–2004. Gut, in press.
[12] Sackett DL, Whelan G. Cancer risk in ulcerative colitis: scientific requirements for the study of prognosis. Gastroenterology 1980;78:1632–5.
[13] Collins RH Jr, Feldman M, Fordtran JS. Colon cancer, dysplasia, and surveillance in patients with ulcerative colitis. A critical review. N Engl J Med 1987;316:1654–8.
[14] Eaden JA, Abrams KR, Mayberry JF. The risk of colorectal cancer in ulcerative colitis: a meta-analysis. Gut 2001;48:526–35.
[15] Eaden JA, Mayberry JF. Colorectal cancer complicating ulcerative colitis: a review. Am J Gastroenterol 2000;95:2710–9.
[16] Ekbom A, Helmick C, Zack M, et al. Ulcerative colitis and colorectal cancer. A population-based study. N Engl J Med 1990;323:1228–33.
[17] Lennard-Jones JE, Melville DM, Morson BC, et al. Precancer and cancer in extensive ulcerative colitis: findings among 401 patients over 22 years. Gut 1990;31:800–6.
[18] Bernstein CN, Blanchard JF, Kliewer E, et al. Cancer risk in patients with inflammatory bowel disease: a population-based study. Cancer 2001;91:854–62.
[19] Winther KV, Jess T, Langholz E, et al. Long-term risk of cancer in ulcerative colitis: a population-based cohort study from Copenhagen County. Clin Gastroenterol Hepatol 2004;2: 1088–95.
[20] Lakatos L, Mester G, Erdelyi Z, et al. Risk factors for ulcerative colitis-associated colorectal cancer in a Hungarian cohort of patients with ulcerative colitis: results of a population-based study. Inflamm Bowel Dis 2006;12:205–11.
[21] Rutter MD, Saunders BP, Wilkinson KH, et al. Thirty-year analysis of a colonoscopic surveillance program for neoplasia in ulcerative colitis. Gastroenterology 2006;130: 1030–8.
[22] Rubio CA, Befrits R, Ljung T, et al. Colorectal carcinoma in ulcerative colitis is decreasing in Scandinavian countries. Anticancer Res 2001;21:2921–4.
[23] Karlen P, Lofberg R, Brostrom O, et al. Increased risk of cancer in ulcerative colitis: a population-based cohort study. Am J Gastroenterol 1999;94:1047–52.
[24] Rubin DT. The changing face of colorectal cancer in inflammatory bowel disease: progress at last! Gastroenterology 2006;130:1350–2.

[25] Connell WR, Lennard-Jones JE, Williams CB, et al. Factors affecting the outcome of endoscopic surveillance for cancer in ulcerative colitis. Gastroenterology 1994;107:934–44.

[26] Lindberg J, Stenling R, Palmqvist R, et al. Efficiency of colorectal cancer surveillance in patients with ulcerative colitis: 26 years' experience in a patient cohort from a defined population area. Scand J Gastroenterol 2005;40:1076–80.

[27] Jess T, Loftus EV, Velayos FS, et al. Incidence and prognosis of colorectal dysplasia in inflammatory bowel disease: a population-based study from Olmsted County, Minnesota. Inflamm Bowel Dis, in press.

[28] Delaunoit T, Limburg PJ, Goldberg RM, et al. Colorectal cancer prognosis among patients with inflammatory bowel disease. Clin Gastroenterol Hepatol 2006;4:335–42.

[29] Rubin DT, Huo D, Rothe JA, et al. Increased inflammatory activity is an independent risk factor for dysplasia and colorectal cancer in ulcerative colitis: a case-control analysis with blinded prospective pathology review [abstract]. Gastroenterology 2006;130:A2.

[30] Itzkowitz SH, Present DH. Consensus conference: colorectal cancer screening and surveillance in inflammatory bowel disease. Inflamm Bowel Dis 2005;11:314–21.

[31] Broome U, Lindberg G, Lofberg R. Primary sclerosing cholangitis in ulcerative colitis—a risk factor for the development of dysplasia and DNA aneuploidy? Gastroenterology 1992;102:1877–80.

[32] D'Haens GR, Lashner BA, Hanauer SB. Pericholangitis and sclerosing cholangitis are risk factors for dysplasia and cancer in ulcerative colitis. Am J Gastroenterol 1993;88:1174–8.

[33] Broome U, Lofberg R, Veress B, et al. Primary sclerosing cholangitis and ulcerative colitis: evidence for increased neoplastic potential. Hepatology 1995;22:1404–8.

[34] Bansal P, Sonnenberg A. Risk factors of colorectal cancer in inflammatory bowel disease. Am J Gastroenterol 1996;91:44–8.

[35] Brentnall TA, Haggitt RC, Rabinovitch PS, et al. Risk and natural history of colonic neoplasia in patients with primary sclerosing cholangitis and ulcerative colitis. Gastroenterology 1996;110:331–8.

[36] Loftus EV Jr, Sandborn WJ, Tremaine WJ, et al. Risk of colorectal neoplasia in patients with primary sclerosing cholangitis. Gastroenterology 1996;110:432–40.

[37] Marchesa P, Lashner BA, Lavery IC, et al. The risk of cancer and dysplasia among ulcerative colitis patients with primary sclerosing cholangitis. Am J Gastroenterol 1997;92:1285–8.

[38] Kornfeld D, Ekbom A, Ihre T. Is there an excess risk for colorectal cancer in patients with ulcerative colitis and concomitant primary sclerosing cholangitis? A population based study. Gut 1997;41:522–5.

[39] Nuako KW, Ahlquist DA, Sandborn WJ, et al. Primary sclerosing cholangitis and colorectal carcinoma in patients with chronic ulcerative colitis: a case-control study. Cancer 1998;82:822–6.

[40] Shetty K, Rybicki L, Brzezinski A, et al. The risk for cancer or dysplasia in ulcerative colitis patients with primary sclerosing cholangitis. Am J Gastroenterol 1999;94:1643–9.

[41] Bergquist A, Ekbom A, Olsson R, et al. Hepatic and extrahepatic malignancies in primary sclerosing cholangitis. J Hepatol 2002;36:321–7.

[42] Loftus EV, Harewood GC, Loftus CG, et al. PSC-IBD: a unique form of inflammatory bowel disease associated with primary sclerosing cholangitis. Gut 2005;54:91–6.

[43] Broome U, Lofberg R, Lundqvist K, et al. Subclinical time span of inflammatory bowel disease in patients with primary sclerosing cholangitis. Dis Colon Rectum 1995;38:1301–5.

[44] Lundqvist K, Broome U. Differences in colonic disease activity in patients with ulcerative colitis with and without primary sclerosing cholangitis: a case control study. Dis Colon Rectum 1997;40:451–6.

[45] Tung BY, Emond MJ, Haggitt RC, et al. Ursodiol use is associated with lower prevalence of colonic neoplasia in patients with ulcerative colitis and primary sclerosing cholangitis. Ann Intern Med 2001;134:89–95.

[46] Pardi DS, Loftus EV Jr, Kremers WK, et al. Ursodeoxycholic acid as a chemopreventive agent in patients with ulcerative colitis and primary sclerosing cholangitis. Gastroenterology 2003;124:889–93.

[47] Nuako KW, Ahlquist DA, Mahoney DW, et al. Familial predisposition for colorectal cancer in chronic ulcerative colitis: a case-control study. Gastroenterology 1998;115:1079–83.

[48] Eaden J, Abrams K, Ekbom A, et al. Colorectal cancer prevention in ulcerative colitis: a case-control study. Aliment Pharmacol Ther 2000;14:145–53.

[49] Askling J, Dickman PW, Karlen P, et al. Family history as a risk factor for colorectal cancer in inflammatory bowel disease. Gastroenterology 2001;120:1356–62.

[50] Velayos FS, Loftus EV, Jess T, et al. Predictive and protective factors associated with colorectal cancer in ulcerative colitis: a case-control study. Gastroenterology 2006;130:1941–9.

[51] Edwards FC, Truelove SC. The course and prognosis of ulcerative colitis. Part IV: carcinoma of the colon. Gut 1964;5:15–22.

[52] Pinczowski D, Ekbom A, Baron J, et al. Risk factors for colorectal cancer in patients with ulcerative colitis: a case-control study. Gastroenterology 1994;107:117–20.

[53] Rutter M, Saunders B, Wilkinson K, et al. Severity of inflammation is a risk factor for colorectal neoplasia in ulcerative colitis. Gastroenterology 2004;126:451–9.

[54] Rutter MD, Saunders BP, Wilkinson KH, et al. Cancer surveillance in longstanding ulcerative colitis: endoscopic appearances help predict cancer risk. Gut 2004;53:1813–6.

[55] Crohn BB, Rosenak BD. A combined form of ileitis and colitis. JAMA 1936;106:1–7.

[56] Heuschen UA, Hinz U, Allemeyer EH, et al. Backwash ileitis is strongly associated with colorectal carcinoma in ulcerative colitis. Gastroenterology 2001;120:841–7.

[57] Haskell H, Andrews CW, Reddy SI, et al. Pathologic features and clinical significance of "backwash" ileitis in ulcerative colitis. Am J Surg Pathol 2005;29:1472–81.

Gastroenterol Clin N Am 35 (2006) 533–552

GASTROENTEROLOGY CLINICS
OF NORTH AMERICA

Pathology of Dysplasia and Cancer in Inflammatory Bowel Disease

Robert D. Odze, MD, FRCPC

Department of Pathology, Brigham and Women's Hospital, Harvard Medical School Boston, 15 Francis Street, MA 02115, USA

In ulcerative colitis (UC) and Crohn's disease (CD), there is abundant evidence to support the theory that cancer develops through an inflammation-dysplasia-carcinoma sequence [1,2].Recent studies confirmed that the risk for cancer is similar in UC and CD [3–7]. In addition, the pathologic features of dysplasia and cancer in UC are similar to CD [1,4,5,8].

Morphologic identification of dysplasia in mucosal biopsies is the best and most reliable marker of an increased risk for malignancy in patients who have inflammatory bowel disease (IBD), and it forms the basis of the recommended endoscopic surveillance strategies that are in practice for patients who have this illness [2,9,10]. In UC and CD, dysplasia is defined as unequivocal neoplastic epithelium that is confined to the basement membrane, without invasion into the lamina propria [9]. Unfortunately, unlike in UC, only a few studies have evaluated the pathologic features and biologic characteristics of dysplasia and carcinoma in CD specifically, and all are retrospective in design [1,2,5,10,11]. As a result, this article focuses mainly on the pathologic features, adjunctive diagnostic methods, and differential diagnosis of dysplasia in UC.

CLASSIFICATION OF DYSPLASIA IN INFLAMMATORY BOWEL DISEASE

From an endoscopic (gross) point of view, dysplasia may be classified as flat or elevated [12–15]. Elevated lesions are referred to by the acronym DALM (dysplasia-associated lesion or mass) [16]. In some aspects, the term "DALM" is not ideal because some types of DALMs do not show aggressive behavior as often is inferred by use of the terms "lesion" or "mass" [14]. Nevertheless, this classification system is important because the treatment of flat versus elevated dysplasia may be different (see later discussion and elsewhere in this issue) [14,17]. Unfortunately, there are inconsistencies in the literature and controversy among investigators regarding the criteria that are used to designate a particular dysplastic lesion as "flat" or "elevated" [12,14–23]. For instance,

E-mail address: rodze@partners.org

0889-8553/06/$ – see front matter
doi:10.1016/j.gtc.2006.07.007
© 2006 Elsevier Inc. All rights reserved.
gastro.theclinics.com

with the advent of newer, more sensitive endoscopic techniques, such as chromoendoscopy, dysplastic lesions that previously were considered "flat" based on the fact that they were undetectable endoscopically, may be detectable endoscopically with these newer endoscopic methods [12,13,15]. Some studies designate dysplastic lesions as "flat" only if they are undetectable endoscopically, and other lesions as "elevated" (DALM) for lesions that are detectable endoscopically. Clearly, some "endoscopically detectable" lesions may, in fact, be "flat" (eg, those that grow as a plaque-like lesion, slightly irregular thickened mucosa, or velvety mucosa) [13,15,24]. Thus, endoscopically detectable lesions may be diagnosed as "flat" by some investigators or "elevated" by others. As a result, the definition of flat dysplasia is controversial and is in transition. Finally, although most, if not all, elevated dysplastic lesions begin as flat, endoscopically undetectable areas of dysplasia, this has never been investigated thoroughly. In fact, rarely, cancers in IBD may appear as endoscopically undetectable lesions.

Nevertheless, regardless of the gross appearance of the neoplastic lesion, flat and elevated dysplastic lesions in IBD are graded similarly at the microscopic level [9,14,21]. Dysplasia is separated into three distinct categories: negative for dysplasia (which implies normal mucosa or mucosa with regenerative changes), indefinite for dysplasia, and positive for dysplasia (low or high grade). This classification system was developed originally in 1983 by a group of expert gastrointestinal (GI) pathologists often referred to as the IBD Dysplasia Morphology Study Group [9]. This classification system is the one that is used most often by pathologists in the United States and by many in Western Europe. In 1988, an alternative classification system for dysplasia in the GI tract was developed by a collective group of European, American, and Japanese pathologists, which was termed the "Vienna" classification [25]. This classification system is used by many pathologists in Europe, and by most in Japan, but has not been accepted commonly by physicians in the United States. It was developed originally with the hope that it would help to standardize the terminology and resolve well-known differences in interpretation between Western and Japanese pathologists with regard to dysplasia and carcinoma. For instance, Western and Japanese pathologists often place a different degree of importance with regard to cytologic and architectural features that are used to diagnose dysplastic lesions in the GI tract [26]. Although most Western pathologists diagnose carcinoma only when there is unequivocal evidence of invasion of cells into the lamina propria, or muscularis mucosa, many Japanese pathologists diagnose carcinoma based solely on the degree of nuclear atypia without a requirement to show definitive morphologic evidence of invasion into the lamina propria.

The Vienna System uses five categories of neoplasia (negative, indefinite, noninvasive low-grade, noninvasive high-grade, and invasive neoplasia), similar to the one that was proposed by the IBD Dysplasia Morphology Study Group. In the former system, the term "noninvasive neoplasia" is used instead of "low or high-grade dysplasia," and the term "suspicious for invasive carcinoma" is used as a separate category for neoplastic lesions that have some, but not all, of the morphologic features of invasion. In addition, the Vienna System subcategorizes invasive cancers into intramucosal and submucosal types. Nevertheless, despite some advantages of the Vienna System, the system has not been adopted widely among GI pathologists in the United States.

PATHOLOGIC FEATURES OF FLAT DYSPLASIA IN INFLAMMATORY BOWEL DISEASE

General Comments

IBD-related neoplasia almost always develops in areas of previous or current, chronic or chronic active inflammation [2,27,28]. In some instances, neoplastic lesions may develop in areas of mucosa that appear histologically unremarkable; however, a reasonable explanation for this phenomenon is that the histologic features of inflammation, both chronic and active, may reverse completely as a result of oral or enema medical therapy [19,29–31]. Of course, sporadic non-IBD–related neoplasms may occur coincidentally in patients who have IBD as well [14,21]. For instance, patients who have left-sided UC may develop right-sided colon cancer that is easy to recognize as "sporadic" because of the location of the tumor in relationship to the most proximal extent of inflammatory disease. Furthermore, rarely, cancer may develop in patients who have IBD without any evidence of previous or current dysplasia, or in patients who have only low-grade dysplasia. This suggests that some tumors develop outside of the stepwise chronic inflammation–low-grade dysplasia–high-grade dysplasia–carcinoma sequence [19,29–31]. In other instances, carcinoma may develop within mucosa that contains extremely well-differentiated, nondysplastic-appearing epithelium without the traditional morphologic features of dysplasia (see later discussion) [9,20]. In general, however, dysplasia is present in more than 90% of cases of IBD with carcinoma, and is more common in UC compared with CD [4,32,33]. Although dysplasia is found adjacent to carcinomas more often, it also may be found in areas distant from the primary tumor [4]. Dysplasia may occur in any portion of the colon in IBD, but often parallels the location of cancer. It may occur as an isolated focus, but more often it is multiple or, rarely, diffuse in nature [4,32,33].

Microscopic Features

The morphologic criteria for dysplasia are based on a combination of cytologic (nuclear and cytoplasmic) and architectural aberrations of the crypt epithelium [9,21]. Cytologic features that pathologists use to evaluate the presence or absence and degree of dysplasia include the nuclear/cytoplasmic (N/C) ratio of the cells; loss of cell polarity; an increase in the number and location of mitoses (typical and atypical); the degree of nuclear stratification within the epithelium; the degree of chromasia of the nuclei (an increase is referred to as "hyperchromasia"); the presence, size, and multiplicity of nucleoli; the size and regularity (or lack thereof) of the contour of nuclei; and the variation in the size and shape

of nuclei between different cells (nuclear pleomorphism). Cytoplasmic characteristics include the degree of mucinous depletion; the number, location, and
shape (normal or dystrophic) of goblet cells; and the presence or absence of surface maturation, which is defined as the progressive acquisition of cytoplasmic
mucin, a decrease in the size of nuclei, and the degree of stratification of the
cells, from the crypt base to the mucosal surface. Architectural features that
are important for the determination of dysplasia include villiform change of
the epithelium and the presence or absence and degree of crypt budding,
branching, and crowding; the latter is referred to commonly as a "back-
to-back" glandular growth pattern. In addition, the contour of the crypts, the
degree of irregularity, and the presence or absence of intraluminal bridges
("cribriforming") are important architectural features that are used to evaluate
dysplasia in IBD.

Negative for Dysplasia

"Negative for dysplasia" applies to epithelium that is regenerative in nature. In
the presence of active inflammation, cryptitis, crypt abscesses, or ulceration, all
of which are common in the active phase of IBD, epithelium can undergo
marked reactive changes that, in some circumstances, may mimic some of
the "atypical" features of dysplasia (see later discussion). In general, nondysplastic ("reactive") epithelium in IBD exhibits only mild or moderate cytologic
atypia coupled with preservation of crypt architecture; however, a significant
degree of atypia may be present in markedly reactive epithelium adjacent to
ulcerated mucosa, an area in which the architecture of the crypts may be altered as well. Thus, pathologists need to exercise caution when evaluating dysplasia in ulcerated mucosa, and these areas should be avoided by the
endoscopist when obtaining mucosal biopsies.

Cytologically, regenerating cells often contain nuclei with a smooth membrane, normal N/C ratio, and a variable number of "normal" mitoses, but
they also may show prominent nucleoli, although without significant enlargement (Fig. 1). Common dysplasia features, such as nuclear pleomorphism,
loss of cell polarity, and elevated N/C ratio, are not typically present in
regenerating epithelium that is considered negative for dysplasia. Although
cytoplasmic mucin usually is depleted, particularly in areas of inflammation,
regenerating crypt cells usually show a progressive increase in the content of
mucin in epithelium close to, or at, the luminal surface, which is indicative
of surface maturation. The presence of surface maturation is the most characteristic feature of nondysplastic "regenerating" epithelium in IBD, and its presence usually, but not always, implies that the epithelium is nondysplastic.
Nuclear stratification, when present, may be prominent at the bases of the
crypts, but this feature normally becomes less prominent in the upper portions
of the crypts and surface epithelium. Architectural aberrations, such as crypt
budding, branching, and cribriforming, are not typical features of regenerating
epithelium, and, as such, their presence suggests dysplasia; however, regenerating epithelium may show villiform change.

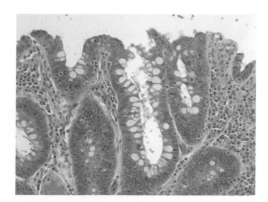

Fig. 1. Typical appearance of chronic active colitis with regenerative changes considered negative for dysplasia. The crypts show basally oriented, slightly hyperchromatic nuclei but without loss of polarity, pleomorphism, or atypical mitosis (hematoxylin-eosin, original magnification ×200).

Indefinite for Dysplasia

Given the subtle gradation of changes, the progressive acquisition of molecular mutations that occurs in the progression of dysplasia in IBD [2,10,29], and the wide range of morphologic patterns of atypia that is related to epithelial regeneration and repair, regenerating epithelium, particularly in the setting of active inflammation or ulceration, may reveal a level of atypia that occasionally is difficult to distinguish from true dysplasia (Fig. 2) [29]. In these situations, pathologists use the "indefinite for dysplasia" diagnostic category. In reality, this diagnostic category is used most often as a result of one of the following circumstances: the presence of technical (tangential sectioning) or staining issues

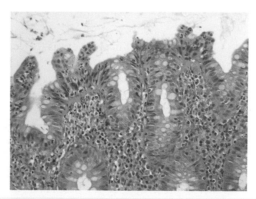

Fig. 2. Patient who has UC with an area considered indefinite for dysplasia. Cytologically, the nuclei show hyperchromaticity and stratification at the surface of the lesion. Based on the amount of acute and chronic inflammation in the biopsy, it is difficult to be certain whether the atypical changes represent the extreme of regeneration or dysplasia (hematoxylin-eosin, original magnification ×200).

that makes interpretation of cytologic or architectural features difficult, atypia related to inflammation or ulceration, or for the rare instances in which dysplasia-like changes are present only in the crypt bases. Naturally, the frequency of the use of this diagnostic category is directly proportional to the "comfort" level and experience of the reviewing pathologist, and is one of the reasons why it is highly recommended to confirm any potential diagnosis of dysplasia with at least one other experienced IBD pathologist before definitive treatment [2,34].

Low-Grade Dysplasia

Low-grade dysplasia is characterized by epithelium that contains cells with significant nuclear hyperchromaticity, enlargement, and elongation; the last is referred to as "pencil-shaped" or "adenomatous" nuclei (Fig. 3). Nuclei in low-grade dysplasia often show a clumped chromatin pattern, multiple nucleoli, or a single large nucleolus. Typically, the cytoplasm is mucin depleted, and, as a result, is hypereosinophilic. A decrease in the number of goblet cells and unusually oriented goblet cells, referred to as "dystrophic" goblet cells, also may be observed. Dysplastic cells usually are organized in a stratified manner, but in general, the nuclei are limited to the basal half of the cell cytoplasm, without full thickness stratification. Mitotic figures may be prominent, but atypical mitotic figures usually are few. Most importantly, dysplastic epithelium usually does not show surface maturation, except in rare circumstances. A minor degree of architectural aberration may occur in low-grade dysplasia, but significant architectural aberration normally is diagnostic of high-grade dysplasia.

High-Grade Dysplasia

With progression to high-grade dysplasia, the degree of cytologic or architectural aberration is more prominent (Fig. 4). Cytologically, full-thickness nuclear

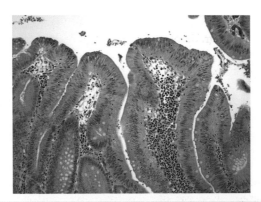

Fig. 3. Typical features of low-grade dysplasia in UC. The mucosa shows elongated pencil-shaped hyperchromatic nuclei, with stratification, increased mitosis, and lack of surface maturation. For the most part, the nuclei are limited to the basal half of the cell cytoplasm without full-thickness stratification (hematoxylin-eosin, original magnification ×200).

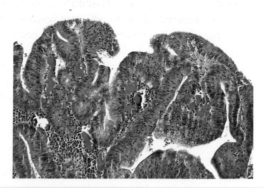

Fig. 4. High-grade dysplasia in UC. In contrast to low-grade dysplasia, the nuclei in high-grade dysplasia show an increased degree of atypia with a higher degree of stratification, mitoses, and loss of polarity. Full-thickness nuclear stratification is present. In addition, the crypts show distortion and a back-to-back configuration (hematoxylin-eosin, original magnification ×200).

stratification, significant loss of cell polarity, nuclear pleomorphism, and an increase in the number of normal appearing and atypical mitoses, often at the level of the surface epithelium, are characteristic features of high-grade dysplasia. In some instances, high-grade nuclei are more round or oval in contour, and show a higher N/C ratio as well. Architectural aberrations, such as a complex crypt budding or branching, or a back-to-back growth pattern that is characterized by dysplastic crypts that show little or no intervening lamina propria, also may be present. Cystic change, villiform surface change, and cribriforming also are features of high-grade dysplasia [20,35,36].

Low-Grade Dysplasia Versus High-Grade Dysplasia

In general, the overall grade of dysplasia is determined by the features of the most atypical portion of the mucosa; however, there is significant variability and controversy among GI pathologists regarding the specific number of high-grade dysplastic crypts that is necessary to upgrade a particular biopsy from low grade to high grade [9,29]. The IBD Dysplasia Morphology Study Group did not offer specific guidelines; it only suggested that a biopsy should not be considered high-grade "based solely on the presence of high-grade dysplasia in one or two crypts" [9]. Unfortunately, the clinical and prognostic significance of the extent of dysplasia, both low- and high-grade, has not been tested in patients who have IBD. Thus, the histologic distinction between low- and high-grade dysplasia often is subjective, and is a major reason for the high level of interobserver disagreement among pathologists (see later discussion). There is an increasing trend among GI pathologists to provide clinicians with objective information regarding the extent of low- and high-grade dysplasia in biopsy reports from individuals who have IBD.

Intramucosal/Invasive Adenocarcinoma

In contrast to dysplasia, in which neoplastic cells are confined to the basement membrane, carcinomas are defined by the infiltration of neoplastic cells or glands into the surrounding lamina propria or muscularis mucosa (both considered "intramucosal carcinoma") or submucosa ("submucosal carcinoma"). Adenocarcinoma is characterized most often by the presence of single cells or small glands that infiltrate the lamina propria. Infiltrating glands may appear large, irregular, or variable in size and shape and may show intraluminal necrosis. The presence of desmoplasia is a diagnostic feature of invasive carcinoma and usually signifies at least submucosal extension.

Unusual Patterns of Dysplasia

In rare instances, dysplasia may reveal a prominent villous growth pattern that is composed of elongated, predominantly mucinous epithelium with numerous goblet cells, and without significant cytologic atypia; these features may be difficult to recognize as neoplastic in origin [20,35,36]. This type of neoplastic proliferation has been termed "villous dysplasia" or "villous hypermucinous mucosa," and it has been reported in UC and CD [20,35]. In addition, dysplastic epithelium in IBD may appear serrated in contour, which mimics some of the features of hyperplastic polyps or serrated adenomas of the colon [36]. In other instances, a mixture of villous, serrated, and traditional dysplasia may be present in the same patient. In one study by Rubio and colleagues [36], the histologic phenotype of dysplasia adjacent to carcinoma was assessed in 100 colectomy specimens: 50 were IBD related and 50 were not IBD related. Of the IBD cases, more than 50% showed a villous pattern and nearly 30% showed a serrated morphologic phenotype.

Rarely, patients who have IBD develop numerous (hundreds) dysplastic polyps, many of which show a hyperplastic or serrated adenomatous appearance that resembles the hyperplastic/serrated polyposis syndrome. In one small series that was reported only in abstract form, Srivastava and colleagues [37] showed that patients who had IBD who had hundreds of hyperplastic/serrated polyps probably had dysplasia that was derived from the underlying IBD, rather than the simultaneous existence of two separate diseases.

Dysplasia in Crohn's Disease

Most studies also support the dysplasia-carcinoma sequence in CD, similar to that which occurs in UC [1,2,8]; 2% to 16% of patients who have CD have dysplasia detected during the course of their illness. For instance, in a study by Friedman and colleagues [3], a screening and surveillance program detected dysplasia or cancer in 16% of 259 patients who had follow-up for a mean of 24 months. The reported frequency of dysplasia in patients who had CD and colorectal carcinoma ranged from 40% to 100% [4,5]. Dysplasia in CD occurs more often in areas close to, rather than distant from, the primary tumor mass. In a study by Sigel and colleagues [1], dysplasia was found adjacent to carcinoma in 87% of cases and distant from carcinoma in 41% of cases. In this study of 30 CD-related adenocarcinomas, 27% occurred in the small intestine and 73% occurred in the colon. In a population-based study from Sweden, the relative risk of colon cancer was 2.5 in patients who had CD and 5.6 in patients who had CD with disease restricted to the colon [6]. The relative risk was even greater in patients who were younger than 30 years of age at the time of diagnosis.

Differential Diagnosis

There is a significant degree of variability in the interpretation of dysplasia in IBD, even among experienced GI pathologists, primarily because cancer develops on a progressive (continuous) scale rather than in discrete intervals [9,38–41]. Therefore, there is overlap at the two ends of the spectrum in each of the different categories of dysplasia. Common areas of diagnostic difficulty include (1) differentiation of reactive epithelium from low-grade dysplasia, (2) separation of low-grade dysplasia from high-grade dysplasia, and (3) determination as to whether a biopsy shows unequivocal evidence of invasion in a patient who has high-grade dysplasia. In Riddell and colleagues' [9] original study of dysplasia in IBD in 1983, the mean interobserver variability discrepancy score was 0.6 grade units, which represents a moderate to poor level of interobserver agreement. Since Riddell's study, several other interobserver studies have been performed, and all have shown only a moderate level of interobserver agreement, at best [38–40]. For instance, in an interobserver study by Odze and colleagues [38], there was only a fair level of agreement ($\kappa = 0.4$) among four experienced GI pathologists in interpreting cases of UC-related dysplasia by evaluation of static electronically transmitted computer images. In general, levels of agreement between pathologists are highest for lesions at the ends of the dysplasia spectrum (ie, negative or high-grade) and lowest for biopsies that fall within the indefinite/low-grade dysplasia range.

Adjunctive Diagnostic Markers

Many studies have been published in an effort to help identify sensitive and specific immunohistochemical or molecular markers that may aid in the differentiation of dysplastic from reactive epithelium in IBD. Most of the markers that were evaluated previously have been linked, in some capacity, to the development of cancer, and include those involved in control of cell proliferation (eg, Ki67, cyclin D1), intercellular adhesion (β-catenin, e-cadherin), DNA content, mucin or glycoprotein histochemistry, and tumor suppression (p53) [10,42–60]. Of these, p53 and Ki67 have been studied the most extensively.

The p53 gene shows an increase in the frequency of mutations in the dysplasia-carcinoma progression in IBD [42,44–49]. p53 is a common early mutation in the dysplasia-carcinoma sequence in IBD, and, as a result, many investigators have evaluated the role of p53 in helping to differentiate reactive from dysplastic epithelium. For instance, in a study by Wong and colleagues [42], a moderate degree of p53 staining was detected in almost 50% of reactive cases, but strong p53 staining was seen only in cases of true dysplasia. Unfortunately, although p53 expression increases progressively from low- to high-grade dysplasia and carcinoma, some studies showed that epithelium that is considered indefinite, or even negative, for dysplasia, may be p53 positive; this diminishes its usefulness as a marker of true dysplasia [10,42,44]. Furthermore, p53 overexpression can be detected in a small proportion of cases that is considered morphologically negative for dysplasia [42,44,46,47]. In addition, several studies in other tissues have revealed a high rate of false-positive staining in the absence of p53 mutations, and a high frequency of false-negative staining as well [58,59]. Nonspecific binding of p53 to non-p53 mutation-related antigens also may lead to false positive results. Furthermore, p53 results may vary substantially depending on the specific type of antibody used. For instance, some p53 mutations result in the production of a protein that does not bind to some antibodies that are directed against the wild-type protein. Finally, there is no known antibody, or combination of antibodies, in use that can detect all p53 mutations [58]. For these reasons, p53 immunostaining is not used in routine practice to help differentiate reactive from dysplastic epithelium in IBD.

Several studies showed that dysplasia expresses markers of cell proliferation at higher levels of the crypt, and in the surface epithelium, compared with biopsies that are considered negative for dysplasia [42,43,57]. Unfortunately, there is much overlap between reactive epithelium and dysplasia in this regard, so evaluation of cell proliferation is not useful in individual cases to distinguish these lesions.

Recently, immunostaining for alpha-methylocyl–CoA racemase (AMACR), an antibody that is used often in the assessment of diagnostically difficult atypical, and potentially neoplastic, lesions of the prostate, was shown to have a high degree of specificity for detection of dysplasia in the GI tract, such as in Barrett's esophagus and IBD [61]. AMACR is a mitochondrial and peroxisomal enzyme that catalyzes the racemation of a wide spectrum of α-methyl branched carboxylic coenzyme A thioesters [62]. The protein is expressed in peroxisomes and mitochondria of normal liver and kidney cells, where it is believed to play a role in the β-oxidation of branched chain fatty acids [63]. It is overexpressed commonly in prostate, gastric, and colon cancers, including sporadic adenomas [64,65]. In a recent study by Dorer and Odze [61], AMACR was not expressed in any mucosal biopsy in UC that was considered negative for dysplasia; however, it was increased significantly in foci of low-grade dysplasia (96%), high-grade dysplasia (80%), and adenocarcinoma (71%) with a specificity for neoplasia of 100%. Thus, AMACR is a new, potentially useful immunohistochemical marker that pathologists may use in their arsenal when trying to differentiate reactive from dysplastic epithelium in IBD.

PATHOLOGIC FEATURES OF ELEVATED DYSPLASIA IN INFLAMMATORY BOWEL DISEASE

The term "DALM" was coined by Blackstone and colleagues [16] in 1981. In that study, 12 of 112 patients who had long-standing UC had a DALM, and, of these, 58% had carcinoma. Given their finding of a strong association between

DALM and cancer, the investigators concluded that the presence of a DALM constituted a strong indication for colectomy, which, until recently, had become the standard of therapy for this type of IBD-related lesion. Furthermore, since Blackstone and colleagues' publication, several studies have confirmed a high association of DALM with cancer. In retrospect, this probably relates to the fact that biopsies of the DALM lesions in many of these studies probably represented the surface of an underlying invasive adenocarcinoma [18–23]; however, it is now apparent that DALMs are, in fact, a heterogenous population of tumors in which the cancer risk is not equal among the various subtypes [14,17]. Recent studies suggest that DALMs may be separated broadly into those that appear similar endoscopically to non-IBD–related sporadic adenomas, referred to as "adenoma-like," and those that do not resemble adenomas, which are referred to as "nonadenoma-like" [66–69]. This classification system is useful clinically and pathologically because it helps to separate DALMs into two groups of lesions, each with a different natural history, risk for malignancy, and treatment [66–68]. For instance, adenoma-like DALMs possess a low risk for synchronous or metachronous neoplasia, and, thus, may be treated conservatively by polypectomy and continued surveillance. Nonadenoma-like DALMs have a high risk for concurrent and subsequent malignancy, and, as a result, often require colectomy as the definitive form of treatment [66,68]. Some recent data suggest that most elevated dysplastic lesions in IBD are, in fact, adenoma-like. For instance, in a study by Rutter and colleagues [13], 56 patients who had UC who developed dysplasia (flat or elevated) in the course of a 14-year surveillance program at St. Mark's Hospital in London were evaluated. In this group, 110 neoplastic areas were detected, of which 77% were visible at colonoscopy. Eighty-seven percent of the visible lesions were adenoma-like. Overall, 70% of dysplastic lesions were visible endoscopically and 30% were invisible.

Grossly, adenoma-like DALMs represent well-circumscribed smooth or papillary, nonnecrotic, sessile or pedunculated polyps that, similar to sporadic adenomas, usually are readily accessible to removal by routine endoscopic methods [14,66]. Nonadenoma-like lesions include velvety patches, plaques, irregular bumps and nodules, wartlike thickenings, stricturing lesions, and broad-based masses [13,16,22,23]. These lesions usually are not amenable to removal by colonoscopy, and, thus, often require surgical resection as the primary method of treatment.

Microscopically, adenoma-like and nonadenoma-like DALMs may show a similar morphologic appearance [21,70,71]. Both types of DALMs usually are composed of a tubular, tubulovillous, or villous "adenomatous"-type dysplastic epithelium similar to flat dysplasia (Fig. 5). Superficial biopsies from nonadenoma-like DALMs may show only fragments of dysplastic epithelium; however, deeper portions of tissue from nonadenoma-like DALMs often reveal characteristic features of invasive adenocarcinoma.

The microscopic features of adenoma-like DALMs are similar to those of sporadic adenomas that are unrelated to IBD [21]. Differentiation of sporadic

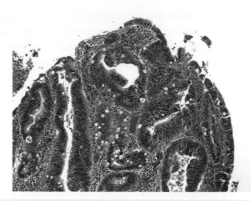

Fig. 5. Medium-power photograph of an adenoma-like DALM with high-grade dysplasia. This patient had an adenoma-like lesion identified endoscopically, but did not have any evidence of flat dysplasia elsewhere in the colon. This lesion was removed endoscopically, and the patient underwent continued surveillance with no further dysplastic lesions identified after 5 years of follow-up (hematoxylin-eosin, original magnification ×200).

from IBD-related adenoma-like DALMs may be difficult or impossible; however, several studies have evaluated morphologic, immunohistochemical, and molecular methods in this regard. For instance, in one case-control study by Torres and colleagues [21], 89 adenoma-like DALMs from 59 patients who had UC were evaluated morphologically. Patients who had UC-related adenoma-like DALMs had a statistically significant longer duration of disease (>10 years), a higher proportion of polyps with tubulovillous or villous architecture, a mixture of normal and dysplastic epithelium at the surface of the polyp, and a higher degree of mononuclear inflammation in the lamina propria compared with non-UC–related sporadic adenomas. In addition, the median age of UC-related lesions was significantly less (48 years) compared with patients who had sporadic adenomas (mean age 63.5 years). In the study by Torres and colleagues [21], stalk dysplasia, which has been suggested anecdotally to represent a feature indicative of an IBD-related lesion, rather than a sporadic adenoma, did not show a significantly different prevalence rate among the two types of lesions. Most importantly, however, patients who had DALMs (adenoma-like or nonadenoma-like) often showed areas of flat (endoscopically invisible or visible) dysplasia in mucosa adjacent to or distant from the dysplastic polyp; this is almost never found in patients who have sporadic adenomas. This finding emphasizes the fact that in the process of working up a patient who has a DALM, it is critical to obtain biopsies from flat mucosa adjacent to and distant from the elevated lesion. The presence of flat dysplasia in a patient who has an adenoma-like DALM provides strong evidence that the lesion is IBD related [21].

Taking into account the different timing and sequence of molecular events in IBD-related versus sporadic colon carcinogenesis, some investigators have evaluated immunohistochemical or molecular methods to differentiate adenoma-like DALMs from sporadic adenomas [53,72–78]. For instance, in a retrospective immunohistochemical study by Walsh and colleagues [76], p53 and β-catenin expression was evaluated in 17 patients who had UC with adenoma-like DALMs, 21 patients who had UC with sporadic adenomas, and 13 control patients who did not have UC but who had sporadic adenomas. In their study, UC-associated adenoma-like DALMs showed a significant increase in the prevalence (29%) and degree of p53 staining compared with sporadic adenomas. In contrast, only 8% of UC-associated adenoma-like DALMs showed nuclear β-catenin expression compared with 40% of UC-related sporadic adenomas. Finally, in a retrospective study, Odze and colleagues [72] evaluated loss of heterozygosity (LOH) of 3p, adenomatus polyposis coli, and p16 in 21 patients who had UC with an adenoma-like DALM, 8 patients who had UC with a nonadenoma-like DALM, and 23 patients who had a sporadic adenoma. UC-associated nonadenoma-like DALMs showed a significantly higher rate of LOH of 3p (50%) and LOH of p16 (56%), compared with UC-associated adenoma-like DALMs or non-UC–related sporadic adenomas. No differences were detected between UC-associated adenoma-like DALMs and non-UC–related sporadic adenomas.

Because several recent follow-up studies and one long-term prospective follow-up study confirmed a low incidence of dysplasia and carcinoma in patients who had UC or CD with an adenoma-like DALM that was treated by polypectomy and continued surveillance, it has become less important for pathologists to differentiate UC-related from sporadic adenoma-like lesions in IBD [66–68]. In both cases, recent studies suggest that these patients can be treated adequately and safely by polypectomy and continued surveillance if there is no other evidence of flat or endoscopically undetectable dysplasia in the patient's colon. In addition, the presence of high-grade dysplasia in an adenoma-like DALM has not been shown to be an adverse predictor of outcome in patients who have IBD who are treated by polypectomy, so the degree of dysplasia is irrelevant when faced with a management decision for patients who have IBD with a DALM [66–68,79].

Of course, the basis of this treatment algorithm relies heavily on the capacity of endoscopists to categorize elevated dysplastic lesions in UC adequately as adenoma-like or nonadenoma-like. In a recent study by Farraye and colleagues [80], 38 gastroenterologists (12 private practice, 13 academic, 13 IBD experts) were asked a series of questions on the diagnosis and management of UC-associated polypoid lesions by an Internet survey of 13 endoscopic images of DALMs. IBD experts showed a significantly higher proportion of correct diagnoses (75%) and interobserver agreement (κ = 0.64) compared with other non-IBD expert gastroenterologists. This suggests that general practice gastroenterologists need to be educated regarding objective endoscopic criteria that can help to separate adenoma-like DALMs from nonadenoma-like DALMs. Nevertheless, regardless of the endoscopic appearance of the lesion, published evidence suggests that UC-related polypoid dysplastic lesions that are amenable to removal by endoscopic resection may, in fact, be treated safely by this method [66–68]. Thus, regardless of the ability of the endoscopist to classify a lesion in UC accurately as adenoma-like or nonadenoma-like, the ability to remove the lesion completely by endoscopic methods is an objective alternative way of determining whether a patient can be treated safely by polypectomy.

PATHOLOGIC FEATURES OF CARCINOMA IN INFLAMMATORY BOWEL DISEASE

The clinical, epidemiologic, and pathologic characteristics of IBD-related cancers are, in many aspects, different from those that occur sporadically in the general population. For instance, cancers that occur in IBD, and particularly UC, tend to be distributed more evenly throughout the length of colon, are more likely to be multiple in number and tend to be of higher histologic grade compared with sporadic carcinomas [29,81]. In some studies, up to 27% of IBD-related cancers are multiple in number [82,83]. In addition, there is a higher prevalence of mucinous carcinomas in IBD [74,81,84,85]. More recently, there has been a shift to a higher incidence of early-stage tumors (stage I–II) compared with IBD-related cancers from previous decades [29,81,82,86]. Contemporary studies show that 50% to 60% of newly diagnosed IBD-related cancers are stages I or II. Of course, this may be due to a combination of many factors, such as increased level of awareness and early detection by colonoscopic surveillance. In one recent study, by Delaunoit and colleagues [81], of 290 patients who had IBD (241 with UC and 49 with CD) and an equal number of age- and sex-matched patients who had sporadic colorectal cancer, UC-related carcinomas were diagnosed at a younger age and tended to be distributed more evenly in the colon compared with sporadic tumors.

Pathologically, IBD-related tumors often grow in a more diffuse fashion compared with sporadic cancers, and may be more difficult to recognize grossly because they may be raised only minimally above the level of the surrounding mucosa [29,81]. The gross appearance of cancers in IBD is heterogenous. They may be strictured, ulcerated, irregular, polypoid (pedunculated or sessile), or nodular or they may appear as an irregular plaque or bump [29,84,87]. Some tumors may be entirely microscopic, without any grossly evident mucosal abnormality [22,88]. A disproportionately higher percentage of cancers in IBD, including UC, occurs in strictured segments of colon [11,29,89].

Microscopically, most IBD-related carcinomas are adenocarcinomas. Mucinous carcinomas make up a high proportion, up to 50% in some studies [10]. In addition, signet ring cell adenocarcinomas are 10 times more common in IBD compared with the general population [29,90]. Rarely, IBD-related adenocarcinomas may be extremely well differentiated and consist of widely separated, regularly arranged, bland appearing glandular profiles that contain only mildly atypical unilayered neoplastic epithelium with low-grade cytologic atypia, and without desmoplasia [29]. These tumors may arise from mucosa that shows little or no definite evidence of dysplasia. Other types of carcinomas, such as neuroendocrine carcinomas, mixed adenocarcinoma/squamous cell carcinoma, undifferentiated carcinoma, and even pure squamous cell carcinoma (particularly in the distal rectum and anal canal in CD), have been encountered in IBD; some occur with increased frequency [10,11,29,89–95]. These tumors are rare, however, and often are reported as single case reports or as small series.

Regarding CD cancers specifically, recent evidence suggests that the risk for cancer in CD is similar to that in UC, particularly for patients who have long-standing and extensive colonic disease [2,6,7,10,96]. In contrast to UC, patients who develop cancer in CD often are older in age, but are much younger than patients who develop sporadic colon cancer in the general population [5,29,82,97]. Some early reports cited a higher left-sided predominance for cancers in CD compared with UC; however, several contemporary studies showed a more equal distribution of tumors in the colon in CD, similar to UC [11,81,98]. Earlier studies may have been biased by the fact that cancers in CD often occur in and around the anal canal related to fissures or fistulas [5,98–100]. As a result, there is an increase in the incidence of pure squamous cell carcinomas in CD compared with UC. Although most cancers in CD are believed to occur within inflamed portions of intestine [10,101–103], in some studies, up to 42% of patients who had CD developed tumors in areas of mucosa devoid of endoscopic or pathologic evidence of inflammation [4,5,11,96,98–100]; however, this may be due to treatment effect [31]. Finally, surgically excluded segments of colon or small bowel also are considered particularly prone to the development of carcinoma in CD, but this is postulated to be related to the fact that excluded segments of inflamed bowel remain at risk for carcinogenesis for longer periods of time over the course of the patient's life [10,29,81,98,104]. Because surgical procedures that result in preservation of inflamed but excluded segments of bowel are performed only infrequently in patients who have CD, cancers in surgically excluded segments of bowel are now uncommon.

References

[1] Sigel JE, Petras RE, Lashner BA, et al. Intestinal adenocarcinoma in Crohn's disease: report of 30 cases with a focus on coexisting dysplasia. Am J Surg Pathol 1999;23(6):651–5.

[2] Ullman TA. Dysplasia and colorectal cancer in Crohn's disease. J Clin Gastroenterol 2003;36(5 Suppl):S75–8.

[3] Itzkowitz SH, Harpaz N. Diagnosis and management of dysplasia in patients with inflammatory bowel diseases. Gastroenterology 2004;126:1634–48.

[4] Friedman S, Rubin PH, Bodian C, et al. Screening and surveillance colonoscopy in chronic Crohn's colitis. Gastroenterology 2001;120(4):820–6.

[5] Connell WR, Sheffield JP, Kamm MA, et al. Lower gastrointestinal malignancy in Crohn's disease. Gut 1994;35:347–52.

[6] Hamilton SR. Colorectal carcinoma in patients with Crohn's disease. Gastroenterology 1985;89:398–407.

[7] Ekbom A, Helmick C, Zack M, et al. Increased risk of large-bowel cancer in Crohn's disease with colonic involvement. Lancet 1990;336:357–9.

[8] Greenstein AJ, Sachar DB, Smith H, et al. Comparison of cancer risk in Crohn's disease and ulcerative colitis. Cancer 1981;48:2742.

[9] Riddell RH, Goldman H, Ransohoff DF, et al. Dysplasia in inflammatory bowel disease: standardized classification with provisional clinical applications. Hum Pathol 1983;14:931–68.

[10] Judge TA, Lewis JD, Lichtenstein GR. Colonic dysplasia and cancer in inflammatory bowel disease. Gastrointest Endosc Clin N Am 2002;12:495–523.

[11] Sjodahl RI, Myrelid P, Soderholm JD. Anal and rectal cancer in Crohn's disease. Colorectal Dis 2003;5(5):490–5.

[12] Itzkowitz S, Ullman T. The world isn't flat. Gastro Endoscop 2004;60:426–7.

[13] Rutter MD, Saunders BP, Wilkinson KH, et al. Most dysplasia in ulcerative colitis is visible at colonoscopy. Gastrointest Endosc 2004;60:334–9.

[14] Odze RD. Adenomas and adenoma-like DALMs in chronic ulcerative colitis: a clinical, pathological, and molecular review. Am J Gastroenterol 1999;94:1746–50.

[15] Rutter M, Bernstein C, Matsumoto T, et al. Endoscopic appearance of dysplasia in ulcerative colitis and the role of staining. Endoscopy 2004;36(12):1109–14.

[16] Blackstone MO, Riddell RH, Rogers BGH, et al. Dysplasia-associated lesion or mass (DALM) detected by colonoscopy in long-standing ulcerative colitis: an indication for colectomy. Gastroenterology 1981;80:366–74.

[17] Odze RD. Recent advances in inflammatory bowel disease. Mod Pathol 2003;16(4):347–58.

[18] Bernstein CN, Shanahan F, Weinstein WM. Are we telling patients the truth about surveillance colonoscopy in ulcerative colitis? Lancet 1994;343:71–4.

[19] Lennard-Jones JE, Melville DM, Morson BC, et al. Precancer and cancer in extensive ulcerative colitis: findings among 401 patients over 22 years. Gut 1990;31:800–6.

[20] Rubio CA, Johansson P, Slezak U, et al. Villous dysplasia. An ominous histologic sign in colitic patients. Dis Colon Rectum 1984;27:283–7.

[21] Torres C, Antonioli D, Odze RD, et al. Polypoid dysplasia and adenomas in inflammatory bowel disease. Am J Surg Pathol 1998;22:275–84.

[22] Butt JH, Konishi F, Morson DM, et al. Macroscopic lesions in dysplasia in carcinoma complicating ulcerative colitis. Dig Dis Sci 1983;28:18–26.

[23] Rosenstock E, Farmer RG, Petras R, et al. Surveillance for colonic carcinoma in ulcerative colitis. Gastroenterology 1985;89:1342–6.

[24] Morson BC, Pang LS. Rectal biopsy as an aid to cancer control in ulcerative colitis. Gut 1967;8:423–34.

[25] Schlemper RJ, Riddell RH, Kato Y, et al. The Vienna classification of gastrointestinal epithelial neoplasia. Gut 2000;47:251–5.

[26] Schlemper RJ, Itabashi M, Kato Y, et al. Differences in diagnostic criteria used by Japanese and Western pathologists to diagnose colorectal carcinoma. Cancer 1998;82:60–9.

[27] Goldman H. Significance and detection of dysplasia in chronic colitis. Cancer 1996;78:2261–3.

[28] Riddell RH. Premalignant and early malignant lesions in the gastrointestinal tract: definitions, terminology, and problems. Am J Gastroenterol 1996;91:864–72.

[29] Harpaz N, Talbot IC. Colorectal cancer in idiopathic inflammatory bowel disease. Semin Diagn Pathol 1996;13:339–57.

[30] Ullman TA, Croog T, Harpaz N, et al. Progression of flat low-grade dysplasia to advanced neoplasia in patients with ulcerative colitis. Gastroenterology 2003;125:1311–9.

[31] Odze R, Antonioli D, Peppercorn M, et al. Effect of topical 5-aminosalicylic acid (5-ASA) therapy on rectal mucosal biopsy morphology in chronic ulcerative colitis. Am J Surg Pathol 1993;17:864–75.

[32] Webb BW, Petras RE, Bozdech JM, et al. Carcinoma and dysplasia in mucosal ulcerative colitis: a clinicopathologic study of 44 patients. Am J Clin Pathol 1991;96:403–7.

[33] Taylor BA, Pemberton JH, Carpenter HA, et al. Dysplasia in chronic ulcerative colitis: implications for colonoscopic surveillance. Dis Colon Rectum 1992;32:950–6.

[34] Itskowitz SH, Present DH, Odze RD, et al. Consensus conference: colorectal cancer screening and surveillance in inflammatory bowel disease. Inflamm Bowel Dis 2005;11(3):314–21.

[35] Anderson SN, Lovig T, Clausen OPF, et al. Villous, hypermucinous mucosa in long standing ulcerative colitis shows high frequency of K-ras mutation. Gut 1999;45:686–92.

[36] Rubio CA, Befrits R, Jaramillo E, et al. Villous and serrated adenomatous growth bordering carcinomas in inflammatory bowel disease. Anticancer Res 2000;20:4761–2.

[37] Srivastava A, Redston M, Odze MD. Hyperplastic/serrated polyposis in inflammatory bowel disease: a case series of a previously undescribed entity. Mod Pathol 2006;19(s1):120A.

[38] Odze RD, Goldblum J, Noffsinger A, et al. Interobserver variability in the diagnosis of ulcerative colitis-associated dysplasia by telepathology. Mod Pathol 2002;4:379–86.

[39] Eaden J, Abrams K, McKay H, et al. Inter-observer variation between general and specialists gastrointestinal pathologists when grading dysplasia in ulcerative colitis. J Pathol 2001;194:152–7.

[40] Melville DM, Jass JR, Morson BC, et al. Observer study of the grading of dysplasia in ulcerative colitis: comparison with clinical outcome. Hum Pathol 1989;20:1008–14.

[41] Dundas SAC, Kay R, Beck S, et al. Can histopathologist reliably assess dysplasia in chronic inflammatory bowel disease? J Clin Pathol 1987;40:1282–6.

[42] Wong NACS, Mayer NJ, MacKell S, et al. Immunohistochemical assessment of Ki67 and p53 expression assists the diagnosis and grading of ulcerative colitis- related dysplasia. Histopathology 2000;37:108–14.

[43] Anderson SN, Rognum TO, Bakka A, et al. Ki-67: a useful marker for the evaluation of dysplasia in ulcerative colitis. Mod Pathol 1998;51:327–32.

[44] Wong NACS, Harrison DJ. Colorectal neoplasia in ulcerative colitis—recent advances. Histopathology 2001;39.221-34.

[45] Burmer GC, Rabinovitch PS, Haggitt RC, et al. Neoplastic progression in ulcerative colitis: histology, DNA content, and loss of a p53 allele. Gastroenterology 1992;103:1602.

[46] Lofberg R, Brostom O, Karlen P, et al. DNA aneuploidy in ulcerative colitis: reproducibility, topographic distribution, and relation to dysplasia. Gastroenterology 1992;102:1149.

[47] Itzkowitz SH, Young E, Dubois D, et al. Sialosyl-Tn antigen is prevalent and precedes dysplasia in ulcerative colitis: a retrospective case-control study. Gastroenterology 1996;110:694.

[48] Itzkowitz SH, Greenwald B, Meltzer SJ. Colon carcinogenesis in inflammatory bowel disease. Inflamm Bowel Dis 1995;1:142.

[49] Greenwald BD, Harpaz N, Yin J, et al. Loss of heterozygosity affecting the p53, Rh, and mmc/apc tumor supressor gene loci in dysplastic and cancerous ulcerative colitis. Cancer Res 1992;52:741.

[50] Sato A, Machinami R. p53 immunohistochemistry of ulcerative colitis-associated with dysplasia and carcinoma. Pathol Int 1998;49:858–68.

[51] Noffsinger AE, Belli JM, Miller MA, et al. A unique basal pattern of p53 expression in ulcerative colitis is associated with mutation in the p53 gene. Histopathology 2001;39:482–92.

[52] Harpaz N, Peck AL, Yin J, et al. p53 protein expression in ulcerative colitis—associated colorectal dysplasia and carcinoma. Hum Pathol 1994;25:1069–74.

[53] Kern SE. p53: tumor suppression through control of the cell cycle. Gastroenterology 1994;106:1708–11.

[54] Chaubert P, Benhattar J, Saraga E, et al. K-ras mutations and p53 alterations in neoplastic and nonneoplastic lesions associated with longstanding ulcerative colitis. Am J Pathol 1994;144:767–75.

[55] Walsh S, Murphy M, Silverman M, et al. p27 expression in inflammatory bowel disease-associated neoplasia. Further evidence of a unique molecular pathogenesis. Am J Pathol 1999;155:1511–8.

[56] Fogt F, Vortmeyer AO, Goldman H, et al. Comparison of genetic alterations in colonic adenoma and ulcerative colitis-associated dysplasia and carcinoma. Hum Pathol 1998;29:131–6.

[57] Noffsinger AE, Miller MA, Cusa MV, et al. The pattern of cell proliferation in neoplastic and nonneoplastic lesions of ulcerative colitis. Cancer 1996;78:2307–12.

[58] Younes M, Lebovitz RM, Lechago LV, et al. p53 protein accumulation in Barrett's metaplasia, dysplasia, and carcinoma: a follow-up study. Gastroenterology 1993;105:1637–42.

[59] Greenblatt MS, Bennett WP, Hollstein MC, et al. Mutations in the p53 tumor suppressor gene: clues to cancer etiology and molecular pathogenesis. Cancer Res 1994;54: 4855–78.

[60] Rubin CE, Haggitt RC, Burmer GC, et al. DNA aneuploidy in colonic biopsies predicts future development of dysplasia in ulcerative colitis. Gastroenterology 1992;103:1611.

[61] Dorer R, Odze RD. AMACR immunostaining is useful in detecting dysplasia epithelium in Barrett's esophagus, ulcerative colitis and Crohn's disease. Am J Surg Pathol 2006;30: 871–7.

[62] Schmitz W, Albers C, Fingerhut R, et al. Purification and characterization of an alpha-methylacyl-CoA racemase from human liver. Eur J Biochem 1995;231:815–22.

[63] Kotti TJ, Savolainen K, Helander HM, et al. In mouse alpha-methylacyl-CoA racemase, the same gene product is simultaneously located in mitochondria and peroxisomes. J Biol Chem 2000;275:20887–95.

[64] Jiang Z, Woda BA, Rock KL, et al. P504S: a new molecular marker for the detection of prostate carcinoma. Am J Surg Pathol 2001;25:1397–404.

[65] Jiang Z, Fanger GR, Woda BA, et al. Expression of alpha-methylacyl-CoA racemase (P504s) in various malignant neoplasms and normal tissues: a study of 761 cases. Hum Pathol 2003;34:792–6.

[66] Odze RD, Farraye FA, Hecht JL, et al. Long-term follow-up after polypectomy treatment for adenoma-like dysplastic lesions in ulcerative colitis. Clin Gastroenterol Hepatol 2004;2: 534–41.

[67] Englesjerd M, Farraye FA, Odze RD. Polypectomy may be adequate treatment for adenoma- like dysplastic lesions in chronic ulcerative colitis. Gastroenterology 1999;117: 1288–94.

[68] Rubin PH, Friedman S, Harpaz N, et al. Colonoscopic polypectomy in chronic colitis: conservative management after endoscopic resection of dysplastic polyps. Gastroenterology 1999;117:11295–300.

[69] Friedman S, Odze RD, Farraye FA. Management of neoplastic polyps in inflammatory bowel disease. Inflamm Bowel Dis 2003;9:260–6.

[70] Schneider A, Stolte M. Differential diagnosis of adenomas and dysplastic lesions in patients with ulcerative colitis. Z Gastroenterol 1993;31:653–6.

[71] Suzuki K, Muto T, Shinozaki M, et al. Differential diagnosis of dysplasia- associated lesion or mass and coincidental adenoma in ulcerative colitis. Dis Colon Rectum 1998;41: 322–7.

[72] Odze RD, Brown CA, Hartmann CJ, et al. Genetic alterations in chronic ulcerative colitis-associated adenoma-like DALMs are similar to non-colitic sporadic adenomas. Am J Surg Pathol 2000;24:1209–16.

[73] Fogt F, Vortmeyer AO, Stolte M, et al. Loss of heterozygosity of the von Hippel Lindau gene locus in polypoid dysplasia but not flat dysplasia in ulcerative colitis or sporadic adenomas. Hum Pathol 1998;29:961–4.

[74] Fogt F, Vortmeyer AO, Goldman H, et al. Comparison of genetic alterations in colonic adenoma and ulcerative colitis-associated dysplasia and carcinoma. Hum Pathol 1998;29: 131–6.

[75] Mueller E, Vieth M, Stolte M, et al. The differentiation of true adenomas from colitis-associated dysplasia in ulcerative colitis: a comparative immunohistochemical study. Hum Pathol 1999;30:898–905.

[76] Walsh SV, Loda M, Torres CM, et al. p53 and β catenin expression in chronic ulcerative colitis-associated polypoid dysplasia and sporadic adenomas. Am J Surg Pathol 1999;23:963–9.

[77] Mikami T, Mitomi H, Atsuko H, et al. Decreased expression of CD44, alpha-catenin, and deleted colon carcinoma and altered expression of beta-catenin in ulcerative colitis-associated dysplasia and carcinoma, as compared with sporadic colon neoplasms. Cancer 2000;89:733–40.

[78] Selaru FM, Xu Y, Yin J, et al. Artificial neural networks distinguish among subtypes of neoplastic colorectal lesions. Gastroenterology 2002;122:606–13.

[79] Kundu R, Blonski W, Su C, et al. High-grade dysplasia in adenoma-like mass lesions is not an indication for colectomy in patients with ulcerative colitis. Am J Gastroenterol 2005;100(9)(Suppl 1):S303.

[80] Farraye FA, Waye JD, Moscandrew M, et al. Variability in the endoscopic diagnosis and clinical management of adenoma-like and non adenoma-like DALMS in patients with ulcerative colitis. Gastrointest Endosc 2005;61:AB250.

[81] Delaunoit T, Limburg PJ, Goldberg RM, et al. Colorectal cancer prognosis among patients with inflammatory bowel disease. Clin Gastroenterol Hepatol 2006;4:335–42.

[82] Sugita A, Greenstein AJ, Ribeiro MB, et al. Survival with colorectal cancer in ulcerative colitis. A study of 102 cases. Ann Surg 1993;218:189–95.

[83] Greenstein AJ, Slater G, Heimann TM, et al. A comparison of multiple synchronous colorectal cancer in ulcerative colitis, familial polyposis coli, and de novo cancer. Ann Surg 1986;203:123–8.

[84] Nugent FW, Haggitt RC, Colcher H, et al. Malignant potential of chronic ulcerative colitis: preliminary report. Gastroenterology 1979;76:1–5.

[85] Cook MG, Goligher JC. Carcinoma and epithelial dysplasia complicating ulcerative colitis. Gastroenterology 1975;68:1127–36.

[86] van Heerden JA, Beart RW Jr. Carcinoma of the colon and rectum complicating chronic ulcerative colitis. Dis Colon Rectum 1980;23:155–9.

[87] Greenstein AJ, Sachar D, Puccilo A, et al. Cancer in universal and left-sided ulcerative colitis: clinical and pathologic features. Mt Sinai J Med 1979;46:25–32.

[88] Richards ME, Rickert RR, Nance FC. Crohn's disease-associated carcinoma. A poorly recognized complication of inflammatory bowel disease. Ann Surg 1989;209:764–73.

[89] Yamazaki Y, Ribeiro MB, Sachar DB. Malignant colorectal strictures in Crohn' disease. Am J Gastroenterol 1991;86:882–5.

[90] Nakahara H, Ishikawa T, Itabashi M, et al. Diffusely infiltrating primary colorectal carcinoma of linitis plastica and lymphangiosis types. Cancer 1992;69:901–6.

[91] Sigel JE, Goldblume JR. Neuroendocrine neoplasms arising in inflammatory bowel disease: a report of 14 cases. Mod Pathol 1998;11(6):537–42.

[92] Michelassi F, Montag AG, Block GE. Adenosquamous cell carcinoma in ulcerative colitis. Report of a case. Dis Colon Rectum 1988;31:323–6.

[93] Hock YL, Scott KW, Grace RH. Mixed adenocarcinoma/carcinoid tumour of large bowel in a patient with Crohn's disease. J Clin Pathol 1993;46:183–5.

[94] Palazzo JP, Mittal KR. Lymphoepithelioma-like carcinoma of the rectum in a patient with ulcerative colitis. Am J Gastroenterol 1996;91:398–9.

[95] Kulaylat MN, Doerr R, Butttler B, et al. Squamous cell carcinoma complicating idiopathic inflammatory bowel disease. J Surg Oncol 1995;59:48–55.

[96] Weedon DD, Shorter RG, Ilstrup DM, et al. Crohn's disease and cancer. N Engl J Med 1973;289(21):1099–103.

[97] Korelitz BI. Carcinoma of the intestinal tract in Crohn's disease: results of a survey conducted by the National Foundation for Ileitis and Colitis. Am J Gastroenterol 1983;78:44–6.

[98] Stahl TJ, Schoetz DJ, Roberts PL, et al. Crohn's disease and carcinoma: increased justification for surveillance? Dis Colon Rectum 1992;35:850–6.

[99] Nikias G, Eisner T, Katz S, et al. Crohn's disease and colorectal carcinoma: rectal cancer complicating longstanding active perianal disease. Am J Gastroenterol 1995;90:216–9.

[100] Walgenbach S, Junginger T, Rothmund M, et al. Crohn's disease and squamous cell carcinoma of the anorectal transition. Chirurg 1987;58:248–51.

[101] Ribeiro MB, Greenstein AJ, Sachar BD, et al. Colorectal adenocarcinoma in Crohn's disease. Ann Surg 1996;223:186–93.

[102] Gyde SN, Prior P, Macartney JC, et al. Malignancy in Crohn's disease. Gut 1980;21(12): 1024–9.

[103] Choi PM, Zelig MP. Similarity of colorectal cancer in Crohn's disease and ulcerative colitis: implications for carcinogenesis and prevention. Gut 1994;35(7):950–4.

[104] Greenstein AJ, Sachar DB, Smith II, et al. Patterns of neoplasia in Crohn's disease and ulcerative colitis. Cancer 1980;46:403–7.

GASTROENTEROLOGY CLINICS
OF NORTH AMERICA

Molecular Biology of Dysplasia and Cancer in Inflammatory Bowel Disease

Steven H. Itzkowitz, MD

The Dr. Henry D. Janowitz Division of Gastroenterology, PO Box 1069, Mount Sinai School of Medicine, One Gustave Levy Place, New York, NY 10029, USA

Colorectal cancer (CRC) develops from a dysplastic precursor lesion, regardless of whether it arises sporadically, in the setting of high-risk hereditary conditions, or in the context of chronic inflammation like inflammatory bowel disease (IBD). In most clinical settings, the dysplastic lesion is an adenomatous polyp. In IBD, however, dysplasia can be polypoid or flat. In fact, the rather unusual macroscopic appearance and biologic behavior of dysplasia in IBD have stimulated a good deal of research into the natural history and molecular pathogenesis of CRC in patients with IBD. This review focuses on the molecular alterations associated with CRC pathogenesis in IBD. Although none of the molecular alterations to be discussed have yet been integrated into clinical practice, there is potential for molecular diagnostics to enhance the management of patients with long-standing IBD. Most of our current understanding of the molecular alterations involved in colitis-associated carcinogenesis (CAC) comes from studies of patients with ulcerative colitis (UC) rather than Crohn's disease (CD). Because Crohn's colitis carries essentially the same CRC risk as UC of similar disease duration and anatomic extent [1], it is possible that the molecular changes discussed here apply to both types of IBD; however, this must await further proof.

CAUSATION: GENES VERSUS ENVIRONMENT

Although CAC accounts for less than 1% of all CRC cases, patients with IBD are among the highest risk groups for developing CRC. It is assumed that the increased risk of CRC in patients with IBD relates to the many years of colonic inflammation. Indeed, recent evidence confirms that patients with more severe degrees of histologic and endoscopic inflammation are at increased risk of CAC [2]. How much of the cancer predisposition is genetic as opposed to environmental is not known, however. A potential role for hereditable factors is suggested by the observation that patients with IBD who have a family history

This work was supported in part by a grant from the Crohn's and Colitis Foundation of America.

E-mail address: steven.itzkowitz@msnyuhealth.org

0889-8553/06/$ – see front matter   © 2006 Elsevier Inc. All rights reserved.
doi:10.1016/j.gtc.2006.07.002   gastro.theclinics.com

of CRC have an approximate twofold greater risk of developing CRC than a patient with IBD with no such family history [3]. A similar degree of familial risk for CRC has been observed in cotton-top tamarins—animals that develop CRC in a setting of chronic inflammation [4]. It is not yet known which hereditable genes, if any, may contribute to increased CRC risk in IBD.

Environmental factors can modify colon cancer risk. For example, aspirin and nonsteroidal anti-inflammatory drugs (NSAIDs) can decrease the risk of sporadic CRC [5] and rectal adenomatous polyps in patients with familial adenomatous polyposis (FAP) [6]. Likewise, the use of the anti-inflammatory agent 5-aminosalicylic acid seems to lower the risk of CRC in patients with IBD [7]. Although the mechanisms underlying any chemopreventive effect of anti-inflammatory agents remain to be elucidated, they may, in part, inhibit cyclooxygenase-2 (COX-2), a gene that is not expressed in normal colonic mucosa but is induced in premalignant and malignant lesions of the colon, including those from patients with IBD [8]. In a rat model of colon cancer, folate deficiency induced progressive DNA strand breaks within exons 5 through 8 of the *p53* gene (but did not affect the *APC* gene) and folate supplementation increased the steady-state levels of *p53* transcript [9]. Likewise, in a handful of patients with UC who demonstrated microsatellite instability (MSI) in non-neoplastic colonic mucosa, serum and colonic tissue folate levels tended to be lower than in those without MSI, and in one patient, folate supplementation for 6 months resulted in an altered pattern of some microsatellite markers [10]. Thus, although environmental factors, such as medications, diet, and vitamins, might interact with certain genes responsible for colon carcinogenesis, more work is needed in this area. Much more is known about the molecular genetic events involved in the development of colon carcinogenesis.

MOLECULAR PATHWAYS OF SPORADIC COLON CARCINOGENESIS

To place the molecular pathogenesis of colitis-associated neoplasia in proper perspective, it is important to appreciate the molecular events involved in the development of sporadic colorectal neoplasia. CRCs arise as a result of genomic instability. There are two main types of genomic instability that contribute to colon carcinogenesis: chromosomal instability (CIN) and MSI. Most (80%–85%) of sporadic CRCs seem to arise via the CIN pathway. This results in abnormal segregation of chromosomes and abnormal DNA content (aneuploidy). As a result, loss of chromosomal material (loss of heterozygosity [LOH]) often occurs, and this contributes to the loss of key tumor suppressor genes, such as *APC* and *p53*. In addition to undergoing LOH, these genes can be rendered nonfunctional by mutations of the genes themselves. In the development of sporadic CRC, loss of *APC* function is typically an early event. For this reason, the *APC* gene has been considered the "gatekeeper" of the colon. If the APC protein is mutated or lost, this allows β-catenin to gain access to the cell nucleus, where it complexes with specific transcription factors to turn on genes that, in turn, contribute to adenoma formation by altering critical cellular functions, such as proliferation, apoptosis (programmed cell death), and cell-cell adhesion. Once sporadic adenomas form, other changes in genetic regulation occur, such as induction of *k-ras* oncogene and loss of function of tumor suppressor genes on chromosome 18q in the region of the *DCC* (deleted in colon cancer) and *DPC4* genes. Loss of *p53* gene function occurs late and is believed to be the defining event that drives the adenoma to carcinoma.

Tumors that arise via the CIN/tumor suppressor gene pathway are typically microsatellite stable (MSS). Approximately 15% of sporadic CRCs arise through the MSI pathway, however. The MSI pathway involves loss of function of genes that normally repair the mismatches between DNA base pairs that occur during the normal process of DNA replication in dividing cells. Several DNA mismatch repair (MMR) genes cooperate to repair these mismatches. Two of these genes, *hMLH1* and *hMSH2*, are most commonly affected by loss of function in CRC, but mutation or loss of other members of the DNA MMR system can also result in DNA replication errors throughout the genome. This replication error phenomenon is what is detected as the MSI phenotype. The MSI phenotype is detected in tissues using a panel of markers that recognize microsatellite sequences in various parts of the genome. Some colon cancers manifest high degrees of MSI (MSI-H), whereas others demonstrate low levels of MSI (MSI-L), depending on the number of markers showing instability using a standardized marker panel [11]. The MSI phenotype can occur when a DNA MMR gene is mutated (eg, hereditary nonpolyposis colorectal cancer) or if the gene is methylated (eg, sporadic colon cancer).

Epigenetic alterations can also contribute to altered gene expression in colon carcinogenesis. The CpG island methylator phenotype (CIMP) occurs when cytosines in the promoter region of genes become extensively methylated [12]. This is associated with promoter silencing, and hence loss of gene expression. Many genes involved in cell cycle control, cell adhesion, and DNA repair can be methylated in colon cancer. So-called "type A methylation," for example, the estrogen receptor (ER), occurs as a function of age and is found in normal colon and colon cancer. Type C methylation, however, is cancer associated, leading to pathogenic silencing of genes, such as *hMLH1*, *MGMT*, *p16*, *p14*, and *HPP1/TPEF*. In general, there is little overlap between CIN and MSI; tumors manifest one phenotype or the other. There can be overlap between the CIMP phenotype and MSI, however. The process of methylation is an area of intense investigation, and it is anticipated that this line of research should help to define further the molecular pathways involved in CRC in a variety of clinical settings.

GENOMIC INSTABILITY AND CLONAL EXPANSION IN INFLAMMATORY BOWEL DISEASE

Like sporadic CRC, colon carcinogenesis in IBD is a consequence of sequential episodes of somatic genetic mutation and clonal expansion. Unlike sporadic colonic neoplasia, however, where only one or two dysplastic lesions arise in extremely focal areas of the colon, it is not unusual for dysplasia or cancer to be multifocal in colitic mucosa, reflecting a broader "field change." This is best exemplified by careful mapping studies that used DNA aneuploidy as a molecular marker to gain insights into temporal and topographic molecular changes in patients with UC. On the basis of DNA indices, individual cell populations were observed in the same locations of the colon on repeated examinations and became more widely distributed over time, occupying larger areas of the mucosa [13,14]. Moreover, within an aneuploid area, additional subclones of aneuploidy emerged from their predecessors [13]. Indeed, whereas only a handful of different aneuploid cell populations have been detected in aneuploid areas without dysplasia, up to 46 different aneuploid populations may be found in areas of aneuploidy that show dysplastic changes [13]. This indicates that substantial genomic alterations can occur in colonic mucosa without disturbing morphology. The fact that genetically abnormal cells have been observed in histologically nondysplastic mucosa adjacent to or even remote from dysplasia suggests that the dysplastic cells arise from the preexisting mutant clones [13,14].

ROLE OF CHRONIC INFLAMMATION IN INFLAMMATORY BOWEL DISEASE NEOPLASIA

Because CAC arises in the setting of chronic inflammation, it is logical to assume that factors associated with inflammation, such as oxidative stress, contribute to the molecular alterations seen in IBD tissues [15]. Support for this theory comes from a study showing a high frequency of *p53* mutations in inflamed tissues more so than in uninflamed tissues of patients with UC [16]. This study also revealed that reactive oxygen species, which are common byproducts of inflammation, contributed to the *p53* mutations. Others have observed increased p53 expression in actively inflamed UC tissues compared with mucosa in histologic remission not only in patients with long-standing UC but even in those with shorter disease duration [17]. Additional support comes from in vitro studies demonstrating that oxidative stress can interfere with the function of the DNA MMR enzymes, thereby contributing to the development of MSI [18]. Even in vivo, the induction of chronic inflammation by dextran sulfate sodium (DSS) results in more frequent development of low-grade dysplasia (LGD) and high-grade dysplasia (HGD) in *Msh2* knockout mice compared with wild-type controls, and colonic mucosa remote from dysplastic lesions in the DNA MMR-deficient animals also demonstrates MSI [19]. In animal models of CAC, the bacterial flora seems to contribute to carcinogenesis. For example, transforming growth factor (TGF)-β1–deficient mice on an immunodeficient background develop colon adenocarcinoma in association with inflammation [20]. When raised under germ-free conditions, neoplasia does not develop in these mice, but when the animals are recolonized with enteric flora, neoplasms occur in association with colitis [21]. In this model, colitis is required but is not sufficient for cancer formation; a genetic predisposition to cancer seems to contribute. The role of bacteria in human CAC is an area that has not been easy to study.

MOLECULAR PATHWAYS OF COLITIS-ASSOCIATED COLON CARCINOGENESIS

Many of the molecular alterations responsible for sporadic CRC development also play a role in colitis-associated colon carcinogenesis. In fact, the emerging evidence suggests that the two major pathways of CIN and MSI also apply to colitis-associated CRCs and with roughly the same frequency (85% CIN, 15% MSI) (Table 1) [22,23]. As discussed in the following sections, however, the timing of these genomic alterations seems to differ between colitis-associated and sporadic neoplasms (Fig. 1). For example, *APC* loss of function, considered to be a common early event in sporadic colon carcinogenesis, is much less frequent and occurs later in the colitis-associated dysplasia-carcinoma sequence [24–26]. Conversely, *p53* mutations in sporadic neoplasia usually occur late in the adenoma-carcinoma sequence, whereas in patients with colitis, *p53*

Table 1			
Genetic alterations in colitis-associated and sporadic colorectal cancer (CRC)			
	Colitis-associated CRC	Sporadic CRC	References
Chromosomal instability			
Overall CIN	85%	85%	[22,33]
APC-related alterations			
5q loss	56%	26%	[33]
APC LOH	0–33%	31%	[50,51,52]
APC mutation	6%	74%	[24]
Beta-catenin LOH	7%	34%	[51]
p53-related alterations			
17p loss	44%	57%	[33]
p53 LOH	47%–85%	50%	[27,52]
p53 mutation	33–100%	75–80%	[28,47,55]
Chromosome 18q genes			
18q loss	78%	69%	[33]
DCC LOH	54%	39%	[51]
DPC4 mutation	0% (1 case)	—	[59] (58)
K-ras mutation	8–24%	40–50%	[50,55,60–62]
E-cadherin			
LOH	0%	17%	[51]
Protein decrease	43%	37%	[84]
CDH1 methylation	57%	36%	[85]
Microsatellite instability			
Overall MSI-positive	15–40%	15–20%	[23,66,69,70]
HMLH1 methylation[a]	46%	76%	[71,75]
TGFβRII mutation[a]	17%	81%	[76]
Hypermethylation			
p16INK4a	100%	40%	[80]
p14ARF	50%	28–33%	[78,79,81]
HPP1	50%	84%	[82,83]
EYA4	87%	83%	[87]

Abbreviations: LOH, lass of heterozygosity; MSI; microsatellite instability; TGF; transforming growth factor.
  [a]In MSI tumors only.

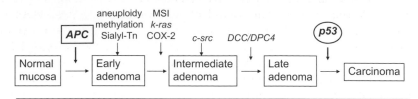

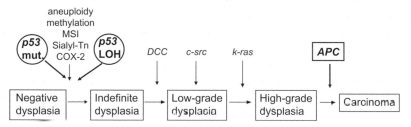

Fig. 1. Comparison of molecular alterations in sporadic colon cancer and colitis-associated colon cancer. Mut, mutation.

mutations occur early and are often detected in mucosa that is nondysplastic or indefinite for dysplasia [27–30]. Indeed, the fact that nondysplastic mucosa from patients with UC demonstrates abnormalities in p53 and DNA MMR function strongly suggests that genomic instability occurs quite early in carcinogenesis.

The model presented in Fig. 1 suggests that colitic mucosa progresses in a systematic fashion in the following way: no dysplasia, indefinite dysplasia, LGD, HGD, and, finally, carcinoma. Although this is a useful paradigm that facilitates the study of cancer risk markers in IBD, it is important to realize that the natural history of dysplasia in IBD is often unpredictable. For example, LGD may progress to cancer without demonstrating HGD, and cancers can arise in colitic colons without any apparent prior dysplasia [31,32]. These caveats should be kept in mind when interpreting the results of studies describing the predictive value of dysplasia or molecular markers in IBD.

CHROMOSOMAL INSTABILITY

Just as with sporadic CRC, CIN represents the major pathway by which cancers seem to arise in patients with IBD. The technique of comparative genomic hybridization demonstrates that a similar number of chromosomal alterations occur in UC-associated and sporadic CRCs, and the frequency of losses and gains of various chromosomal arms is quite similar between the two types of neoplasms [33]. Using probes specific for chromosomes 8, 11, 17, and 18, studies employing fluorescent in situ hybridization noted that patients with UC who had a neoplasm (HGD or cancer) in their colon demonstrated abnormalities in these chromosomal arms not only in the neoplastic lesions themselves but even in nondysplastic rectal mucosa remote from the neoplastic areas [34]. Normal mucosa from control subjects without UC and nondysplastic mucosa of patients with UC who did not harbor a neoplasm in their colon did not exhibit CIN. This observation was reinforced by studies in which DNA fingerprinting demonstrated substantial genomic instability in the dysplastic as well as nondysplastic mucosa of patients with UC harboring a neoplasm [35]. This instability, which was not present in organs outside the colon or in the colon of normal controls, remained at a steady state in precancerous and cancerous biopsies from the same patient, suggesting that genomic instability had reached the maximum level early in neoplastic progression. Thus, widespread genomic instability seems to occur in patients with UC who develop colonic neoplasia but not in patients with UC who have not yet developed neoplasia despite comparable disease duration.

A possible mechanism to explain the CIN associated with UC is telomere shortening. Telomeres are the protective ends of chromosomes that shorten with age and inflammation. Shorter telomeres become sticky, predisposing chromosomal ends to indiscriminately fuse together, forming bridges that subsequently cause the chromosomal arms to break [35]. In biopsies of nondysplastic mucosa from patients with UC with dysplasia or cancer, chromosomal losses were greater and telomeres were shorter than in similar biopsies from patients with UC without neoplasia or from non-UC controls [36]. Support for this comes from a limited study in which telomerase activity was detected in neoplastic as well as nondysplastic colonic mucosa of patients with UC [37].

Aneuploidy

Aneuploidy (abnormal DNA content) occurs as a consequence of CIN. Of all the molecular markers studied in IBD colon carcinogenesis, aneuploidy is the best studied, with observations dating back almost 2 decades. Usually measured by flow cytometry on fresh biopsies, aneuploidy occurs in approximately 14% to 33% of patients with long-standing UC [14,38–40], and its presence has been associated with a longer duration of colitis [41,42]. Aneuploidy correlates directly with dysplasia; approximately 20% to 50% of dysplastic lesions and 50% to 90% of cancers demonstrate aneuploidy [27,39,42–45]. Some studies suggest that aneuploidy is more frequent in HGD than LGD lesions [43,46], whereas others have not confirmed this finding [27,41,47]. Importantly, up to 35% of histologically nondysplastic mucosal biopsies already demonstrate aneuploidy [27,39,41,42,44,45,47]. Thus, aneuploidy is a relatively early event. Curiously, there are examples in which diploid colon cancer occurs in a background of aneuploid mucosa [41]. Moreover, despite intensive repeated surveillance biopsies, colon cancers may arise without preceding dysplasia or aneuploidy [48]. Thus, although aneuploidy as a surrogate measure of CIN seems to be a useful marker of the high-risk colon, aneuploidy may not be universally present or required for progression to the malignant phenotype. This suggests that other pathways also contribute.

Loss of Tumor Suppressor Genes

Tumor suppressor genes are normal cellular genes that control cell proliferation, death, and differentiation. Loss of function of both copies of tumor suppressor genes impairs their function and predisposes to cancer. Inactivation occurs typically by two separate mechanisms; allelic deletion (LOH) of one allele and mutation of the other. The classic tumor suppressor genes *APC*, *p53*, and *DCC/DPC4*, which are important for sporadic colon carcinogenesis, have also been implicated in CAC.

APC *tumor suppressor gene*

As noted previously, *APC* mutations are rare in UC and occur late in the progression from dysplasia to carcinoma (see Fig. 1). Mutations in *APC* are rarely if ever encountered in colitic mucosa that is negative or indefinite for dysplasia [25], and fewer than 14% of tissues manifesting LGD harbor *APC* mutations [25,49]. Indeed, fewer than 14% of UC cancers demonstrate *APC* mutations [25,26,50]. The frequency of *APC* mutations in HGD lesions has been reported to be as high as 50% to 100% [25,49], but this is based on only a few cases. With respect to allelic deletion of *APC*, two studies observed a 33% rate of *APC* LOH [51,52], whereas a third study found no *APC* LOH [50]. Although the APC protein was reported to be abnormally expressed in 76% of UC cancers by immunohistochemistry [53], the overall data suggest that the *APC* gene is rarely involved in CAC.

P53 *tumor suppressor gene*

The normal p53 protein is considered to be an important guardian of the genome and acts to prevent clonal expansion of mutant cells by not allowing cells that have acquired damaged DNA to progress through the cell cycle. Allelic deletion of *p53* occurs in approximately 47% to 85% of UC-associated CRC [27,30,52]. Burmer and colleagues [27] found that *p53* LOH correlated with malignant progression, detecting this molecular change in 6% of biopsies without dysplasia, 9% with indefinite dysplasia, 33% with LGD, 63% with HGD, and 85% with cancer. They also noted that *p53* LOH was restricted to biopsies that were aneuploid, suggesting that aneuploidy precedes *p53* LOH. Further studies from these investigators indicated that *p53* mutations were distributed more extensively than *p53* LOH in carefully mapped colectomy specimens and that mutation but not LOH of *p53* was found in diploid nondysplastic mucosa, suggesting that *p53* mutation was an early molecular change that occurred before aneuploidy, which, in turn, preceded *p53* LOH (see Fig. 1) [28]. Other investigators found a more variable association between *p53* mutation and aneuploidy but confirmed that *p53* mutations occurred in 19% of biopsies without dysplasia, with a steady increase in frequency among biopsies that showed progressive degrees of dysplasia [47]. In fact, using tissues from patients with UC who did not have cancer, Hussain and coworkers [16] demonstrated a high frequency of *p53* mutations in inflamed mucosa, suggesting that chronic inflammation itself may predispose to these early mutations. Additional evidence from immunohistochemical studies links altered p53 expression with dysplasia in UC; with this technique, biopsies that are negative for dysplasia do not often demonstrate p53 staining [29,54–56]. Thus, considerable evidence implicates *p53* as playing an instrumental role in UC carcinogenesis, apparently at an early stage.

Tumor suppressor genes on 18q (DCC/DPC4)

Allelic losses of 18q, particularly 18q21.1, are common in sporadic and colitis-associated CRC. Allelic loss of 18q has been reported to occur in 78% of UC-associated CRC compared with 69% of sporadic CRC [33]. Moreover, three (60%) of five dysplastic lesions and one (20%) of five nondysplastic samples manifested 18q allelic deletion [57]. Candidate tumor suppressor genes that reside in this location include *DCC* and *DPC4*. LOH at *DCC* has been reported to occur in 54% of CAC compared with 39% of sporadic CRC [51]. One study of 10 cases of CAC found 18q LOH in 3 cases, one of which also demonstrated mutation in *DPC4* [58]. Others were unable to detect any DPC4 mutations among 10 cases of colitis-associated CRC [59].

Activation of Proto-Oncogenes

Proto-oncogenes are normal cellular genes that, when activated by mutation of one allele, can disrupt normal cell growth and differentiation and enhance the progression to neoplastic transformation. With regard to colitis-associated CRC, two proto-oncogenes have received the most attention: *k-ras* and *c-src*.

K-ras *oncogene*

K-ras mutations typically are not found in UC mucosa that is negative for dysplasia. In fact, most studies also indicate that *k-ras* mutations are rare even in LGD [47,50,60–62], although one study using a highly sensitive assay detected *k-ras* mutations in 36% and 14% of lesions that were indefinite for dysplasia and LGD, respectively [25]. When *k-ras* mutations occur, they tend to be found in HGD or cancerous lesions. Early studies suggested that the 8% to 24% frequency of *k-ras* mutations in UC cancers was lower than the approximately 40% to 50% rate in sporadic CRC [50,55,60–62], but more recent studies suggest that 40% to 50% of UC-associated CRC cases demonstrate *k-ras* mutations [25,47,49,63].

Src *oncogene*

The cellular oncogene, *c-src*, is a tyrosine kinase that is associated with malignant transformation in a variety of tumors. Elevated *c-src* levels have been reported in sporadic colon adenomas and carcinomas [64]. In patients with UC, *c-src* activity was low in areas of inflammation but demonstrated a progressive increase in activity in LGD, HGD, a dysplastic-associated lesion or mass (DALM), and cancer lesions [65].

MICROSATELLITE INSTABILITY

MSI is not found in normal colonic mucosa from healthy controls or from patients with other types of benign inflammatory colitis [66,67]. MSI is also quite rare in colonic mucosa from patients with Crohn's colitis [68].

As many as 15% to 40% of patients with UC demonstrate MSI in cancer tissues, however (see Table 1). In some studies, UC-associated cancers were more likely to express MSI-L rather than MSI-H [50,69,70], but other studies indicate that the two types of instability can occur with similar frequency [22,23,66,71]. Some of this difference may relate to the fact that not all studies applied the National Institutes of Health (NIH) consensus microsatellite marker panel. Curiously, MSI has been detected as an early event, occurring in non-dysplastic mucosa even from patients with disease of rather short duration [66,67]. The DNA MMR system is important for repairing frameshift mutations that can be induced by oxidative stress accompanying chronic inflammation. Cells that are deficient in MMR, but even cells that are MMR proficient, accumulate frameshift mutations, suggesting that oxidative stress acts as a mutagen [72]. Also, oxidative stress can functionally impair the protein components of the MMR system without necessarily causing genetic mutations [18]. This may contribute to the MSI-L phenotype seen in nonneoplastic and neoplastic mucosa of patients with IBD. A germline hMSH2 mutation was reported to be more frequent in patients with UC who developed HGD and cancer than in those who did not [73], but this finding was not substantiated by other investigators [74]. In sporadic CRC, hypermethylation of hMLH1 is an important mechanism for silencing the function of this gene resulting in MSI-H tumors [75]. Likewise, in UC-associated neoplasms, hypermethylation of hMLH1 was detected in almost half of MSI-H cancers and dysplasias [71].

Impairment of Type II Transforming Growth Factor-β1 Receptor
Mutations of the TGF-β1 receptor permit colonic cells to escape growth control. The type II TGF-β1 receptor (TGFβRII) has two microsatellites within its coding region that predispose this gene to replication errors in cells that have abnormal DNA MMR. Thus, as a target gene for MSI, TGFβRII instability has been demonstrated in as many as 81% of cases of MSI sporadic CRC [76]. In contrast, among 18 UC neoplasms that demonstrated MSI, only 3 (17%) demonstrated instability of TGFβRII [76], indicating that this same phenomenon occurs in CAC but with lesser frequency.

PROMOTER METHYLATION
Methylation of CpG islands in several genes seems to precede and be more widespread than dysplasia [77]. In colitis-associated neoplasms, hMLH1 hypermethylation was observed in 6 (46%) of 13 MSI-H, 1 (16%) of 6 MSI-L, and 4 (15%) of 27 MSS specimens, implicating this epigenetic change as a cause of MSI [71]. The cell cycle inhibitor, $p16^{INK4a}$, loss of which has been implicated in sporadic CRC [78,79], is commonly hypermethylated in UC neoplasms [80]. Approximately 10% of biopsies without dysplasia already demonstrate $p16$ promoter hypermethylation, with the rate increasing with higher grades of dysplasia and reaching 100% in cancer specimens. $p14^{ARF}$ is an indirect regulator of $p53$, and it resides at the same locus as $p16^{INK4a}$. Loss of $p14^{ARF}$ function by promoter hypermethylation has been reported in 50% of adenocarcinomas,

33% of dysplastic lesions, and even in 60% of nondysplastic mucosal samples in patients with UC [81]. Another gene, *HPP1*, recently implicated in the hyperplastic polyp-serrated adenoma-carcinoma pathway of colorectal cancer [82] undergoes methylation silencing in 50% and 40% of cases of CAC and dysplasia, respectively [83].

E-cadherin (*CDH1*), a member of the calcium-dependent cell adhesion molecule family, plays an important role in cell-cell contacts, thereby functioning as a tumor suppressor gene. Loss of E-cadherin function has been implicated in various cancers, including diffuse gastric cancer, breast cancer, and prostate cancer. Loss of E-cadherin expression has been reported in approximately 57% of CAC because of hypermethylation of the E-cadherin promoter rather than allelic loss [84,85]. In fact, *CDH1* promoter hypermethylation was detected in 13 (93%) of 14 colonoscopies in which dysplasia was present, compared with only 1 (6%) of 17 colonoscopies without detectable dysplasia, and it is typically the dysplastic lesion itself that manifests reduced E-cadherin protein expression [86].

Methylation of the eyes absent 4 (*EYA4*) gene, a transcription activator involved in apoptosis, seems to be a promising new marker demonstrating hypermethylation in 83% and 67% of cancerous and dysplastic UC tissues but not at all in inflamed mucosa [87].

POTENTIAL CLINICAL APPLICATION OF MOLECULAR MARKERS
Markers of Cancer Progression
Histologic evidence of dysplasia on colonic biopsies is the "gold standard" marker for determining cancer risk and deciding on clinical management. There are many limitations of dysplasia, however, such as variations in pathologic interpretation, focality of dysplasia often making random biopsy detection difficult, and the fact that cancers can arise without any apparent preceding detectable dysplasia. This has raised the question of whether newer molecular markers could be complementary to dysplasia for assigning cancer risk.

To date, most of our knowledge about the types of molecular alterations in colitis-associated neoplasia has come from studies that took a particular marker of interest and analyzed its expression in pathologic lesions at a single time point from several patients representing the pathologic spectrum of no dysplasia, indefinite dysplasia, LGD, HGD, and cancer. In this type of horizontal cross-sectional study design, any genetic alteration that demonstrates a preferential or increased expression in neoplastic (dysplasia or cancer) tissues is considered potentially useful. Many such markers, such as those indicated in Fig. 1, have been evaluated in this way. In many of these studies, when a marker is detected in nondysplastic tissue from a patient who also has dysplasia or cancer elsewhere in the colon, the marker is considered to be expressed "earlier" than dysplasia. Although this concept may be plausible, it is not biologically or clinically accurate to assign a chronologic sequence to marker expression when the tissue derives from a single time point.

Molecular Markers of Future Cancer Risk

An advantage to studying patients with IBD is that they typically undergo periodic surveillance colonoscopies with repeated tissue sampling. IBD is one of the few clinical settings in which multiple repetitive sampling of colonic tissue is routinely performed. This provides a unique opportunity to study histologic and molecular changes chronologically. To date, few studies describing a promising new marker in IBD tissues have used a chronologic study design. The reasons for this are multifactorial but include difficulty in obtaining these tissues (which are often more plentiful in tertiary referral centers), interest of the investigator in studying the marker chronologically, and definition of what a "marker-positive" patient is.

To date, only four molecular markers—aneuploidy, p53, MSI, and the mucin-associated sialyl-Tn (STn) antigen—have been evaluated in a chronologic context, and each has been demonstrated to be a harbinger of subsequent risk of developing dysplasia or cancer. Longitudinal prospective studies have demonstrated that aneuploidy is a marker of subsequent progression to neoplasia in patients with long-standing UC who have not yet demonstrated dysplasia. Among 25 high-risk patients with UC without dysplasia, all 5 who showed aneuploidy progressed to dysplasia within 1 to 2.5 years, whereas 19 (95%) of 20 without aneuploidy did not progress to dysplasia or aneuploidy over a 2- to 9-year period [13]. Likewise, among 34 patients with UC without dysplasia, 3 (75%) of 4 patients with aneuploidy progressed to LGD, whereas only 2 (7%) of 30 without aneuploidy progressed to LGD over a 10-year period [38]. These and other studies indicate that when aneuploidy is detected, it usually is found before or at the same time as dysplasia [13,14,38,40]. In the largest study with the longest follow-up, all the 10 patients who developed HGD or cancer had aneuploidy detected before or simultaneously with these histologically more advanced neoplastic lesions, whereas 5 (42%) of 12 patients with LGD had aneuploidy detected after LGD [40]. Aneuploidy following dysplasia has also been reported by others [14]. Thus, it seems that finding aneuploidy may be a useful marker of cancer risk, but not finding it does not offer reassurance.

Little is known about whether p53 expression in surveillance biopsies predicts the future development of dysplasia or cancer. One study suggested that abnormal p53 immunostaining may precede LGD, HGD, and cancer by 8, 26, and 38 months, respectively [88]. Other reports in a handful of patients also suggest that p53 expression may precede cancer by 2 to 4 years [89,90].

Another study retrospectively analyzed biopsy specimens for MSI and *k-ras* mutations before surgical resection [69]. The presence of MSI in the biopsies did not predict the presence of MSI in the resection specimens. There were three cases in which *k-ras* mutations were detected in dysplastic presurgical biopsies, and two of them demonstrated the identical mutation in the resection specimen. MSI-H was reported to be present in chronic colitis tissue 2 to 12 years before the development of MSI-H CAC in four patients [91].

STn is a mucin-associated carbohydrate antigen whose expression has been studied in cross-sectional and longitudinal study designs, and it fulfills the criteria of being more widespread and appearing chronologically earlier than dysplasia [92,93]. In fact, STn expression was noted as early as 2 to 9 years before the first detection of dysplasia. Importantly, STn expression does not just overlap with dysplasia but is complementary to it. Moreover, STn expression is also independent of aneuploidy, thereby adding information beyond what dysplasia or aneuploidy provides [93].

There is no consensus as to how, or even whether, these markers of cancer risk should be incorporated into clinical management of patients with long-standing IBD. Given our current knowledge, no one is likely to recommend colectomy to a patient solely on the basis of marker positivity without some evidence of dysplasia, even if the patient's tissue demonstrated marker positivity on several colonoscopies. Perhaps more intensive surveillance should be offered to such patients. These issues should be considered as more research is conducted in this field.

PROBLEM OF POLYPOID DYSPLASIA IN INFLAMMATORY BOWEL DISEASE

One dilemma that worries clinicians is the finding of dysplasia in a polypoid lesion of a patient with long-standing IBD. If the lesion is considered a sporadic adenoma, it can be removed endoscopically and the patient continued under surveillance. If it is a more ominous DALM, however, this usually prompts a recommendation for total proctocolectomy because of the high synchronous and metachronous rate of CRC. Recent studies suggest that if the polypoid lesion can be completely removed by endoscopic polypectomy and if numerous biopsies of mucosa adjacent to the polyp base and throughout the rest of colon are negative for dysplasia, the polypectomy alone is sufficient and colectomy can be deferred while the patient continues to undergo surveillance [94,95]. A study using global gene expression profiles suggested that an artificial neural network may be able to distinguish between a sporadic adenoma and a polypoid dysplastic lesion in a patient with UC [96]. Whether this technology is applied for future molecular diagnostics in IBD remains to be seen.

NEW MOLECULAR SCREENING APPROACHES

Most efforts to date have understandably focused on studying tissues from patients with IBD to identify molecular markers that might be helpful for understanding cancer pathogenesis or possibly assigning risk. A more comprehensive technique applied to tissues is molecular profiling using microarrays, which, in a recent study, identified 699 transcripts that differed between benign mucosa and HGD and 242 transcripts that differed between benign mucosa and CAC. Additional studies are needed to confirm these findings and sort out their relevance to the biology of neoplasia in UC [97]. Other investigators used DNA extracted from serum and detected *k-ras* mutations in two of four patients with UC but not in any of three patients with CD or in healthy controls [98].

Another approach worth considering is to examine the stool of patients with IBD for molecular alterations. This technology, which uses markers associated with the more common molecular alterations associated with CIN, MSI and abnormal apoptosis, has already been shown to have reasonable sensitivity and rather high specificity for sporadic CRC and adenomas [99]. Because the DNA shed into stool should theoretically provide a more comprehensive sampling of abnormal cells than random pinch biopsies, stool DNA testing could significantly contribute to the management of patients with long-standing IBD who are at risk for developing CRC. Molecular markers have also been studied in colonic lavage fluid taken at the time of colonoscopy. One such study analyzed *p53* and *k-ras* mutations in colonic effluent and noted mutations in either gene in up to 19% of patients with UC, particularly in those with longer disease duration [100]. In addition, 15% of patients with Crohn's colitis but not ileitis had a positive mutation. Mutations were also found in 2% of noninflammatory controls and in only 50% of patients with sporadic colon cancer. In several patients, the molecular alteration could not be confirmed on subsequent lavage samples, and only one patient who repeatedly had a *p53* mutation in the fluid had the same mutation discovered in biopsy tissues. The appealing concept behind stool- or lavage-based molecular diagnostics is the potential to sample a much larger surface area of the colon than the multiple random pinch biopsies currently performed. As this technology becomes further developed and newer more specific molecular markers become available, this approach may assume greater importance.

References

[1] Canavan C, Abrams KR, Mayberry J. Meta-analysis: colorectal and small bowel cancer risk in patients with Crohn's disease. Aliment Pharmacol Ther 2006;23:1097–104.

[2] Rutter M, Saunders B, Wilkinson K, et al. Severity of inflammation is a risk factor for colorectal neoplasia in ulcerative colitis. Gastroenterology 2004;126:451–9.

[3] Nuako KW, Ahlquist DA, Mahoney DW, et al. Familial predisposition for colorectal cancer in chronic ulcerative colitis: a case-control study. Gastroenterology 1998;115:1079–83.

[4] Bertone ER, Giovannucci EL, King NW Jr, et al. Family history as a risk factor for ulcerative colitis-associated colon cancer in cotton-top tamarin. Gastroenterology 1998;114:669–74.

[5] Janne PA, Mayer RJ. Chemoprevention of colorectal cancer. N Engl J Med 2000;342: 1960–8.

[6] Cruz-Correa M, Hylind LM, Romans KE, et al. Long-term treatment with sulindac in familial adenomatous polyposis: a prospective cohort study. Gastroenterology 2002;122:641–5.

[7] Velayos FS, Terdiman JP, Walsh JM. Effect of 5-aminosalicylate use on colorectal cancer and dysplasia risk: a systematic review and metaanalysis of observational studies. Am J Gastroenterol 2005;100:1345–53.

[8] Agoff SN, Brentnall TA, Crispin DA, et al. The role of cyclooxygenase 2 in ulcerative colitis-associated neoplasia. Am J Pathol 2000;157:737–45.

[9] Kim YI, Shirwadkar S, Choi SW, et al. Effects of dietary folate on DNA strand breaks within mutation-prone exons of the *p53* gene in rat colon. Gastroenterology 2000;119:151–61.

[10] Cravo ML, Albuqueurque CM, Salazar de Sousa L, et al. Microsatellite instability in non-neoplastic mucosa of patients with ulcerative colitis: effect of folate supplementation. Am J Gastroenterol 1998;93:2060–4.

[11] Boland CR, Thibodeau SN, Hamilton SR, et al. A National Cancer Institute workshop on microsatellite instability for cancer detection and familial predisposition: development of international criteria for the determination of microsatellite instability in colorectal cancer. Cancer Res 1998;58:5248–57.

[12] Ahuja N, Mohan AL, Li Q, et al. Association between CpG island methylation and micro-satellite instability in colorectal cancer. Cancer Res 1997;57:3370–4.
[13] Rubin CE, Haggitt RC, Burmer GC, et al. DNA aneuploidy in colonic biopsies predicts future development of dysplasia in ulcerative colitis. Gastroenterology 1992;103: 1611–20.
[14] Lofberg R, Brostrom O, Karlen P, et al. DNA aneuploidy in ulcerative colitis: reproducibility, topographic distribution, and relation to dysplasia. Gastroenterology 1992;102:1149–54.
[15] Itzkowitz SH, Yio X. Inflammation and cancer. IV. Colorectal cancer in inflammatory bowel disease: the role of inflammation. Am J Physiol Gastrointest Liver Physiol 2004;287(1): G7–17.
[16] Hussain SP, Amstad P, Raja K, et al. Increased p53 mutation load in noncancerous colon tissue from ulcerative colitis: a cancer-prone chronic inflammatory bowel disease. Cancer Res 2000;60:3333–7.
[17] Arai N, Mitomi H, Ohtani Y, et al. Enhanced epithelial cell turnover associated with p53 accumulation and high p21WAF1/CIP1 expression in ulcerative colitis. Mod Pathol 1999;12:604–11.
[18] Chang CL, Marra G, Chauhan DP, et al. Oxidative stress inactivates the human DNA mis-match repair system. Am J Physiol Cell Physiol 2002;283:C148–54.
[19] Kohonen-Corish MRJ, Daniel JJ, te Riele H, et al. Susceptibility of Msh2-deficient mice to inflammation-associated colorectal tumors. Cancer Res 2002;62:2092–7.
[20] Engle SJ, Hoying JB, Boivin GP, et al. Transforming growth factor beta-1 suppresses non-metastatic colon cancer at an early stage of tumorigenesis. Cancer Res 1999;59: 3379–86.
[21] Engle SJ, Ormsby I, Pawlowski S, et al. Elimination of colon cancer in germ-free transform-ing growth factor beta 1-deficient mice. Cancer Res 2002;62:6362–6.
[22] Willenbucher RF, Aust DE, Chang CG, et al. Genomic instability is an early event during the progression pathway of ulcerative colitis-related neoplasia. Am J Pathol 1999;154: 1825–30.
[23] Suzuki H, Harpaz N, Tarmin L, et al. Microsatellite instability in ulcerative colitis-associated colorectal dysplasias and cancers. Cancer Res 1994;54:4841–4.
[24] Tarmin L, Yin J, Harpaz N, et al. Adenomatous polyposis coli gene mutations in ulcerative colitis-associated dysplasias and cancers versus sporadic colon neoplasms. Cancer Res 1995;55:2035–8.
[25] Redston MS, Papadopoulos N, Caldas C, et al. Common occurrence of APC and K-ras gene mutations in the spectrum of colitis-associated neoplasias. Gastroenterology 1995;108:383–92.
[26] Aust DE, Terdiman JP, Willenbucher RF, et al. The APC/β-catenin pathway in ulcerative co-litis-related colorectal carcinomas. Cancer 2002;94:1421–7.
[27] Burmer GC, Rabinovitch PS, Haggitt RC, et al. Neoplastic progression in ulcerative colitis: histology, DNA content, and loss of a p53 allele. Gastroenterology 1992;103:1602–10.
[28] Brentnall TA, Crispin DA, Rabinovitch PS, et al. Mutations of the p53 gene: an early marker of neoplastic progression in ulcerative colitis. Gastroenterology 1994;107: 369–78.
[29] Klump B, Holzmann K, Kuhn A, et al. Distribution of cell populations with DNA aneuploidy and p53 protein expression in ulcerative colitis. Eur J Gastroenterol Hepatol 1997;9: 789–94.
[30] Yin J, Harpaz N, Tong Y, et al. p53 Point mutations in dysplastic and cancerous ulcerative colitis lesions. Gastroenterology 1993;104:1633–9.
[31] Lennard-Jones JE, Morson BC, Ritchie JK, et al. Cancer surveillance in ulcerative colitis. Ex-perience over 15 years. Lancet 1983;II:149–52.
[32] Rosenstock E, Farmer RG, Petras R, et al. Surveillance for colonic carcinoma in ulcerative colitis. Gastroenterology 1985;89:1342–6.

[33] Aust DE, Willenbucher RF, Terdiman JP, et al. Chromosomal alterations in ulcerative colitis-related and sporadic colorectal cancers by comparative genomic hybridization. Hum Pathol 2000;31:109–14.

[34] Rabinovitch PS, Dziadon S, Brentnall TA, et al. Pancolonic chromosomal instability precedes dysplasia and cancer in ulcerative colitis. Cancer Res 1999;59:5148–53.

[35] Brentnall TA. Molecular underpinnings of cancer in ulcerative colitis. Curr Opin Gastroenterol 2003;19:64–8.

[36] O'Sullivan JN, Bronner MP, Brentnall TA, et al. Chromosomal instability in ulcerative colitis is related to telomere shortening. Nat Genet 2002;32:280–4.

[37] Holzmann K, Klump B, Weis-Klemm M, et al. Telomerase activity in long-standing ulcerative colitis. Anticancer Res 2000;20:3951–6.

[38] Befrits R, Hammarberg C, Rubio C, et al. DNA aneuploidy and histologic dysplasia in long-standing ulcerative colitis: a 10-year follow-up study. Dis Colon Rectum 1994;37:313–20.

[39] Melville DM, Jass JR, Shepherd NA, et al. Dysplasia and deoxyribonucleic acid aneuploidy in the assessment of precancerous changes in chronic ulcerative colitis. Gastroenterology 1988;95:668–75.

[40] Lindberg JO, Stenling RB, Rutegard JN. DNA aneuploidy as a marker of premalignancy in surveillance of patients with ulcerative colitis. Br J Surg 1999;86:947–50.

[41] Fozard JBJ, Quirke P, Dixon MF, et al. DNA aneuploidy in ulcerative colitis. Gut 1986;27:1414–8.

[42] Hammarberg C, Slezak P, Tribukait B. Early detection of malignancy in ulcerative colitis; a flow cytometric DNA study. Cancer 1984;53:291–5.

[43] Cuvelier CA, Morson BC, Roels HJ. The DNA content in cancer and dysplasia in chronic ulcerative colitis. Histopathology 1987;11:927–39.

[44] Lofberg R, Tribukait B, Ost A, et al. Flow cytometric DNA analysis in longstanding ulcerative colitis: a method of prediction of dysplasia and carcinoma development? Gut 1987;28:1100–6.

[45] Meling GI, Clausen OPF, Bergan A, et al. Flow cytometric DNA ploidy pattern in dysplastic mucosa, and in primary and metastatic carcinomas in patients with longstanding ulcerative colitis. Br J Cancer 1991;64:339–44.

[46] Suzuki K, Muto T, Masaki T, et al. Microspectrophotometric DNA analysis in ulcerative colitis with special reference to its application in diagnosis of carcinoma and dysplasia. Gut 1990;31:1266–70.

[47] Holzmann K, Klump B, Borchard F, et al. Comparative analysis of histology, DNA content, p53, and Ki-ras mutations in colectomy specimens with long-standing ulcerative colitis. Int J Cancer 1998;76:1–6.

[48] Lofberg R, Lindquist K, Veress B, et al. Highly malignant carcinoma in chronic ulcerative colitis without preceding dysplasia or DNA aneuploidy. Dis Colon Rectum 1992;35:82–6.

[49] Kern SE, Redston M, Seymour AB, et al. Molecular genetic profiles of colitis associated neoplasms. Gastroenterology 1994;107:420–8.

[50] Umetani N, Sasaki S, Watanabe T, et al. Genetic alterations in ulcerative colitis-associated neoplasia focusing on APC, K-ras gene and microsatellite instability. Jpn J Cancer Res 1999;90:1081–7.

[51] Tomlinson I, Ilyas M, Johnson V, et al. A comparison of the genetic pathways involved in the pathogenesis of three types of colorectal cancer. J Pathol 1998;184:148–52.

[52] Greenwald BD, Harpaz N, Yin J, et al. Loss of heterozygosity affecting the p53, Rb, and mcc/apc tumor suppressor gene loci in dysplastic and cancerous ulcerative colitis. Cancer Res 1992;52:741–5.

[53] Aust DE, Terdiman JP, Willenbucher RF, et al. Altered distribution of β-catenin, and its binding proteins E-cadherin and APC, in ulcerative colitis-related colorectal cancers. Mod Pathol 2001;14:29–39.

[54] Harpaz N, Peck AL, Yin J, et al. P53 protein expression in ulcerative colitis-associated colorectal dysplasia and carcinoma. Hum Pathol 1994;25:1069–74.

[55] Chaubert P, Benhattar J, Saraga E, et al. K-ras mutations and p53 alterations in neoplastic and nonneoplastic lesions associated with longstanding ulcerative colitis. Am J Pathol 1994;144:767–75.

[56] Wong NACS, Mayer NJ, MacKell S, et al. Immunohistochemical assessment of Ki67 and p53 expression assists the diagnosis and grading of ulcerative colitis-related dysplasia. Histopathology 2000;37:108–14.

[57] Willenbucher RF, Zelman SJ, Ferrell LD, et al. Chromosomal alterations in ulcerative colitis-related neoplastic progression. Gastroenterology 1997;113:791–801.

[58] Hoque ATMS, Hahn SA, Schutte M, et al. DPC4 gene mutation in colitis associated neoplasia. Gut 1997;40:120–2.

[59] Lei J, Zou TT, Shi YQ, et al. Infrequent DPC4 gene mutation in esophageal cancer, gastric cancer and ulcerative colitis-associated neoplasms. Oncogene 1996;13:2459–62.

[60] Burmer GC, Levine DS, Kulander BG, et al. c-Ki-ras mutations in chronic ulcerative colitis and sporadic colon carcinoma. Gastroenterology 1990;99:416–20.

[61] Meltzer SJ, Mane SM, Wood PK, et al. Activation of c-Ki-ras in human gastrointestinal dysplasias determined by direct sequencing of polymerase chain reaction products. Cancer Res 1990;50:3627–30.

[62] Bell SM, Kelly SA, Hoyle JA, et al. c-Ki-ras gene mutations in dysplasia and carcinomas complicating ulcerative colitis. Br J Cancer 1991;64:174–8.

[63] Chen J, Compton C, Cheng B, et al. c-Ki-ras mutations in dysplastic fields and cancer in ulcerative colitis. Gastroenterology 1992;102:1983–7.

[64] Cartwright CA, Meisler AI, Eckhart W. Activation of the pp60 c-src protein kinase is an early event in colonic carcinogenesis. Proc Natl Acad Sci USA 1990;87:558–62.

[65] Cartwright CA, Coad CA, Egbert BM. Elevated c-src tyrosine kinase activity in premalignant epithelia of ulcerative colitis. J Clin Invest 1994;93:509–15.

[66] Brentnall TA, Crispin DA, Bronner MP, et al. Microsatellite instability in nonneoplastic mucosa from patients with chronic ulcerative colitis. Cancer Res 1996;56:1237–40.

[67] Heinen CD, Noffsinger AE, Belli J, et al. Regenerative lesions in ulcerative colitis are characterized by microsatellite mutation. Genes Chromosomes Cancer 1997;19:170–5.

[68] Noffsinger A, Kretschmer S, Belli J, et al. Microsatellite instability is uncommon in intestinal mucosa of patients with Crohn's disease. Dig Dis Sci 2000;45:378–84.

[69] Lyda MH, Noffsinger A, Belli J, et al. Microsatellite instability and K-ras mutations in patients with ulcerative colitis. Hum Pathol 2000;31:665–71.

[70] Cawkwell L, Sutherland F, Murgatroyd H, et al. Defective hMSH2/hMLH1 protein expression is seen infrequently in ulcerative colitis associated colorectal cancers. Gut 2000;46:367–9.

[71] Fleisher AS, Esteller M, Harpaz N, et al. Microsatellite instability in inflammatory bowel disease-associated neoplastic lesions is associated with hypermethylation and diminished expression of the DNA mismatch repair gene, hMLH1. Cancer Res 2000;60:4864–8.

[72] Gasche C, Chang CL, Rhees J, et al. Oxidative stress increases frameshift mutations in human colorectal cancer cells. Cancer Res 2001;61:7444–8.

[73] Brentnall TA, Rubin CE, Crispin DA, et al. A germline substitution in the human MSH2 gene is associated with high-grade dysplasia and cancer in ulcerative colitis. Gastroenterology 1995;109:151–5.

[74] Noffsinger AE, Belli J, Fogt F, et al. A germline hMSH2 alteration is unrelated to colonic microsatellite instability in patients with ulcerative colitis. Hum Pathol 1999;30:8–12.

[75] Cunningham JM, Christensen ER, Tester DJ, et al. Hypermethylation of the hMLH1 promoter in colon cancer with microsatellite instability. Cancer Res 1998;58:3455–60.

[76] Souza RF, Lei J, Yin J, et al. A transforming growth factor beta 1 receptor type II mutation in ulcerative colitis-associated neoplasms. Gastroenterology 1997;112:40–5.

[77] Issa JPJ, Ahuja N, Toyota M, et al. Accelerated age-related CpG island methylation in ulcerative colitis. Cancer Res 2001;61:3573–7.

[78] Esteller M, Tortola S, Toyota M, et al. Hypermethylation-associated inactivation of $p14^{ARF}$ is independent of $p16^{INK4a}$ methylation and $p53$ mutational status. Cancer Res 2000;60: 129–33.

[79] Burri N, Shaw P, Bouzourene H, et al. Methylation silencing and mutations of the $p14ARF$ and $p16INK4a$ genes in colon cancer. Lab Invest 2001;81:217–29.

[80] Hsieh CJ, Klump B, Holzmann K, et al. Hypermethylation of the p16INK4a promoter in colectomy specimens of patients with long-standing and extensive ulcerative colitis. Cancer Res 1998;58:3942–5.

[81] Sato F, Harpaz N, Shibata D, et al. Hypermethylation of the $p14^{ARF}$ gene in ulcerative colitis-associated colorectal carcinogenesis. Cancer Res 2002;62:1148–51.

[82] Young J, Biden KG, Simms LA, et al. HPP1: a transmembrane protein-encoding gene commonly methylated in colorectal polyps and cancers. Proc Natl Acad Sci USA 2001;98: 265–70.

[83] Sato F, Shibata D, Harpaz N, et al. Aberrant methylation of the HPP1 gene in ulcerative colitis-associated colorectal carcinoma. Cancer Res 2002;62:6820–2.

[84] Ilyas M, Tomlinson IP, Hanby A, et al. Allele loss, replication errors and loss of expression of E-cadherin in colorectal cancers. Gut 1997;40:654–9.

[85] Wheeler JMD, Kim HC, Efstathiou JA, et al. Hypermethylation of the promoter region of the E-cadherin gene (CDH1) in sporadic and ulcerative colitis associated colorectal cancer. Gut 2001;48:367–71.

[86] Azarschab P, Porschen R, Gregor M, et al. Epigenetic control of the E-cadherin gene (CDH1) by CpG methylation in colectomy samples of patients with ulcerative colitis. Genes Chromosomes Cancer 2002;35:121–6.

[87] Osborn NK, Zou H, Molina JR, et al. Aberrant methylation of the eyes absent 4 gene in ulcerative colitis-associated dysplasia. Clin Gastroenterol Hepatol 2006;4:212–8.

[88] Lashner BA, Shapiro BD, Husain A, et al. Evaluation of the usefulness of testing for p53 mutations in colorectal cancer surveillance for ulcerative colitis. Am J Gastroenterol 1999;94:456–62.

[89] Sato A, Machinami R. p53 Immunohistochemistry of ulcerative colitis-associated with dysplasia and carcinoma. Pathol Int 1999;49:858–68.

[90] Ilyas M, Talbot IC. p53 Expression in ulcerative colitis: a longitudinal study. Gut 1995;37: 802–4.

[91] Tahara T, Inoue N, Hisamatsu T, et al. Clinical significance of microsatellite instability in the inflamed mucosa for the prediction of colonic neoplasms in patients with ulcerative colitis. J Gastroenterol Hepatol 2005;20:710–5.

[92] Itzkowitz SH, Young E, Dubois D, et al. Sialosyl-Tn antigen is prevalent and precedes dysplasia in ulcerative colitis: a retrospective case-control study. Gastroenterology 1996;110: 694–704.

[93] Karlen P, Young E, Brostrom O, et al. Sialyl-Tn antigen as a marker of colon cancer risk in ulcerative colitis: relation to dysplasia and DNA aneuploidy. Gastroenterology 1998; 115:1395–404.

[94] Rubin PH, Friedman S, Harpaz S, et al. Colonoscopic polypectomy in chronic colitis: conservative management after endoscopic resection of dysplastic polyps. Gastroenterology 1999;117:1295–300.

[95] Odze RD, Farraye FA, Hecht JL, et al. Long-term follow-up after polypectomy treatment for adenoma-like dysplastic lesions in ulcerative colitis. Clin Gastroenterol Hepatol 2004;2: 534–41.

[96] Selaru FM, Xu Y, Yin J, et al. Artificial neural networks distinguish among subtypes of neoplastic colorectal lesions. Gastroenterology 2002;122:606–13.

[97] Colliver DW, Crawford NP, Eichenberger MR, et al. Molecular profiling of ulcerative colitis-associated neoplastic progression. Exp Mol Pathol 2006;80:1–10.

[98] Borchers R, Heinzlmann M, Zahn R, et al. K-ras mutations in sera of patients with colorectal neoplasia and long-standing inflammatory bowel disease. Scand J Gastroenterol 2002;37:715–8.

[99] Imperiale TF, Ransohoff DF, Itzkowitz SH, et al. Fecal DNA versus fecal occult blood for colorectal-cancer screening in an average-risk population. N Engl J Med 2004;351: 2704–14.

[100] Heinzlmann M, Lang SM, Neynaber S, et al. Screening for p53 and k-ras mutations in whole-gut lavage in chronic inflammatory bowel disease. Eur J Gastroenterol Hepatol 2002;14:1061–6.

Gastroenterol Clin N Am 35 (2006) 573–579

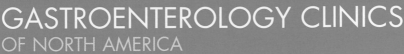

Natural History and Management of Flat and Polypoid Dysplasia in Inflammatory Bowel Disease

Charles N. Bernstein, MD

Department of Internal Medicine and Inflammatory Bowel Disease Clinical and Research Centre, University of Manitoba, 804F-715 McDermot Avenue, Winnipeg, Manitoba, R3E 3P4, Canada

THE INCIDENCE OF DYSPLASIA IN ULCERATIVE COLITIS

In 1994, a synthesis of all dysplasia studies reported that 12% of subjects had dysplasia or cancer already present at presentation for initial screening endoscopy [1]. For those who did not have a neoplasm at initial screening endoscopy, the overall incidence of an advanced lesion (high-grade dysplasia, a dysplasia-associated lesion or mass [DALM], or cancer) over the period of the surveillance was low (2.4%). In that same year, the St. Mark's Hospital group published a report with similar outcomes; it assessed 332 subjects who participated in a screening program and found that 13.2% had dysplasia at the initial presentation [2]. Of patients who had a negative initial colonoscopy, 13.9% developed any form of neoplasm, including flat or mass-related dysplasia (including low-grade dysplasia) or cancer. Over an average follow-up period of 15 years, only 3.3% developed cancer. Hence, initial endoscopic surveillance identifies approximately 10% to 15% of subjects who already have neoplasia; however, over time follow-up surveillance colonoscopies rarely (~3% of the time) identify a lesion that is highly likely to already harbor a cancer, or to be at high risk for transforming into cancer.

In 2000, Eaden and colleagues [3] published a meta-analysis of dysplasia surveillance studies. They reported that by 20 years 8% of participants would have colorectal cancer, and by 30 years 18% would have colorectal cancer. Since then few comprehensive studies on the incidence of dysplasia have been published. The largest and most recent study updated the St. Mark's Hospital experience [4]. In this report, 600 subjects who had ulcerative colitis (UC) underwent dysplasia surveillance colonoscopies between 1971 and 2001. There was a median of three colonoscopies per patient and a median of only eight biopsies per patient. Excluding sporadic adenomas, 74 patients had definite neoplasia, including 30 colorectal cancers. The actuarial cumulative incidence of neoplasia was 7.7% at 20 years, 15.8% at 30 years, and 22.7% at 40 years.

E-mail address: cbernst@cc.umanitoba.ca

0889-8553/06/$ – see front matter
doi:10.1016/j.gtc.2006.07.010

© 2006 Elsevier Inc. All rights reserved.
gastro.theclinics.com

The cumulative incidence of colorectal cancer was 2.5% at 20 years, 7.6% at 30 years, and 10.8% at 40 years of disease.

The incidence of dysplasia is low in UC, in that most subjects who have UC do not get dysplasia—either because they undergo colectomy, which removes the at-risk mucosa before its occurrence or because it is a minority of subjects that truly is at risk for dysplasia. Although primary sclerosing cholangitis, a positive family history of sporadic colon cancer, and disease duration are well-established risk factors for dysplasia progression, other predictors are lacking [5]. Although active inflammation confers a risk [6] (and neoplasia is mostly likely to arise in the rectosigmoid, the area that is affected in UC most uniformly), the value of chronic anti-inflammatory therapy is controversial. Some studies have suggested a risk reduction with 5-aminosalicyclin acid (5-ASA) [7,8], whereas others have not [6,9]. Hence, we are left to consider dysplasia surveillance in all patients who have UC, and in most centers this is undertaken. Although the Eaden [3] meta-analysis suggested a linear relationship between disease duration and dysplasia incidence, most subjects with more than 30 years of disease likely do not develop dysplasia. In fact, the recent St. Mark's report suggested somewhat of a plateau in actuarial cancer incidence after 30 years of disease [4]. It remains unknown, however, if the incidence curve flattens at some point, such that if dysplasia has not arisen, it simply will not, regardless of further follow-up, or whether there remains a steady upward incidence curve that mandates some type of ongoing surveillance.

THE INCIDENCE OF CANCER AFTER FLAT DYSPLASIA IS DIAGNOSED

It has been argued that if dysplasia is diagnosed—either unifocal or multifocal, low grade or high grade—then colectomy should be pursued [5]. In the 1994 synthesis analysis, high-grade dysplasia was associated with cancer already being present in 42% of patients. There has been little debate as to the value and rationale of pursuing colectomy in the setting of high-grade dysplasia. The recommendation for colectomy in the setting of low-grade dysplasia still garners some debate. The rationale for pursuing colectomy includes the evolution to high-grade dysplasia or cancer in 35% to 50% of cases over 5 years [2,10–12]; that low-grade dysplasia can be the only grade of dysplasia adjacent to or at a distance from frank cancers in colon specimens; and that the interpretation of what is low-grade dysplasia versus high-grade dysplasia is an inexact science with considerable interobserver disagreement among experts [5,13].

One report from the Leeds group [14] suggested that the incidence of at least low-grade dysplasia was 25% by 17 years of disease duration and 50% by 25 years. This group has a skeptical view of dysplasia surveillance because they found that of 40 patients who initially had low-grade dysplasia, 50% had no further dysplasia found at subsequent endoscopies. This casts serious doubt on the initial diagnoses of dysplasia by this group, because no other center has reported that degree of dysplasia disappearance over time. In the same report, 9 of 180 (5%) subjects ultimately developed colorectal cancer at a mean disease duration of 18 years. Of these 9 subjects, 4 subjects were lost to the surveillance follow-up program, 3 did not fulfill eligibility criteria, 1 defaulted, and 1 was picked up successfully by the surveillance program. The investigators argued that dysplasia surveillance was not productive at detecting early colorectal cancer. Although their data reflect that their dysplasia surveillance program was not successful, it also reflects that colorectal cancer is as significant a problem among their population that had UC as elsewhere, and that some form of enhanced program might be beneficial.

The Leeds' group then reported on a follow-up study of 29 subjects who had low-grade dysplasia [15]. Over 10 years, 3 subjects (10%) developed high-grade dysplasia or cancer, including 1 subject who died at age 44 from carcinomatosis, 7 years after low-grade dysplasia was diagnosed. In their discussion the investigators argued that patients who have low-grade dysplasia and progress will progress quickly, whereas others may be at no increased risk for developing a more sinister lesion. If we accept that such a dichotomy exists among subjects who have low-grade dysplasia, no marker can identify clearly which patients have the "more sinister low-grade dysplasia." This is the underpinning of the recommendation to pursue colectomy for all subjects who have low-grade dysplasia [5]. The Leeds' group argued that the interobserver agreement on low-grade dysplasia was so poor that it is too unstable a diagnosis to use as an independent predictor for surgery. Even with their dataset there was a 3% death rate by 7 years by not having acted on low-grade dysplasia.

In the synthesis analysis where surgery for low-grade dysplasia was advocated [1], the rate of progression was only 8%; however, the studies that were included in this analysis included cases that antedated more modern interpretations of low-grade dysplasia. Studies have shown that many cases that are interpreted previously as low-grade dysplasia become downgraded to indefinite or no dysplasia on re-review [2,15].

Recently, two large surveillance series were published: one from the St. Mark's Hospital in the United Kingdom and one from Sweden. In the St. Mark's study 46 patients were diagnosed with low-grade dysplasia [4]. Ten patients underwent colectomy and 2 patients had colorectal cancer at resection. In the other 36 patients, 7 patients developed colorectal cancer and 9 patients developed high-grade dysplasia on follow-up. Overall, 19 of 46 patients who had low-grade dysplasia (39%) developed high-grade dysplasia or colorectal cancer; however, the investigators did not segregate flat low-grade dysplasia from DALM-associated low-grade dysplasia. Sixteen of the 30 patients in this study who presented with colorectal cancer presented with interval cancers. In 13 patients, these cancers involved local lymph nodes or dissemination and presented at a median of 1.5 years from the previous surveillance colonoscopy. Although there seems to be a great concern regarding interval cancers, these also occurred in a program where a median of only eight biopsies was taken per endoscopy.

In the Swedish study, 41 of 204 patients who were followed during a 25-year period (up until 2002) were diagnosed with low-grade dysplasia [16]. Low-grade dysplasia was diagnosed simultaneously with high-grade dysplasia or DALM in 8 patients, and it preceded high-grade dysplasia, DALM, or cancer in 10 patients. The time to diagnosis from low-grade dysplasia to findings of high-grade dysplasia, DALM, or cancer varied from 1 to 11 years. This study also presented a patient who had a DALM who was surveyed for 18 years before a carcinoma was diagnosed. Another patient was still under surveillance for 15 years after a diagnosis of flat high-grade dysplasia was made. Some investigators who advocate ongoing surveillance use these published anecdotes as evidence where cancer is not found for years into a surveillance program. Conversely, there is evidence, including from this Swedish study, that cancer will occur within the year or even years after a dysplasia diagnosis. Hence, patients will have to decide how much uncertainty they can live with, and whether rates of not progressing to a more significant lesion (estimated at 50%–75%) are sufficiently reassuring.

In summary, the decision of pursuing colectomy for flat low-grade dysplasia is one to be made by the patient after being armed with the facts as best as they are available. If patients decide that they prefer to opt for annual colonoscopy and accept the risk that cancer may be present already, it should be their prerogative. Some practitioners can point to the anecdotes where patients can harbor low-grade dysplasia for years. At Mt. Sinai Hospital in New York, practitioners have had conflicting views on whether low-grade dysplasia should mandate a colectomy. It is reasonable to discuss the data from Mt Sinai Hospital with patients; 53% of 46 patients who had low-grade dysplasia progressed to an advanced lesion (high grade-dysplasia, DALM, or cancer) within 5 years (Fig. 1). Only the patient can decide what level of uncertainty he or she can tolerate and how much impact an ileoanal pouch may have on quality of life, particularly if the disease is in complete remission when dysplasia is diagnosed.

THE POLYPOID DYSPLASTIC LESION

The initial description of the polypoid dysplastic lesion was made more than 20 years ago when the term "dysplasia-associated lesion or mass" (DALM) was coined. This referred mostly to a lesion that was irregular and ominous [17]. Gastroenterologists feared this lesion [18], and recommended colectomy at its discovery nearly uniformly. In 1999, two prospective series addressed the issue of less ominous looking raised lesions in the setting of colitis [19,20]. Lesions that appeared within the colitis mucosa and looked like routine adenomas—had they occurred in patients who did not have colitis—were referred to as adenoma-like masses (ALMs). Some debate ensued as to whether it was truly safe to pursue a polypectomy plus survey flat adjacent mucosa approach as opposed to colectomy [21]. In one report from Boston, 24 subjects harbored ALMs within the colitis mucosa that were treated by polypectomy with multiple surveillance biopsies of ALM-adjacent flat mucosa. After a mean follow-up of 4.5 years 58% had recurrent ALMs and 4% developed flat dysplasia [19]. In a second report from New York, 48 subjects harbored 60 ALMs within the colitis

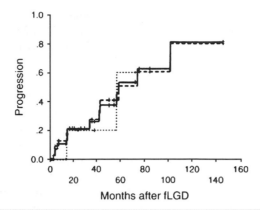

Fig. 1. Kaplan-Meier curve comparing the cumulative progression to advanced neoplasia in patients with any focal low grade dysplasia (fLGD) (solid line), unifocal fLGD (dashed line), and multifocal fLGD (dotted line). Cross-hatches (+) indicate censoring of patients for no further follow-up or colectomy without evidence of progression. Vertical lines (|) represent progression events. (*From* Ullman TA, Croog T, Harpaz N, et al. Progression of flat low-grade dysplasia to advanced neoplasia in patients with ulcerative colitis. Gastroenterology 2003;125:1316; with permission.)

mucosa; after a mean follow-up of 4.1 years 48% had recurrent ALMs and none developed flat dysplasia [20]. At issue was long-term follow-up. Although these groups clearly proved that in the short term, the approach to pursuing polypectomy—taking multiple biopsies from the adjacent flat mucosa and repeating colonoscopy at annual intervals—was safe, it remained to be proved that subjects were not at risk for returning with more advanced neoplasia.

The Boston group updated their experience in 2004 [22]. In this report, 24 patients who had UC with ALMs were studied. Six underwent colectomy within 6 months of ALM diagnosis, including 1 patient who also had flat low-grade dysplasia. Eighteen patients were followed for an average of nearly 7 years; 5 of these patients were lost to follow-up. Of the remaining 13 patients, 1 developed a cecal adenocarcinoma. The cancer occurred 7.5 years after the ALM was found, and in a distant location from the ALM. Hence, a recurrent ALM may not occur at the site of the original ALM, but rather can serve as a marker of predisposition to neoplasia.

Polyps on stalks are uncommon in UC, but they can be approached in the same fashion and likely with more confidence that the entire lesion has been removed. Most investigators believe that adenomas that arise in normal mucosa proximal to the colitis zone can be treated with polypectomy, as with sporadic adenoma. One of the challenges in this category of lesion is determining whether the adenoma has arisen in a truly noncolitic zone. For instance, biopsies from the right colon often can be misinterpreted as colitis, even in health; hence, the endoscopist may have to make a special point of conferring with the pathologist to be sure that the adenoma is sporadic.

In summary, polypoid dysplasia or ALM lesions that arise within the colitis mucosa can be approached with polypectomy, biopsy of flat mucosa adjacent to the ALM site, and follow-up. Annual surveillance–at least over the ensuing 5 years–is mandatory to ensure that dysplasia is not being missed. For young patients with many years of colonoscopy ahead of them or patients who have grumbling disease, the finding of an ALM in colitis mucosa can be added to the rationale for pursuing colectomy.

SUMMARY

Dysplasia can be a marker that cancer is already present or is coming in the near future. Hence, physicians should not be cavalier in approach to finding it or in approach after it is found, whether it is in flat mucosa or raised mucosa. Low-grade dysplasia should garner similar respect to high-grade dysplasia, if for no other reason than the difficulty that expert pathologists have with distinguishing low-grade dysplasia from high-grade dysplasia. There is no sure way to reduce the likelihood that dysplasia will arise in UC. Some investigators have promoted the use of 5-ASA. This topic is covered in greater detail elsewhere in this issue (see article by Rubin and Kavitt elsewhere in this issue); however, there is no definitive evidence that 5-ASA can reduce cancer incidence.

References

[1] Bernstein CN, Shanahan F, Weinstein WM. Are we telling patients the truth about surveillance colonoscopy in ulcerative colitis? Lancet 1994;343:71–4.

[2] Connell WR, Lennard-Jones JE, Williams CB, et al. Factors affecting the outcome of endoscopic surveillance for cancer in ulcerative colitis. Gastroenterology 1994;107:934–44.

[3] Eaden J, Abrams KR, Mayberry JF. The risk of CRC in ulcerative colitis: a meta-analysis. Gut 2001;48:526–35.

[4] Rutter MD, Saunders BP, Wilkinson KH, et al. Thirty-year analysis of a colonoscopic surveillance program for neoplasia in ulcerative colitis. Gastroenterology 2006;130:1030–8.

[5] Bernstein CN. Low grade dysplasia in ulcerative colitis. Gastroenterology 2004;127:950–6.

[6] Rutter M, Saunders B, Wilkinson K, et al. Severity of inflammation is a risk factor for colorectal neoplasia in ulcerative colitis. Gastroenterology 2004;126:451–9.

[7] Eaden J, Abrams K, Ekbom A, et al. Colorectal cancer prevention in ulcerative colitis: a case control study. Aliment Pharmacol Ther 2000;14:145–53.

[8] Van Staa TP, Card T, Logan RF, et al. 5-Aminosalicylate use and colorectal cancer risk in inflammatory bowel disease: a large epidemiological study. Gut 2005;54:1573–8.

[9] Bernstein CN, Metge C, Blanchard JF, et al. Does the use of 5-aminosalicylates in inflammatory bowel disease prevent the development of colorectal cancer? Am J Gastroenterol 2003;98:2784–8.

[10] Lindberg B, Persson B, Veress B, et al. Twenty years' colonoscopic surveillance of patients with ulcerative colitis. Scand J Gastroenterol 1996;31:1195–204.

[11] Ullman TA, Loftus EV, Kakar S, et al. The fate of low grade dysplasia in ulcerative colitis. Am J Gastroenterol 2002;97:922–7.

[12] Ullman TA, Croog T, Harpaz N, et al. Progression of flat low-grade dysplasia to advanced neoplasia in patients with ulcerative colitis. Gastroenterology 2003;125:1311–9.

[13] Itzkowitz SH, Harpaz N. Diagnosis and management of dysplasia in patients with inflammatory bowel diseases. Gastroenterology 2004;126:1634–48.

[14] Lynch DAF, Lobo AJ, Sobala GM, et al. Failure of colonoscopic surveillance in ulcerative colitis. Gut 1993;34:1075–80.

[15] Lim DH, Dixon MF, Vail A, et al. Ten year follow up of ulcerative colitis patients with and without low grade dysplasia. Gut 2003;52:1127–32.
[16] Lindberg J, Stenling R, Palmqvist R, et al. Efficiency of colorectal cancer surveillance in patients with ulcerative colitis: 26 years experience in a patient cohort from a defined population area. Scand J Gastroenterol 2005;40:1076–80.
[17] Blackstone MO, Riddell RH, Rogers BHG, et al. Dysplasia associated lesion or mass (DALM) detected by colonoscopy in long standing ulcerative colitis: an indication for colectomy. Gastroenterology 1981;80:366–74.
[18] Bernstein CN, Weinstein WM, Levine DS, et al. Physicians' perceptions of dysplasia and approaches to surveillance colonoscopy in ulcerative colitis. Am J Gastroenterol 1995;90:2106–14.
[19] Engelsgjerd M, Farraye F, Odze RD. Polypectomy may be adequate treatment for adenoma-like dysplastic lesions in chronic ulcerative colitis. Gastroenterology 1999;117:1288–94.
[20] Rubin PH, Friedman S, Harpaz N, et al. Colonoscopic polypectomy in chronic colitis: conservative management after endoscopic resection of dysplastic polyps. Gastroenterology 1999;117:1295–300.
[21] Bernstein CN. ALMs versus DALMs in ulcerative colitis: polypectomy or colectomy? Gastroenterology 1999;117:1488–91.
[22] Odze R, Farraye FA, Hecht JL, et al. Long-term follow-up after polypectomy treatment for adenoma-like dysplastic lesions in ulcerative colitis. Clin Gastroenterol Hepatol 2004;2:534–41.

Gastroenterol Clin N Am 35 (2006) 581–604

GASTROENTEROLOGY CLINICS
OF NORTH AMERICA

Surveillance for Cancer and Dysplasia in Inflammatory Bowel Disease

David T. Rubin, MD[a,b,c],*, Robert T. Kavitt, MD[c]

[a]Section of Gastroenterology, and The MacLean Center for Clinical Medical Ethics, University of Chicago, Chicago, IL, USA
[b]The Reva and David Logan Center for Research in Gastroenterology, University of Chicago, Chicago, IL, USA
[c]Department of Medicine, University of Chicago, Chicago, IL, USA

C olorectal cancer (CRC) remains a feared complication of chronic idiopathic inflammatory bowel disease (IBD). Due to known associated risk factors and the fact that patients who develop this complication are younger than patients without IBD who develop CRC, aggressive prevention strategies are warranted. Although prospective evidence supporting the practice of surveillance colonoscopy with random biopsies does not exist, this practice is of good clinical rationale and has been proposed to be cost-effective.

RISK FACTORS FOR COLORECTAL CANCER IN ULCERATIVE COLITIS

The development of prevention strategies for cancer in IBD depends on the understanding of the risk factors. The association between ulcerative colitis (UC) and CRC was first described in the 1920s and has been confirmed by numerous studies of populations around the globe [1–4]. The risk of CRC in UC is related to the duration of disease, age at diagnosis, and extent of the colitis. Additional risk factors include diagnosis with primary sclerosing cholangitis (PSC), family history of CRC, and the finding of precancerous dysplasia in other parts of the bowel. A more recently described and potentially modifiable risk factor for CRC in UC is the histologic degree of inflammatory activity [5].

There is an increasing risk of CRC with longer duration of disease. A 2001 meta-analysis by Eaden and colleagues [6] found that the cumulative incidence of CRC in UC was 2% at 10 years, 8% at 20 years, and 18% after 30 years of disease. More recently, Rutter and colleagues [7] reported the 30-year results of

Dr. Rubin is a consultant for Procter and Gamble Pharmaceuticals, Salix Pharmaceuticals, and Shire Pharmaceuticals. He is on the speakers' bureaus for Procter and Gamble Pharmaceuticals and Salix Pharmaceuticals.

*Corresponding author. Section of Gastroenterology, University of Chicago, 5841 South Maryland Avenue, MC 4076, Chicago, IL 60637. E-mail address: drubin@medicine.bsd.uchicago.edu (D.T. Rubin).

0889-8553/06/$ – see front matter
doi:10.1016/j.gtc.2006.07.001
© 2006 Elsevier Inc. All rights reserved.
gastro.theclinics.com

the longest prospectively collected surveillance database in patients with UC at the referral-based St. Mark's Hospital in London. Of 600 patients with UC undergoing 2627 colonoscopic examinations in 5932 patient-years of follow-up, the cumulative incidence of CRC was lower than that in the meta-analysis by Eaden and colleagues [6]: 2.5% after 20 years of disease, 7.6% after 30 years, and 10.8% after as long as 40 years of follow-up. When including dysplasia and CRC together, the cumulative incidence of neoplasia in the St. Mark's Hospital program was still lower: 1.5% after 10 years of UC, 7.7% after 20 years, but as high as 27.5% after 45 years of UC [7].

Some studies have suggested that an independent risk factor for the development of CRC is a younger age at UC diagnosis, with one population-based study showing that as age at diagnosis increased, the relative risk of CRC decreased [2]. This observation is independent of duration of disease, which remains a greater risk for CRC in UC than a younger age at diagnosis [8]. It remains unclear whether the more recent evidence demonstrating that the degree of histologic inflammation is an independent risk for neoplasia in UC may offer an explanation for the impact of age at diagnosis on risk of subsequent CRC, because it has been suggested that a younger age at diagnosis is also associated with more severe inflammation [5].

Extent of colitis is an independent risk factor for the development of CRC. Less extensive disease is associated with a lower risk of developing CRC. In one large population-based study, after adjustment for age, patients with ulcerative proctitis had a standardized incidence ratio of developing CRC of 1.7 (95% confidence interval [CI], 0.8–3.2) compared with age-matched population controls without UC, whereas those with left-sided colitis had a standardized incidence ratio of CRC of 2.8 (95% CI, 1.6–4.4). Pancolitis, inflammation of the entire colon, or extensive colitis (variously defined as disease that extends beyond the hepatic flexure) conferred a standardized incidence ratio of CRC of 14.8 (95% CI, 11.4–18.9) [2]. Despite this greater risk associated with greater extent of disease, when CRC occurs in UC, it is more often in the rectum or sigmoid colon [9]. The mechanism for the varied risk based on extent of disease remains incompletely understood, although proposed explanations include the possibilities that greater surface area provides more tissue in which mutations may persist, greater organ involvement overwhelms the body's DNA repair mechanisms, and there is an inherent abnormality or genetic instability of the colorectum that contributes to the development of neoplasia over time (the concept of an organ "field defect"). More recently, there has been interest in proliferation of aberrant stem cells as a possible explanation for the underlying source of genetic instability and multifocal neoplasia in colonic mucosa [10,11].

At least two previous studies have shown that independent of a family history of IBD, a family history of CRC doubles the risk of CRC in a patient with IBD [12,13]. In addition, the finding of a stricture in the colon of a patient with UC is strongly associated with CRC, with one study showing that 24% of such strictures were malignant [14].

Patients with PSC and UC have an increased risk of developing CRC. Shetty and colleagues [15] reviewed a historical cohort of patients with UC with PSC and a control group without PSC and found that 25% of 132 patients with PSC developed dysplasia, compared with 6% of 196 patients without PSC. In addition, they demonstrated that these patients tended to have disease located more proximally in the colon and, when diagnosed, were at an advanced stage compared with controls. Patients with PSC also had a significantly higher mortality rate compared with those without PSC (4.5% versus 0%). A subsequent meta-analysis of 11 studies of CRC or dysplasia risk in patients with UC and PSC has confirmed an odds ratio (OR) of 4.79 (95% CI, 3.58–6.41) and an OR of 4.09 (95% CI, 2.89–5.76) for CRC alone [16]. Theories of the pathogenesis of this increased risk include differences in bile salts in the colon affecting genetic repair mechanisms and putative genetic abnormalities that cause PSC and CRC.

Loftus and colleagues [17] analyzed the risk of CRC in UC after liver transplantation for PSC. Although there was a defined risk of developing dysplasia after transplantation, when compared with patients with PSC who had not received transplants, this was not statistically significant and did not seem to have an impact on patient survival. They concluded that although prophylactic proctocolectomy is not recommended when patients undergo liver transplantation, annual colonoscopic examination with biopsies should be performed. It is because of this profound increased risk that patients with PSC are advised to undergo screening and subsequent surveillance examinations at the time of diagnosis of colitis (rather than waiting 8 years) and to continue doing so even after liver transplantation [18].

There have also been studies that show a lower risk of CRC in some patients with UC. In a retrospective case-control study, Eaden and colleagues [19] in the United Kingdom demonstrated a number of factors associated with a decreased risk of CRC in UC, including mesalazine therapy (1.2 g/d or greater), which reduced cancer risk by 81%, as did regular follow-up with physicians and having at least one colonoscopy. Subsequent work by other investigators has shown additional evidence for chemoprevention [5,20–22].

DYSPLASIA

In chronic IBD, the mucosa undergoes change and development of precancerous cytologic or architectural abnormalities known as dysplasia. In this regard, the neoplastic transformation in IBD is thought to be similar to the adenoma-carcinoma sequence in sporadic CRC. Unlike the sporadic CRC adenomatous polyp-to-cancer pathway, however, dysplasia in IBD is often found in flat mucosa and traditionally has been reported to be invisible to the endoscopist or radiologist, therefore warranting the approach of random biopsy sampling of the involved mucosa in the search for these histologic changes. A standardized classification system of dysplasia in IBD was established in 1983 and divided dysplasia into high-grade dysplasia (HGD), low-grade dysplasia (LGD), and indefinite dysplasia (IND) (which is further broken down into "probably positive IND" and "probably negative IND") based on histologic appearances of the epithelial cells and their nuclei [23,24]. This system continues to be in use today but, unfortunately, has been shown to have a number of important limitations. Its interobserver reproducibility and intraobserver reliability are poor, with the weakest agreement in the classification of IND and LGD, but it does not spare HGD, and even expert gastrointestinal (GI) pathologists often disagree in their interpretation [23]. Therefore, most experts agree that when dysplasia is suspected, more than one experienced GI pathologist should review the biopsies to confirm a diagnosis before making critical treatment decisions, especially in cases of LGD or IND.

The grade and appearance of dysplasia correlates to cancer risk in UC. Patients with a dysplasia-associated lesion or mass (DALM), an endoscopically visible but endoscopically unresectable dysplastic lesion, often have CRC at the time of colectomy. The original description that coined the acronym DALM contained 12 cases that were described as unresectable single polypoid masses, collections of polyps, or flat plaque-like lesions. Of these 12 cases, 7 harbored adenocarcinoma despite multiple biopsies that had not revealed it. Five of the 7 cases were single polypoid masses [25]. In a subsequent more recent review of 10 prospective studies, 43% of patients who underwent colectomy because of a DALM had coexistent CRC. Those with flat HGD had a markedly higher rate of concurrent CRC (42%), and even those with flat LGD also had a significant amount of concurrent CRC (19%). In this review, patients with LGD who did not have an immediate colectomy progressed in a future evaluation to DALM, HGD, or cancer 16% to 29% of the time [26]. Because the identification of dysplasia is associated with the concurrent or subsequent development of CRC, surveillance recommendations for UC (and Crohn's disease [CD]) were developed to detect premalignant dysplasia and to perform a curative colectomy [23–26].

More recently, Ullman and colleagues [27] at Mount Sinai Hospital in New York City performed a retrospective cohort analysis of 46 patients with UC who had flat LGD but did not undergo immediate colectomy. They found that among these 46 patients, 7 were found to have CRC by the time of subsequent colectomy; in addition, 4 of 17 patients undergoing colectomy for flat LGD were found to have unexpected advanced neoplasia. The authors advocate that continued surveillance after finding flat LGD is "at best a risky strategy" because of the fact that they found no clinical features to predict which patients would progress to HGD or CRC, advanced neoplasia was found at colectomy performed for LGD, and patients progressed to advanced CRC while under ongoing surveillance. In fact, in two cases, invasive CRC was identified after an interval examination that was negative for any dysplasia. It is unlikely that the previously identified dysplasia had regressed in the interim period but much more likely that it was simply missed on the interval examination because of the limits of detection technology and sampling techniques. Given these findings, they conclude that even a single biopsy showing LGD should proceed to colectomy [27]. Others have suggested that a physician and a patient willing to perform more careful and frequent follow-up might detect ongoing dysplastic mucosa and allow for surgery sooner; furthermore, it has been suggested that mortality, rather than the presence of dysplasia or cancer, should be the ultimate outcome of interest. Unfortunately, there remains limited evidence of a mortality benefit from cancer surveillance in IBD.

The 30-year experience reported by St. Mark's Hospital in their surveillance database study also found that the outcome of dysplasia was remarkably consistent with previous reports. In the St. Mark's Hospital experience, 20% of patients with LGD who proceeded to colectomy had concurrent adenocarcinoma and 39.1% who had follow-up of the LGD progressed to subsequent HGD or CRC. As with other studies, patients in the St. Mark's Hospital program with HGD had a high rate of concurrent CRC (36.8%) [7].

The traditional teaching that dysplasia is often not visible is based on the historical descriptions of barium radiography and early colonoscopy and the contrast with the polypoid lesions in patients without IBD. Recent retrospective reviews of surveillance examinations using modern endoscopy equipment with improved resolution suggest that dysplasia may, in fact, be endoscopically visible in most patients [28,29]. Furthermore, there is great interest and ongoing work in the evaluation of novel endoscopic techniques, such as chromoendoscopy or magnification endoscopy, which have, in randomized prospective trials, identified a greater number of dysplastic lesions than random nontargeted biopsies [30–32]. Additional technologic advances, such as high-definition colonoscopy and narrow band imaging, are likely to modify our understanding of dysplasia visibility further. This topic is addressed in greater detail in another article in this issue.

BIOMARKERS OF DYSPLASIA

Despite improvements in visualizing dysplasia with endoscopes, the difficulty in diagnosing dysplasia and understanding its significance certainly warrants the identification of improved markers of cancer risk in patients with IBD. Although a number of potential markers have been studied (and are described in another article in this issue), there are currently no markers of dysplasia or CRC in UC that have been sufficiently developed to eliminate the use of colonoscopy with biopsy and pathologic review. It is more likely that if potential biomarkers are identified and prospectively validated, their presence would be incorporated into stratification schemes for surveillance. Such biomarkers would be cost-effective if they identify the subset of patients who should have more frequent surveillance and the subset not requiring the same vigilant monitoring. In addition, markers of genetic risk could influence recommendations for screening at-risk family members and might provide additional clues to the pathogenesis of IBD.

RATIONALE FOR SURVEILLANCE COLONOSCOPY IN ULCERATIVE COLITIS

Recognizing the previously mentioned risk factors and limitations to accurate detection, a strategic approach to detection and prevention has been developed in UC. These guidelines have been composed from expert and consensus opinion and are supported by a solid rationale, an "ethical imperative," but minimal confirmatory evidence (level B). Fig. 1 is a model of current cancer prevention strategies in UC.

In this model, chronic inflammation develops at an early time point and continues in a relapsing and remitting course until dysplasia develops at some time point in the future. Based on existing screening and prevention recommendations, a colonoscopy that is performed before dysplasia develops (A) would not detect the neoplasia. A subsequent examination at some future point in time (B), however, could detect dysplasia. The time during which the screening test is able to detect the finding of interest is defined as the "detectable preclinical phase"; in CRC, this is a period during which an intervention may occur (proctocolectomy) and prevent cancer or prevent invasive cancer and death. In UC, the intervention is a proctocolectomy. The detectable preclinical phase is determined by the length of time between precancerous dysplasia, cancer, and metastasis or death, and it is dependent on the sensitivity and specificity of the colonoscopy and interpretation of the biopsies. Improvements in dysplasia detection or surrogate markers of dysplasia that could identify precancerous changes at an earlier time would therefore expand the detectable preclinical phase.

EVIDENCE FOR SURVEILLANCE COLONOSCOPY IN ULCERATIVE COLITIS

A number of centers have reported their experience with surveillance colonoscopy in the chronic UC population. Most of these reports are limited by

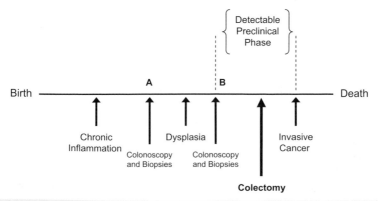

Fig. 1. Cancer in IBD: proposed natural history and secondary prevention strategy.

retrospective analyses, no comparison group, and inconsistent surveillance practices, making generalizability difficult. Nonetheless, a general review of these reports is worthwhile.

In 1985, Rosenstock and colleagues [33] at the Cleveland Clinic published their retrospective review of 248 patients who underwent 370 surveillance examinations with a mean duration of disease 12 years, specifically looking at the diagnosis of HGD or cancer. They identified 16 patients with HGD or CRC, and the most common predictor of these findings was a DALM, which was present in 4 of the 16 patients. Six of seven cancers were recognized by colonoscopy, but the seventh had dysplasia detected on random biopsy (100% per patient sensitivity for cancer).

A number of studies have been performed in the United Kingdom. Jones and colleagues [34] from Wycombe General Hospital in the United Kingdom reviewed the diagnosis and care of all patients with UC in one health district between 1975 and 1984. There were 313 patients with UC (prevalence of 84 per 100,000 population) who were followed for 1168 patient-years, during which three cases of HGD and two asymptomatic (Duke's stage A and B) carcinomas on "routine" colonoscopy and, subsequently, an additional five symptomatic carcinomas were identified (two Duke's stage B, one Duke's stage C, and two Duke's stage D). Based on these retrospective findings, they suggested that an annual colonoscopy should be performed to detect HGD or cancer but were unable to make any claims about a mortality benefit from routine examinations. In 1991, Leidenius and colleagues [35] described their surveillance program at the Helsinki University Central Hospital in Finland. From 1976 to 1989, 66 patients with chronic UC (36 left-sided and 30 extensive) underwent routine colonoscopy and biopsies to detect dysplasia and carcinoma. One hundred eighty-two examinations were performed (mean of 2.8 per patient), with approximately 20 biopsies per examination. Five patients in the extensive colitis group had LGD, and 1 had HGD. In the left-sided colitis group, 3 patients had LGD. None had CRC in follow-up. The conclusion from this study was that surveillance was a safe alternative to prophylactic colectomy.

Lynch and colleagues [36] at the General Infirmary of Leeds Hospital in London subsequently reported the results of a prospective surveillance program in patients with long-standing extensive UC between 1978 and 1990 that included an annual colonoscopy with biopsies. One hundred sixty patients had 739 colonoscopies (mean of 4.6 per patient, 88% right colon intubation). There were no significant procedural complications, and only one case of Duke's stage A cancer was detected. These authors questioned the benefit of a surveillance program given this finding, but there were a number of criticisms of this study, including the fact that there was a substantial drop-out rate in the study (25%); of these, approximately one third of patients were lost to follow-up completely. In contrast, Connell and colleagues [37] at St. Mark's Hospital in London shared the 21-year results of their surveillance program in a 1994 review and suggested that surveillance was successful at diagnosing early-stage cancers and dysplasia. Of 332 patients with extensive colitis and long-standing duration (>10 years), annual sigmoidoscopy and biopsy were performed alternating with colonoscopy and biopsy, more often if dysplasia was detected. Eleven asymptomatic cases of cancer were identified (8 Duke's stage A, 1 Duke's stage B, and 2 Duke's stage C), but 6 cases of symptomatic cancer were detected after a negative colonoscopy (4 Duke's stage C and 2 Duke's stage D). Twelve asymptomatic patients had dysplasia of various degrees and underwent colectomy. A 5-year predictive value for LGD to result in HGD or CRC was 54%. These investigators concluded that the biennial colonoscopy strategy missed some cancers at an earlier stage and that there were difficulties in biopsy interpretation.

At the Tel Aviv Medical Center in Israel, Rozen and colleagues [38] reported their prospective endoscopic study of 154 patients with UC of greater than 7 years' duration between 1976 and 1994. Five patients had 10 dysplasia-associated polypoid lesions managed by polypectomy, and IND was found in 16 patients, none of whom had progression to higher grades of neoplasia on follow-up. LGD was identified in 10 patients, 2 of whom had coexistent HGD and 2 of whom progressed to HGD. HGD was seen in 7 patients, 4 of whom had concurrent cancer (of which three cases were successfully treated. The authors concluded that a surveillance program was successful at identifying treatable cancers. Lindberg and colleagues [39] subsequently reported the experience at the Huddinge University Hospital in Sweden of 20 years of prospective follow-up of 143 patients with extensive UC of greater than 10 years' duration. In this program, patients underwent colonoscopy with random biopsy (two biopsies in each of nine locations) every other year. Fifty-five patients had dysplasia, 7 of whom had CRC, of which two cases were Duke's stage A. LGD was predictive of coexistent HGD or CRC in 41% of the other patients. These investigators concluded that surveillance was effective at identifying neoplasia and was worthwhile.

Unlike the previously described retrospective single-arm studies, there have been three studies and a subsequent Cochrane analysis that have attempted to assess the impact of surveillance examinations in patients with UC compared with no surveillance, all with limited results. Choi and colleagues [40] described a retrospective outcome analysis of 41 patients with UC who developed CRC. They showed that patients undergoing surveillance colonoscopy were diagnosed with CRC at a significantly earlier Duke's stage than those who did not undergo surveillance. These data translated into improved 5-year survival for the surveillance group (77%) compared with that of the patients without surveillance (36%; $P = .26$).

Karlen and colleagues [41] performed a population-based, nested, case-control study in Sweden in 1997. The surveillance exposure of all patients with UC who had died from CRC after 1975 was compared with that of controls matched for disease and demographic information. They identified 2 of 40 patients with UC and 18 of 102 controls who had undergone at least one surveillance colonoscopy who died as a result of CRC (relative risk [RR] = 0.29, 95% CI, 0.06–1.31) Although not statistically significant, the investigators suggested that surveillance colonoscopy with biopsy may have a protective effect against death from CRC.

Lashner and colleagues [42] at the University of Chicago performed a historical cohort study of 91 patients undergoing an annual colonoscopy and biopsies compared with 95 patients who did not and found that 4 of 91 patients in the surveillance group died as a result of CRC compared with 2 of 95 patients in the group that had not undergone surveillance. In addition, 33 patients in the surveillance group had a colectomy on average 4 years later than the 51 patients in the nonsurveillance group who had undergone a colectomy. The results of this study were not significantly in favor of a surveillance program.

A 2004 Cochrane Database systematic pooled data analysis combined the results of the studies by Choi and colleagues [40], Karlen and colleagues [41], and Lashner and colleagues [42], summarizing that 8 of 110 patients who had undergone surveillance died of CRC compared with 13 of 117 patients in the nonsurveillance group (RR = 0.81, 95% CI, 0.17–3.83). The authors concluded that "there is no clear evidence that surveillance colonoscopy prolongs survival in patients with extensive colitis. There is evidence that cancers tend to be detected at an earlier stage in patients who are undergoing surveillance and that these patients have a correspondingly better prognosis, but lead-time bias could contribute substantially to this apparent benefit. There is indirect evidence that surveillance is likely to be effective at reducing the risk of death from IBD-associated colorectal cancer and indirect evidence that it is acceptably cost-effective" (level of evidence B) (Table 1) [43].

SURVEILLANCE IN PATIENTS WHO HAVE ILEOANAL J-POUCH ANASTOMOSIS

Patients with UC who have undergone a proctocolectomy for medically refractory disease or because of the development of neoplasia may have a surgically created ileoanal pouch. It has been suggested that these patients are at increased risk for neoplastic transformation as well, although the evidence is far from convincing. In one study, seven patients with an ileoanal pouch with mucosal atrophy of a severe subtype were compared with controls without mucosal atrophy, and those with atrophy had a statistically significant risk (71%) of developing dysplasia [44]. It has also been reported that a retained rectal cuff or rectal pouch is at risk for neoplastic transformation. Although predominantly case reports, neoplasia of the retained cuff or retained ileum has been reported often enough to lead some to suggest routine surveillance of these patients [45].

WHAT ABOUT CROHN'S DISEASE?

CD also has been shown to confer an increased risk of CRC but has been more difficult to study, given the often patchy nature of the disease and difficulty in controlling for disease extent and separating patients with primarily small bowel CD from those with colonic involvement. Nevertheless, studies that do adjust for location of disease consistently demonstrate an increased risk of CRC in CD of the colon. In one study of patients in Sweden, CD of the

Table 1
Evidence for surveillance colonoscopy in ulcerative colitis

Study	Outcomes of CRC		Statistics
	Surveillance	No Surveillance	
Karlen et al 1998	2/40 deaths	18/102 deaths	RR = 0.28 95% CI, 0.07–1.17
Choi et al 1993	15/19 Duke's stage A–B 5-year survival, 77.2%	9/22 Duke's stage A–B 5-year survival, 36.3%	P = .039
Lashner et al 1990	4/91 deaths	2/95 deaths	RR = 2.09 95% CI, 0.39–11.12
Mpofu et al (Cochrane systematic pooled analysis) 2004	8/110 deaths	13/117 deaths	RR = 0.81 95% CI, 0.17–3.83

Abbreviations: CI, confidence interval; CRC, colorectal cancer; RR, relative risk.

colon alone had a RR of CRC of 5.6 (95% CI, 2.1–12.2), whereas patients with disease of the terminal ileum and colon and terminal ileum alone had RRs of CRC of 3.2 (95% CI, 0.7–9.2) and 1.0 (95% CI, 0.1–3.4), respectively [46]. Similar to patients with UC, patients diagnosed at a younger age (<30 years) had a higher RR (20.9) than those who were older (RR = 2.2) when they were diagnosed with CD. A population-based study from Manitoba, Canada showed similar results [47].

There is much less available evidence, and therefore few published guidelines, for surveillance of neoplasia in CD of the colon. In addition, patients with CD have an increased risk of small bowel adenocarcinoma as well as an increased risk of squamous cell cancer in the perianal areas. A 1999 report by Sigel and colleagues [48] of 30 cases of resected adenocarcinoma in patients with CD concluded that most (86%) of CD-related colorectal adenocarcinomas exhibit dysplasia in adjacent mucosa and that 41% of CRCs exhibit distant dysplasia. They conclude that this finding supports a dysplasia-carcinoma sequence in CD similar to that described in UC and that a prevention strategy using dysplasia as a marker is justified.

There is much less evidence for the benefit (or lack of benefit) of surveillance in CD, but Friedman and colleagues [49] performed a retrospective study at the Mount Sinai Hospital in New York City. A total of 259 patients with a diagnosis of CD for at least 8 years and more than one third of the colon involved (90% with extensive colitis) underwent an initial colonoscopy (14% of these patients also had increased symptoms). The subsequent surveillance colonoscopy interval varied depending on results of the initial screening procedure. Twelve percent of these patients were found to have new neoplasia (LGD, HGD, or CRC) diagnosed on the screening or surveillance colonoscopy. Furthermore, 22% of patients were diagnosed with neoplasia by their fourth surveillance colonoscopy after a negative screening. These numbers are comparable to the UC population with extensive disease. Age greater than 45 years increased the risk of neoplasia, notably including those patients with short-term disease (less than 20 years); increased number of symptoms was also a risk factor for neoplasia on screening colonoscopy.

Risk factors for developing carcinoma in small bowel segments of involved mucosa in patients with CD are poorly defined. Presumably, "at-risk" mucosa would be that with prolonged inflammation. A higher rate of small bowel adenocarcinoma has been consistently reported in patients with CD, although given the rarity of this occurrence overall and the inability to inspect or sample much of the small intestine endoscopically, surveillance has not been defined or recommended [50,51]. There have been numerous case reports of carcinoma arising in strictured mucosa and, more recently, in fistulae (colocolonic, perirectal, and enterocutaneous) [52–54]. The cancers arising in fistulae are sometimes adenomatous and sometimes squamous in origin [55]. Patients with small bowel or fistulous cancers tend to present with pain or disease refractory to therapies. Biopsy of the stricture or fistula, pathologic review of resections, and examination under anesthesia are the techniques usually described in the diagnosis of these lesions. Surgery should be performed if the fistula or stricture cannot be adequately examined.

Patients with CD may develop benign strictures of the colon, whereas in UC, strictures are more likely to be associated with CRC. In one study, nearly 7% of colonic strictures in CD contained a malignancy [56]. Although it can be difficult to pass through a stricture to perform surveillance biopsies proximal to it, use of a pediatric colonoscope has been shown to improve the rate of full colonoscopic examination significantly in patients with CD who have strictures [49].

The now largely retired practice of surgical diversion of loops of bowel has been associated with adenocarcinoma; because surveillance of these loops is not possible, one must consider elective surgical removal of these diverted loops. Although, in theory, bowel-sparing stricturoplasty may increase the risk of adenocarcinoma of the small bowel given the retained segments of chronic inflammation, this has not yet been described. Nevertheless, our surgeons emphasize the importance of obtaining frozen sections of the small bowel during surgery in which stricturoplasty is performed to ensure no neoplasia before leaving these segments in vivo.

Unlike the case in UC, there are not yet data on the utility of chemoprevention of cancer in CD or on the newer techniques of surveillance, such as chromoendoscopy with high-resolution magnification.

TECHNIQUE OF SURVEILLANCE

Itzkowitz and Harpaz [32] note that a typical biopsy samples less than 0.05% of the total surface area of the colon, underscoring the possibility of false-negative results of surveillance. Rubin and colleagues [57] determined that 33 biopsies are necessary to detect dysplasia in UC with 90% probability, whereas 64 biopsies are necessary to detect dysplasia with 95% probability.

Surveillance guidelines have been developed to standardize an approach to mucosal sampling looking for dysplasia or occult malignancy. Most guidelines recommend colonoscopy with four-quadrant biopsies every 10 cm, obtaining a total of at least 30 to 40 biopsy specimens. In our practice, we biopsy all areas, regardless of current or previous disease activity, and pay special attention to mucosal abnormalities or polypoid lesions. In addition, we submit the biopsies in separate jars to distinguish between endoscopically active disease areas and quiescent areas, more for the determination of ongoing specific topical therapies than for utility in dysplasia diagnosis, because dysplasia at any location requires a total colectomy.

APPROACH TO POLYPOID LESIONS IN INFLAMMATORY BOWEL DISEASE

Non-DALM discrete polypoid lesions in the colon of patients with IBD pose a special challenge and, more recently, have been termed *adenoma-like lesions or masses* (ALMs). First, it must be determined whether these raised discrete lesions are dysplastic and, second, whether they are colitis associated or sporadic.

Sporadic adenomas are most common in patients older than 40 to 60 years of age, whereas colitis-associated dysplastic polyps may appear at any age. Colitis-associated dysplastic polyps are uncommon within 10 years of disease diagnosis, are more common among patients with pancolitis, and generally occur in a region of diseased bowel, whereas sporadic adenomas may occur proximal to the area of colitis. Dysplasia in surrounding nonpolypoid mucosa is highly suggestive of colitis-associated dysplasia.

When adenomas appear proximal to diseased mucosa, the recommended approach is to perform a complete polypectomy and to biopsy the surrounding flat mucosa. If the flat biopsies reveal no evidence of chronic UC in a patient whose age suggests the possibility of a sporadic adenoma, follow-up may occur as would with any patient without IBD with an adenoma. If, however, the polypoid lesion is dysplastic and in a field of colitis, available evidence suggests that in the absence of flat dysplasia in the surrounding mucosa or elsewhere in the colon, these patients may be followed without colectomy [58] but perhaps at an increased surveillance schedule. Engelsgjerd and colleagues [59] concluded in a 1999 study that patients with chronic UC with an adenoma-like DALM resembling a sporadic adenoma by endoscopy and histology may be treated with polypectomy and surveillance, regardless of location, because of its "relatively benign course."

Odze and colleagues [60] subsequently reported the long-term outcomes of patients with UC with adenoma-like DALMs treated by polypectomy. The mean follow-up time was 82.1 months in the cohort of patients with UC with an adenoma-like DALM within the area of colitis. One of these patients was found to have flat LGD of the colon, which was resected, and one patient developed CRC in the setting of PSC after orthotopic liver transplant and 7.5 years after initial removal of the adenoma-like DALM. The authors concluded that patients with UC with an adenoma-like DALM may be treated with polypectomy with complete excision and continued surveillance.

Patients younger than 40 years of age with dysplasia-associated polypoid lesions outside of known colitis should be evaluated for a possible genetic or hereditary contribution to their neoplasia, as would occur in patients without IBD. In addition, even if these lesions are solitary and easily resectable in a field of colitis without surrounding flat dysplasia, these lesions may, in fact, represent a higher risk lesion than the sporadic adenoma occurring in an age-appropriate individual with colitis. Although the limited available evidence suggests that these patients may be followed after resection of the polyp, the surveillance intensity should probably be increased. Table 2 outlines the features that distinguish a sporadic adenoma from colitis-associated dysplasia.

PUTTING IT ALL TOGETHER: CURRENT GUIDELINES AND CONSENSUS

A number of guidelines have been published over the past decade in the United States and United Kingdom to assist gastroenterologists in approaching surveillance for CRC in IBD in a uniform manner. The conclusions of these various guidelines are delineated here; however, it is important to note that many of these explanations are guided by expert opinion rather than by the findings of controlled trials. Box 1 contains a detailed summary of existing surveillance guidelines and additional recommendations.

With the goal of developing international standardized consensus guidelines regarding the role of surveillance for CRC in IBD, the Crohn's and Colitis Foundation of America commissioned a group of experts who published their conclusions in 2005 [61]. They state, "Because the risk of CRC becomes greater than that of the general population after 8 to 10 years from the onset

---

Table 2
Features to help distinguish between sporadic adenoma and inflammatory bowel disease–associated dysplasia

	Sporadic adenoma	Inflammatory bowel disease–associated dysplasia
Patient age	>40–60 years	Any
Duration	Any	>8–10 years
Extent	Any	More often pancolitis
Location	Any	In colitic region
Adjacent mucosa	No dysplasia	Colitis ± dysplasia
Other lesions	Sometimes	Often
Architecture	More often tubular	Occasionally villous
Admixed benign and dysplastic epithelium	Absent	May be present
Immunostains	Research tool: not helpful in individual cases	

Box 1: Summary of existing surveillance guidelines and additional recommendations

UC (level of evidence B)

- Who
  - All patients with left-sided or pan-UC for 8 to 10 years[a,c–f]
  - All patients 7 to 8 years after onset of colitis[b]
  - "Whether patients with previously extensive disease whose disease has regressed benefit from surveillance is unknown."[c]
  - "The appropriateness of surveillance should be discussed with patients who have UC or Crohn's colitis and a joint decision made on the balance of benefit to the individual."[c]
  - If patients have proctosigmoiditis (with no colitis proximal to 35 cm), they should be managed based on standard CRC screening guidelines for the general population.[a]
  - Conduct regular surveillance after 8 to 10 years from symptom onset for patients with pancolitis and after 15 to 20 years for patients with left-sided colitis.[e]
  - Conduct surveillance every 1 to 2 years after 8 years of disease in patients with pancolitis and after 15 years in patients with left-sided colitis.[f]

- Technique
  - Four-quadrant biopsies every 10 cm of mucosa; more than 32 biopsies[a,b]; extra focus on nodules, masses, and strictures[f]
  - Multiple biopsies at 10-cm intervals[d]
  - Two to 4 random biopsies every 10 cm from the entire colon, with additional samples from suspicious areas[e]
  - Four random biopsies every 10 cm from the entire colon, with additional samples of suspicious areas[c]
  - Some advocate more biopsies in distal rectosigmoid (approximately every 5 cm).[b]
  - Put each set of four biopsies in separate jars in case of need to re-examine a certain area.[b]
  - Control inflammation medically in patients with moderate to severe colitis symptoms before colonoscopy.[b]

- How often
  - Every 1 to 2 years, avoiding periods of clinical relapse: "Although some data suggest a later onset of cancer risk in left-sided than in more extensive colitis, this evidence is not sufficiently strong to justify different guidelines for surveillance in the two groups."[d]
  - "Patients with longstanding UC may also be offered the option of prophylactic total proctocolectomy, but patients in remission rarely opt for this approach."[d]

- For those with extensive colitis opting for surveillance, conduct surveillance every 3 years during the second decade of disease, every 2 years in the third decade of disease, and annually by the fourth decade of disease.[c,e]
- If no dysplasia is detected, patients with extensive colitis (proximal-to-hepatic flexure) should undergo colonoscopy every 1 to 2 years.[b]
- Patients with left-sided colitis should follow the same schedule as patients with extensive colitis, although some suggest beginning surveillance after 15 years of disease.[b]
- Do not alter the surveillance interval based on disease duration.[b]
- Every 1 to 2 years for patients with UC with extensive colitis or left-sided colitis and a negative screening colonoscopy; after 2 negative examinations, perform surveillance in 1 to 3 years until the patient has had UC for 20 years; at that point, consider surveillance every 1 to 2 years.[a]
- Decrease screening interval with increasing disease duration.[e]

- Outcome (reviewed by a second pathologist)
    - If dysplasia of any grade is detected and confirmed by a second GI pathologist, "then colectomy is usually advisable."[c]

- Approach to HGD
    - HGD in flat mucosa, confirmed by an expert pathologist, is an indication for colectomy.[a,b,d,f]

- Approach to LGD
    - LGD in flat mucosa should prompt consideration of colectomy to prevent progression to a higher grade of neoplasia.[d]
    - A finding of LGD should lead to a discussion with the patient of competing options, with a prophylactic colectomy offered.[a] If flat LGD is multifocal or is repetitive between examinations, strongly encourage prophylactic total proctocolectomy.[a,b,f] If the patient does not undergo surgery, repeat surveillance in 3 to 6 months.[a]
    - If a patient with flat LGD (especially if multifocal) refuses colectomy, repeat surveillance in 3 to 6 months or less; advise the patient of the risk and that negative future examinations do not ensure safety.[b]
    - For LGD in a mass lesion not resembling a sporadic adenoma, a symptomatic stricture, or a stricture that is not passable during colonoscopy, colectomy is advisable.[a,d]

- Approach to IND
    - If IND, have reviewed by an expert GI pathologist and undergo repeat surveillance colonoscopy at a "briefer interval."[d]
    - If IND with high suspicion, repeat biopsy in 3 to 6 months or less.[b]
    - If IND with low suspicion, repeat biopsy every 6 to 12 months.[b]
    - If IND is confirmed, repeat surveillance within 3 to 6 months.[a]

- Approach to polypoid lesions
  - If a patient has long-standing UC and a polypoid mass within a colitic area is found and resembles a typical sporadic adenoma, vigilant follow-up surveillance colonoscopy may suffice (if polyps have a plaque or carpet-like morphology, consider this a DALM, and surgery is required).[d]
  - If LGD or HGD in a resectable polyp with no flat dysplasia adjacent or elsewhere in colon, perform India ink tattoo of polypectomy site for future relocalization, and temporarily increase frequency of surveillance to every 3 to 6 months.[b]
  - If a tubular adenoma is found to have LGD and is found in areas of colitis, with no dysplasia in flat mucosa, consider it a sporadic adenoma and continue surveillance.[f]

Colitis (UC or CD) and PSC (level of evidence B)

- As above, but start surveillance at the time of diagnosis of PSC; do not wait 8 years.[a,b,d]
- All patients with PSC but not known to have IBD should undergo colonoscopy to determine status.[a]
- How often
  - Annual surveillance examination[a,e]
  - Patients with UC and PSC should have "more frequent (perhaps annual) colonoscopy."[c]
  - If patients have other risk factors (eg, family history of CRC), they may require shorter surveillance intervals.[a]
  - Also conduct annual surveillance in patients with PSC who have undergone an orthotopic liver transplant.[e]

Crohn's colitis (level of evidence B)

- Approach as explained previously for UC.
- The risk of CRC is similar to that of UC if disease duration and surface area involved are comparable.[a]
- Who
  - "The appropriateness of surveillance should be discussed with patients who have UC or Crohn's colitis and a joint decision made on the balance of benefit to the individual."[c]

- How often
  - Follow UC surveillance strategies for patients with at least 8 years of Crohn's colitis involving at least one third of the colon.[b]
  - Begin surveillance 8 to 10 years after symptom onset, and if dysplasia or cancer is not found, perform surveillance similar to that stated previously for patients with UC every 1 to 2 years.[a] With two negative examinations, the next examination may be done in 1 to 3 years until Crohn's colitis has been present for 20 years; then perform surveillance every 1 to 2 years.[a]

- Outcome
  - Approach abnormal findings as you would for patients with UC.[a]
  - Confirmed dysplasia of any degree should have surgery; it is unclear whether total colectomy or subtotal colectomy should be performed.
  - It is as yet unclear if patients with dysplasia or cancer in segmental Crohn's colitis can have segmental resection versus a more extensive approach.[a,b]
  - If a stricture is present, it may often be managed conservatively. To conduct surveillance, you may attempt the use of a narrower colonoscope or dilating stricture to view proximal mucosa. Consider brush cytology or a barium enema to assess strictures that are impassable.[a,b]
  - If there is more than 20 years of disease in the presence of a stricture, the CRC risk indicates consideration of total colectomy or segmental resection if you are unable to evaluate the colon proximal to the stricture.[a]

CD of the small bowel (no published guidelines) (level of evidence B)
- Recommend early surgical exploration if there are obstructive symptoms.
- If there is no colonic involvement, manage according to CRC screening guidelines for the general population.[a]

Ileoanal pouch anastomosis (no published guidelines) (level of evidence B)
- Know a patient's anatomy and whether mucosal stripping occurred.
- Retained cuff or residual rectal mucosa should have periodic biopsies and assessment.

[a]Itzkowitz SH, Present DH. Consensus conference: colorectal cancer screening and surveillance in inflammatory bowel disease. Inflamm Bowel Dis 2005;11(3):314–21 [Crohn's and Colitis Foundation of America guidelines].
[b]Itzkowitz SH, Harpaz N. Diagnosis and management of dysplasia in patients with inflammatory bowel diseases. Gastroenterology 2004;126(6):1634–48.
[c]Carter MJ, Lobo AJ, Travis SP. Guidelines for the management of inflammatory bowel disease in adults. Gut 2004;53(Suppl 5):V1–16 [British Society of Gastroenterology guidelines].
[d]Kornbluth A, Sachar DB. Ulcerative colitis practice guidelines in adults (update): American College of Gastroenterology, Practice Parameters Committee. Am J Gastroenterol 2004;99(7):1371–85 [American College of Gastroenterology guidelines].
[e]Eaden JA, Mayberry JF. Guidelines for screening and surveillance of asymptomatic colorectal cancer in patients with inflammatory bowel disease. Gut 2002;51(Suppl 5):V10–2.
[f]Winawer S, Fletcher R, Rex D, et al. Colorectal cancer screening and surveillance: clinical guidelines and rationale—update based on new evidence. Gastroenterology 2003;124(2):544–60.

of disease, the Committee recommends that a screening colonoscopy be performed 8 to 10 years after the onset of symptoms attributable to UC." The authors advocate subsequent surveillance colonoscopies every 1 to 2 years for patients with UC with extensive colitis or left-sided colitis and a negative screening colonoscopy. They further recommend that after two negative examinations, the next surveillance examination can be performed in 1 to 3 years until the patient has had UC for 20 years; at that point, one should consider a surveillance examination every 1 to 2 years. They advocate annual surveillance examinations for patients with concurrent UC and PSC. If a confirmed finding of IND is determined, they recommend repeat surveillance within 3 to 6 months. If a confirmed finding of LGD in flat mucosa is determined, they recommend discussing competing options with the patient and offering the option of prophylactic colectomy, given the possibility of a synchronous adenocarcinoma. They state that patients with UC with multifocal flat LGD or repetitive flat LGD should be strongly encouraged to undergo prophylactic total proctocolectomy. If colectomy is deferred for any patient with flat LGD, they advise repeat surveillance within 3 months and no later than 6 months, with subsequent frequent examinations (less than 6 months apart).

For patients with Crohn's colitis, the authors state that "the risk of CRC is similar to that of UC if there is comparable surface area involvement and disease duration" and that patients with CD with "major colonic involvement (at least one-third of the colon involved)" should undergo screening colonoscopy at 8 to 10 years after symptom onset. If this examination does not find dysplasia or cancer, the authors advocate surveillance in a pattern similar to the approach that they advocate for patients with UC.

In 2004, Itzkowitz and Harpaz [32] from Mount Sinai Hospital in New York advocated a strategy of initial screening colonoscopy 7 to 8 years from the onset of colitis among patients with UC. They recommend that patients lacking dysplasia on screening undergo surveillance every 1 to 2 years if they have extensive colitis (defined as colitis located proximal to the hepatic flexure). They recommend the same for patients with left-sided colitis, although acknowledging that others advocate beginning surveillance for patients with left-sided colitis after 15 years of disease. They also do not recommend altering surveillance patterns based on disease duration. Fig. 2 illustrates their approach to dysplasia identified on colonoscopy.

Itzkowitz and Harpaz [32] recommend that approximately 4 biopsies be taken every 10 cm, with a total of more than 32 biopsies in most patients. They raise the important point that although we follow a UC-based surveillance strategy for patients with Crohn's colitis involving at least one third of the colon, we do not know if patients with dysplasia or CRC and segmental Crohn's colitis can undergo segmental resection or must undergo a more drastic surgical approach.

In 2004, the British Society of Gastroenterology (BSG) released surveillance guidelines that advocate an initial screening colonoscopy after 8 to 10 years of IBD symptoms but that surveillance intervals should vary based on extent of disease, duration of disease, and presence of PSC [62]. They recommend that patients with extensive colitis undergo surveillance every 3 years during the second decade of disease, every 2 years in the third decade of disease, and annually in subsequent years.

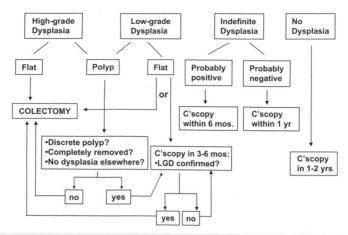

Fig. 2. Suggested surveillance strategy. C'scopy, colonoscopy; mo, month, yr, year. (*From* Itz-kowitz SH, Harpaz N. Diagnosis and management of dysplasia in patients with inflammatory bowel diseases. Gastroenterology 2004;126(6):1642; with permissions from the American Gastroenterological Association.)

The American College of Gastroenterology (ACG) Practice Parameters Committee published a set of practice guidelines regarding UC in 2004 [18]. They advocate annual or biannual surveillance after 8 to 10 years of colitis and state, "Although some data suggest a later onset of cancer risk in left-sided than in more extensive colitis [63], this evidence is not sufficiently strong to justify different guidelines for surveillance in the two groups."

DO CLINICIANS UNDERSTAND THESE GUIDELINES?

Given the confusing and contradictory recommendations as well as the lack of confirmatory evidence, it is understandable that clinicians and patients might be confused or noncompliant with these recommendations.

Bernstein and colleagues [64] surveyed US gastroenterologists in 1993 to determine their understanding of these concepts and found that only 19% were able to identify the correct definition of dysplasia as a neoplastic state. In addition, almost all respondents continued surveillance colonoscopy and did not recommend colectomy when LGD was identified, and nearly one third of respondents recommended continued surveillance colonoscopies and not colectomy when HGD was identified. Although this survey study occurred more than 10 years ago, there remains ongoing confusion regarding the approach to dysplasia in IBD, and a more recently published survey of gastroenterologists in Wales found that 26.1% of them (95% CI, 8.2%–44.0%) believed (contrary to the BSG guidelines [65]) that surveillance in left-sided colitis was unnecessary [66]. The discrepancies between published guidelines and opinions of practicing gastroenterologists have led to nonuniform practice by gastroen-terologists and have probably contributed to confusion among patients. More uniformity and educational efforts need to occur.

IS SURVEILLANCE FOR NEOPLASIA IN ULCERATIVE COLITIS COST-EFFECTIVE?

A number of decision analyses and cost-effectiveness models have been pro-posed that analyze a surveillance approach in UC. They are limited by assump-tions based on the available data; however, in general, they conclude that surveillance is cost-effective. In an admittedly "back of the envelope" analysis, Sonnenberg and El-Serag [67] found that a biannual surveillance colonoscopy of patients with UC was comparable in cost-effectiveness to screening for ade-nocarcinoma annually in patients with Barrett's esophagus and screening for CRC every 5 years in the general population.

In a subsequent review, Provenzale and Onken [68] determined that among a hypothetic cohort of 10,000 patients with UC, the incremental cost-effective-ness ratio of annual surveillance with colonoscopy was $247,200 per life-year gained. They compare this with a value of $250,000 per life-year gained in the practice of screening for cervical cancer every 3 years.

FUTURE RESEARCH AIMS

The best study to assess the mortality benefit of surveillance for dysplasia in IBD would be a prospective trial with patient groups randomized to various surveillance strategies. Such a study would be logistically difficult and possibly unethical, and thus would be challenging to perform. Nevertheless, the Crohn's and Colitis Foundation of America Clinical Alliance is launching a national multicenter prospective registry of dysplasia and cancer in IBD that is expected to shed more light on this complex issue so that future guidelines can more ef-fectively stratify risk and individualize prevention strategies.

SUMMARY

There remain technical challenges to the accurate prediction and diagnosis of neoplasia in IBD; therefore, prevention strategies are based on limited evidence and, instead, consensus opinions and guidelines.

Existing guidelines and published expert opinions are in agreement that given the increased risk of cancer in IBD and well-described associated risks, prevention strategies are warranted. The preponderance of existing prevention is focused on secondary prevention by performance of screening and surveil-lance colonoscopies with random biopsies to identify neoplasia and trigger sur-gical resection for prevention of invasive cancer and death. Substantial technical and practical challenges remain, however, and there is a great need for improved understanding of the compounded risks of neoplasia, the natural history of dysplasia, and more accurate detection and diagnostic techniques. A future approach to prevention is likely to stratify patients based on individualized risks that include, among other things, the histologic degree of inflammation present. In the meantime, existing guidelines should be emphasized and ongoing education of clinicians and patients must occur.

References

[1] Bargan J. Chronic ulcerative colitis associated with malignant disease. Arch Surg 1928;17: 561–76.

[2] Ekbom A, Helmick C, Zack M, et al. Ulcerative colitis and colorectal cancer. A population-based study. N Engl J Med 1990;323(18):1228–33.

[3] Lennard-Jones JE, Melville DM, Morson BC, et al. Precancer and cancer in extensive ulcerative colitis: findings among 401 patients over 22 years. Gut 1990;31(7):800–6.

[4] Lofberg R, Brostrom O, Karlen P, et al. Colonoscopic surveillance in long-standing total ulcerative colitis—a 15-year follow-up study. Gastroenterology 1990;99(4):1021–31.

[5] Rutter MD, Saunders BP, Wilkinson KH, et al. Severity of inflammation is a risk factor for colorectal neoplasia in ulcerative colitis. Gastroenterology 2004;126(2):451–9.

[6] Eaden JA, Abrams KR, Mayberry JF. The risk of colorectal cancer in ulcerative colitis: a meta-analysis. Gut 2001;48(4):526–35.

[7] Rutter MD, Saunders BP, Wilkinson KH, et al. Thirty-year analysis of a colonoscopic surveillance program for neoplasia in ulcerative colitis. Gastroenterology 2006;130(4):1030–8.

[8] Sugita ASD, Bodian C, Ribeiro MB, et al. Colorectal cancer in ulcerative colitis. Influence of anatomical extent and age of onset on colitis-cancer interval. Gut 1991;32:167–9.

[9] Connell WR, Talbot IC, Harpaz N, et al. Clinicopathological characteristics of colorectal carcinoma complicating ulcerative colitis. Gut 1994;35(10):1419–23.

[10] Grimm G, Lee G, Dirisina R, et al. Dose-dependent inhibition of stem cell activation with 5-ASA: a possible explanation for the chemopreventive effect of 5-ASA therapy in colitis-induced cancer. [abstract]. Gastroenterology 2006;130(4 Suppl 2):A-693.

[11] Bjerknes M. Expansion of mutant stem cell populations in the human colon. J Theor Biol 1996;178(4):381–5.

[12] Askling J, Dickman PW, Karlen P, et al. Family history as a risk factor for colorectal cancer in inflammatory bowel disease. Gastroenterology 2001;120(6):1356–62.

[13] Nuako KW, Ahlquist DA, Mahoney DW, et al. Familial predisposition for colorectal cancer in chronic ulcerative colitis: a case-control study. Gastroenterology 1998;115(5): 1079–83.

[14] Gumaste V, Sachar DB, Greenstein AJ. Benign and malignant colorectal strictures in ulcerative colitis. Gut 1992;33(7):938–41.

[15] Shetty K, Rybicki L, Brzezinski A, et al. The risk for cancer or dysplasia in ulcerative colitis patients with primary sclerosing cholangitis. Am J Gastroenterol 1999;94(6):1643–9.

[16] Soetikno RM, Lin OS, Heidenreich PA, et al. Increased risk of colorectal neoplasia in patients with primary sclerosing cholangitis and ulcerative colitis: a meta-analysis. Gastrointest Endosc 2002;56(1):48–54.

[17] Loftus EJ, Aguilar HI, Sandborn WJ, et al. Risk of colorectal neoplasia in patients with primary sclerosing cholangitis and ulcerative colitis following orthotopic liver transplantation. Hepatology 1998;27(3):685–90.

[18] Kornbluth A, Sachar DB. Ulcerative colitis practice guidelines in adults (update): American College of Gastroenterology, Practice Parameters Committee. Am J Gastroenterol 2004;99(7):1371–85.

[19] Eaden J, Abrams K, Ekbom A, et al. Colorectal cancer prevention in ulcerative colitis: a case-control study. Aliment Pharmacol Ther 2000;14(2):145–53.

[20] van Staa TP, Card T, Logan RF, et al. 5-Aminosalicylate use and colorectal cancer risk in inflammatory bowel disease: a large epidemiological study. Gut 2005;54(11): 1573–8.

[21] Bernstein CN, Blanchard JF, Metge C, et al. Does the use of 5-aminosalicylates in inflammatory bowel disease prevent the development of colorectal cancer? Am J Gastroenterol 2003;98(12):2784–8.

[22] Velayos FS, Terdiman JP, Walsh JM. Effect of 5-aminosalicylate use on colorectal cancer and dysplasia risk: a systematic review and metaanalysis of observational studies. Am J Gastroenterol 2005;100(6):1345–53.

[23] Riddell R, Goldman H, Ransohoff DF, et al. Dysplasia in inflammatory bowel disease: standardized classification with provisional clinical applications. Hum Pathol 1983;14(11): 931–68.

[24] Riddell RH. Grading of dysplasia. Eur J Cancer 1995;31A(7/8):1169–70.

[25] Blackstone MO, Riddell RH, Rogers BH, et al. Dysplasia-associated lesion or mass (DALM) detected by colonoscopy in long-standing ulcerative colitis: an indication for colectomy. Gastroenterology 1981;80(2):366–74.

[26] Bernstein CN, Shanahan F, Weinstein WM. Are we telling patients the truth about surveillance colonoscopy in ulcerative colitis? Lancet 1994;343(8889):71–4.

[27] Ullman T, Croog V, Harpaz N, et al. Progression of flat low-grade dysplasia to advanced neoplasia in patients with ulcerative colitis. Gastroenterology 2003;125(5):1311–9.

[28] Rubin DT, Rothe JA, Cohen RD, et al. Is dysplasia and colorectal cancer endoscopically visible in patients with ulcerative colitis?. [abstract]. Gastroenterology 2005;128(4 Suppl. 2): A-122.

[29] Rutter MD, Saunders BP, Wilkinson KH, et al. Most dysplasia in ulcerative colitis is visible at colonoscopy. Gastrointest Endosc 2004;60(3):334–9.

[30] Kiesslich R, Fritsch J, Holtmann M, et al. Methylene blue-aided chromoendoscopy for the detection of intraepithelial neoplasia and colon cancer in ulcerative colitis. Gastroenterology 2003;124(4):880–8.

[31] Kiesslich R, Neurath MF. Chromoendoscopy: an evolving standard in surveillance for ulcerative colitis. Inflamm Bowel Dis 2004;10(5):695–6.

[32] Itzkowitz SH, Harpaz N. Diagnosis and management of dysplasia in patients with inflammatory bowel diseases. Gastroenterology 2004;126(6):1634–48.

[33] Rosenstock E, Farmer RG, Petras R, et al. Surveillance for colonic carcinoma in ulcerative colitis. Gastroenterology 1985;89(6):1342–6.

[34] Jones HW, Grogono J, Hoare AM. Surveillance in ulcerative colitis: burdens and benefit. Gut 1988;29(3):325–31.

[35] Leidenius M, Kellokumpu I, Husa A, et al. Dysplasia and carcinoma in longstanding ulcerative colitis: an endoscopic and histological surveillance programme. Gut 1991;32(12): 1521–5.

[36] Lynch DA, Lobo AJ, Sobala GM, et al. Failure of colonoscopic surveillance in ulcerative colitis. Gut 1993;34(8):1075–80.

[37] Connell WR, Lennard-Jones JE, Williams CB, et al. Factors affecting the outcome of endoscopic surveillance for cancer in ulcerative colitis. Gastroenterology 1994;107(4):934–44.

[38] Rozen P, Baratz M, Fefer F, et al. Low incidence of significant dysplasia in a successful endoscopic surveillance program of patients with ulcerative colitis. Gastroenterology 1995;108(5):1361–70.

[39] Lindberg B, Persson B, Veress B, et al. Twenty years' colonoscopic surveillance of patients with ulcerative colitis. Detection of dysplastic and malignant transformation. Scand J Gastroenterol 1996;31(12):1195–204.

[40] Choi PM, Nugent FW, Schoetz DJ Jr, et al. Colonoscopic surveillance reduces mortality from colorectal cancer in ulcerative colitis. Gastroenterology 1993;105(2):418–24.

[41] Karlen P, Kornfeld D, Brostrom O, et al. Is colonoscopic surveillance reducing colorectal cancer mortality in ulcerative colitis? A population based case control study. [see comments]. Gut 1998;42(5):711–4.

[42] Lashner BA, Kane SV, Hanauer SB. Colon cancer surveillance in chronic ulcerative colitis: historical cohort study. Am J Gastroenterol 1990;85:1083–7.

[43] Mpofu C, Watson AJ, Rhodes JM. Strategies for detecting colon cancer and/or dysplasia in patients with inflammatory bowel disease. Cochrane Database Syst Rev 2004;2: CD000279.
[44] Gullberg K, Stahlberg D, Liljeqvist L, et al. Neoplastic transformation of the pelvic pouch mucosa in patients with ulcerative colitis. Gastroenterology 1997;112(5):1487–92.
[45] Bernstein CN. Ulcerative colitis with low-grade dysplasia. Gastroenterology 2004;127(3): 950–6.
[46] Ekbom A, Helmick C, Zack M, et al. Increased risk of large-bowel cancer in Crohn's disease with colonic involvement. Lancet 1990;336(8711):357–9.
[47] Bernstein CN, Blanchard JF, Rawsthorne P, et al. The prevelence of extraintestinal diseases in inflammatory bowel disease: a population-based study. Am J Gastroenterol 2001;96: 11116–22.
[48] Sigel JE, Petras RE, Lashner BA, et al. Intestinal adenocarcinoma in Crohn's disease: a report of 30 cases with a focus on coexisting dysplasia. Am J Surg Pathol 1999;23(6):651–5.
[49] Friedman S, Rubin PH, Bodian C, et al. Screening and surveillance colonoscopy in chronic Crohn's colitis. Gastroenterology 2001;120(4):820–6.
[50] Ullman TA. Dysplasia and colorectal cancer in Crohn's disease. J Clin Gastroenterol 2003;36(5 Suppl):S75–8 [discussion: S94–6].
[51] Jess T, Loftus EV Jr, Velayos FS, et al. Risk of intestinal cancer in inflammatory bowel disease: a population-based study from Olmsted County, Minnesota. Gastroenterology 2006;130(4):1039–46.
[52] Sjodahl RI, Myrelid P, Soderholm JD. Anal and rectal cancer in Crohn's disease. Colorectal Dis 2003;5(5):490–5.
[53] Ky A, Sohn N, Weinstein MA, et al. Carcinoma arising in anorectal fistulas of Crohn's disease. Dis Colon Rectum 1998;41(8):992–6.
[54] Connell WR, Sheffield JP, Kamm MA, et al. Lower gastrointestinal malignancy in Crohn's disease. Gut 1994;35(3):347–52.
[55] Korelitz B. Carcinoma arising in Crohn's disease fistulae: another concern warranting another type of surveillance. Am J Gastroenterol 1999;94(9):2337–9.
[56] Yamazuki Y, Riberio MB, Sachar DB, et al. Malignant colorectal strictures in Crohn's disease. Am J Gastroenterol 1991;86(7):882–5.
[57] Rubin CE, Haggitt RC, Burmer GC, et al. DNA aneuploidy in colonic biopsies predicts future development of dysplasia in ulcerative colitis. Gastroenterology 1992;103(5):1611–20.
[58] Rubin PH, Friedman S, Harpaz N, et al. Colonoscopic polypectomy in chronic colitis: conservative management after endoscopic resection of dysplastic polyps. Gastroenterology 1999;117(6):1295–300.
[59] Engelsgjerd M, Farraye FA, Odze RD. Polypectomy may be adequate treatment for adenoma-like dysplastic lesions in chronic ulcerative colitis. Gastroenterology 1999;117(6): 1288–94 [discussion: 1488–91].
[60] Odze RD, Farraye FA, Hecht JL, et al. Long-term follow-up after polypectomy treatment for adenoma-like dysplastic lesions in ulcerative colitis. Clin Gastroenterol Hepatol 2004;2(7):534–41.
[61] Itzkowitz SH, Present DH. Consensus conference: colorectal cancer screening and surveillance in inflammatory bowel disease. Inflamm Bowel Dis 2005;11(3):314–21.
[62] Carter MJ, Lobo AJ, Travis SP. Guidelines for the management of inflammatory bowel disease in adults. Gut 2004;53(Suppl 5):V1–V16.
[63] Greenstein AJ, Sachar DB, Smith H, et al. Cancer in universal and left-sided ulcerative colitis: factors determining risk. Gastroenterology 1979;77(2):290–4.
[64] Bernstein CN, Weinstein WM, Levine DS, et al. Physicians' perceptions of dysplasia and approaches to surveillance colonoscopy in ulcerative colitis. Am J Gastroenterol 1995;90(12): 2106–2092.
[65] Eaden JA, Mayberry JF. Guidelines for screening and surveillance of asymptomatic colorectal cancer in patients with inflammatory bowel disease. Gut 2002;51(Suppl 5):V10–2.

[66] Hudson B, Green J. British Society of Gastroenterology guidelines for ulcerative colitis surveillance: creating consensus or confusion? Gut 2006;55(7):1052–3.
[67] Sonnenberg A, El-Serag HB. Economic aspects of endoscopic screening for intestinal precancerous conditions. Gastrointest Endosc Clin N Am 1997;7(1):165–84.
[68] Provenzale D, Onken J. Surveillance issues in inflammatory bowel disease: ulcerative colitis. J Clin Gastroenterol 2001;32(2):99–105.

Gastroenterol Clin N Am 35 (2006) 605–619

GASTROENTEROLOGY CLINICS
OF NORTH AMERICA

ELSEVIER
SAUNDERS

Chromoendoscopy and Other Novel Imaging Techniques

Ralf Kiesslich, MD, PhD*, Markus F. Neurath, MD, PhD

I. Med. Klinik und Poliklinik, Johannes Gutenberg Universität Mainz, Langenbeckstrasse 1,
55131 Mainz, Germany

CANCER RISK AND SURVEILLANCE

Patients with long-standing extensive ulcerative colitis (UC) are at increased risk of developing colorectal cancer [1]. Colonoscopic surveillance is recommended to reduce associated mortality [2]. Surveillance relies on the detection of premalignant dysplastic tissue, and where multifocal dysplasia is detected, proctocolectomy remains the management technique of choice, although there is increasing evidence that adenoma-like dysplastic lesions may safely be resected endoscopically [3–5].

DETECTION OF PREMALIGNANT LESIONS IN ULCERATIVE COLITIS

In patients without UC, the premalignant dysplastic lesion, the adenoma, usually occurs as a clearly delineated and macroscopically visible abnormality. In UC, however, there is no clear-cut adenoma-carcinoma sequence. Colitis-associated neoplasia can occur in addition to adenomas in patients with long-standing UC. These lesions are triggered by inflammation, and the macroscopic appearances are often flat and multifocal [6]. There are no clear-cut endoscopic, histologic, or immunohistochemical discriminators to permit accurate stratification of raised dysplasia in colitis and no universally agreed definition. In accordance with the new Vienna classification, the term *intraepithelial neoplasias* was established, which summarizes adenomas and colitis-associated neoplasia [7].

Currently, multiple, untargeted, random biopsies are recommended to diagnose intraepithelial neoplasia. Four random biopsies per site over nine sites throughout the colon should be undertaken, with increased sampling from the rectosigmoid and with additional biopsies from raised or suspicious lesions [2]. This approach is time-consuming, however, and dysplastic lesions might still be overlooked. Chromoendoscopy can help to identify premalignant and malignant lesions. Magnifying endoscopy enables one to analyze surface structure, whereas confocal laser endomicroscopy facilitates in vivo histology.

*Corresponding author. E-mail address: info@ralf-kiesslich.de (R. Kiesslich).

0889-8553/06/$ – see front matter
doi:10.1016/j.gtc.2006.07.004
© 2006 Elsevier Inc. All rights reserved.
gastro.theclinics.com

CHROMOENDOSCOPY

Intravital staining is the oldest and simplest method used to improve the diagnosis of epithelial changes. Chromoendoscopy, vital staining, and contrast endoscopy are synonyms for the same technique: dye solutions are applied to the mucosa of the gastrointestinal tract, enhancing the recognition of details to uncover mucosal changes not perceivable by purely optical methods before targeted biopsy and histology [8]. In general, there are three classes of dyes that can be used for chromoendoscopy [9,10].

Contrast Dyes

Contrast dyes simply coat the colonic mucosal surface and neither react with nor are absorbed by the mucosa. An example is indigo carmine. Contrast dyes are effective because the colonic mucosa is covered with tiny pits and whorls of parallel "innominate" grooves, similar to a fingerprint. When a dye is sprayed on the surface, this pattern becomes evident, and disruption to these grooves caused by mucosal lesions (which have a different surface topography) is highlighted.

Absorptive Dyes

Absorptive dyes are absorbed by different cells to different degrees, highlighting particular cell types. An example is methylene blue, which avidly stains noninflamed mucosa after a few minutes but is poorly taken up by areas of active inflammation and dysplasia.

Reactive Dyes

The binding of reactive coloring agents with certain mucosal areas is used to identify reactions. Their use is less common, and their diagnostic relevance is rather low.

In patients with UC, the most common dyes are indigo carmine and methylene blue. Chromoendoscopy has two main goals. First, it improves the detection of subtle colonic lesions, raising the sensitivity of the endoscopic examination; this is important in UC, because flat dysplastic lesions can be difficult to detect. Second, once a lesion is detected, chromoendoscopy can improve lesion characterization, increasing the specificity of the examination. This can be further refined with a magnifying colonoscope. Surface analysis of colorectal lesions using magnifying endoscopes allows a new optical impression for endoscopists. Kudo and colleagues [10] described that some of the regular staining patterns are often seen in hyperplastic polyps or normal mucosa, whereas an unstructured surface architecture pattern is associated with malignancy. Also, the kind of adenoma (tubular versus villous) can be seen by detailed inspection (Fig. 1). This work has led to categorization of the different staining patterns in the colon. The so-called "pit-pattern classification" [10] differentiated five types and several subtypes. Types I and II are staining patterns that predict nonneoplastic lesions, whereas types III through V predict neoplastic lesions (Fig. 2). With the help of this classification system, the endoscopist can predict histologic findings with good accuracy [11].

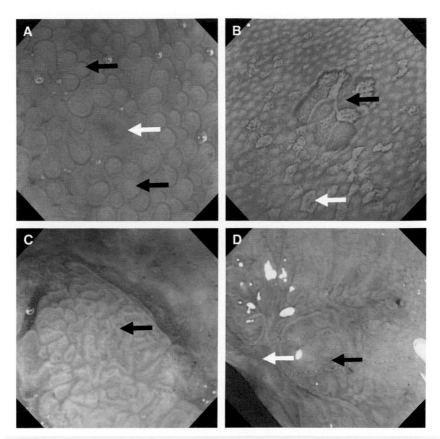

Fig. 1. (A) Chromoendoscopy and magnifying endoscopy of the terminal ileum. Single villi are clearly visible (*black arrows*). A small erosion (<1 mm) is visible in the center of the image. (B) Magnification endoscopy after methylene blue–aided chromoendoscopy. Small inflammatory changes are visible (*white arrow*) surrounded by normal crypt architecture. Chromoendoscopy unmasks aberrant crypt foci (pit-pattern type II; *black arrow*). (C) Tubular staining pattern (type IIIL) is clearly visible after intravital staining. Targeted biopsy revealed low-grade intraepithelial neoplasia. (D) Flat growing cancer with unstructured surface (pit-pattern type V; *black arrow*) with accompanying ulceration (*white arrow*) indicates malignancy.

As recently shown in prospective and randomized trials, panchromoendoscopy with methylene blue– or indigo carmine–aided biopsies is superior in the detection of intraepithelial neoplasia as compared with random biopsies [11–14]. Based on the currently available data, SURFACE guidelines [15] are proposed for the use and standardization of this new technique in patients with UC (Box 1).

Ideally, surveillance colonoscopies should be performed in patients whose symptoms are in remission so as to aid macroscopic and histologic discrimination between inflammatory changes and dysplasia (see Box 1, strict patient selection). Thus, a patient with active symptoms should first have his or her

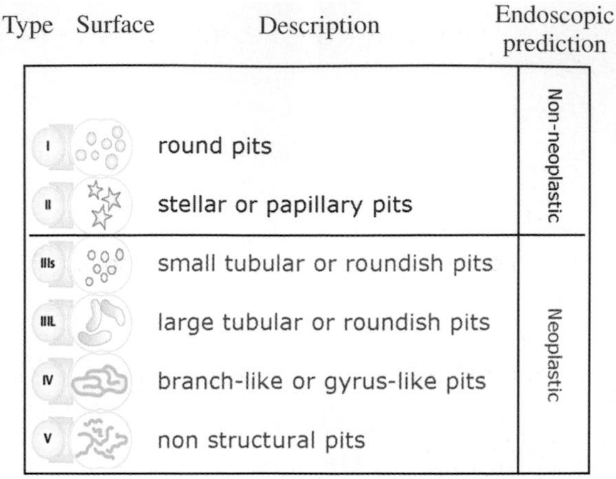

Type	Surface	Description	Endoscopic prediction
I		round pits	Non-neoplastic
II		stellar or papillary pits	Non-neoplastic
IIIs		small tubular or roundish pits	Neoplastic
IIIL		large tubular or roundish pits	Neoplastic
IV		branch-like or gyrus-like pits	Neoplastic
V		non structural pits	Neoplastic

Fig. 2. Pit-pattern classification.

medical therapy optimized to induce remission whenever possible. Because patients with chronic active inflammation are at increased risk of colorectal neoplasia [16], however, the procedure should not be unduly delayed if they fail to respond to therapy.

Examination Technique

Thorough bowel preparation is of crucial importance and is a prerequisite for chromoendoscopy [9]. On insertion, all fecal fluid should be aspirated to ensure optimal mucosal views (see Box 1, unmask the mucosal surface). When the cecal pole has been reached, meticulous inspection of the colonic mucosa is performed on withdrawal. To reduce spasm and haustral fold prominence (thus reducing blind spots), intravenous butyl-scopolamine, 20 mg (or intravenous glucagon, 1 mg) should be given when the cecal pole is reached. Further increments can be given as required (see Box 1, reduce peristaltic waves). Adequate air insufflation is necessary, and if the lumen remains collapsed, the patient should be turned. Inspection is performed by scouring the mucosa in a spiral fashion. Dye spraying of the entire colorectal mucosa (panchromoendoscopy) greatly reduces the risk of overlooking subtle abnormalities (see Box 1, full-length staining of the colon) and adds little to the duration of the procedure. Before the procedure, 0.1% indigo carmine or 0.1% methylene blue (100 mL of either) is prepared and drawn into 50-mL syringes. A dye-spray catheter is inserted down the instrumentation channel, and the tip is protruded 2 to 3 cm. Under the direction of the endoscopist, an assistant firmly squeezes the syringe, generating a fine mist of dye, which is then painted onto the mucosa by withdrawing the colonoscope in a spiral fashion.

Spraying should be done in a segmental fashion (every 20–30 cm). Once a segment has been sprayed, excess dye is suctioned and the colonoscope is

Box 1: SURFACE guidelines for chromoendoscopy in patients with ulcerative colitis

Strict patient selection

Patients with histologically proven UC and at least 8 years' duration in clinical remission; avoid patients with active disease.

Unmask the mucosal surface

Excellent bowel preparation is needed. Remove mucus and remaining fluid in the colon when necessary.

Reduce peristaltic waves

When drawing back the endoscope, a spasmolytic agent should be used (if necessary).

Full-length staining of the colon

Perform full-length staining of the colon (panchromoendoscopy) in UC rather than local staining.

Augmented detection with dyes

Intravital staining with 0.4% indigo carmine or 0.1% methylene blue should be used to unmask flat lesions more frequently than with conventional colonoscopy.

Crypt architecture analysis

All lesions should be analyzed according to the pit-pattern classification. Whereas pit-pattern types I and II suggest the presence of nonmalignant lesions, staining patterns III through V suggest the presence of intraepithelial neoplasias and carcinomas.

Endoscopic targeted biopsies

Perform targeted biopsies of all mucosal alterations, particularly of circumscript lesions with staining patterns indicative of intraepithelial neoplasias and carcinomas (pit-pattern types III–V).

reinserted to the proximal extent of the segment. It is occasionally necessary to wait a few seconds for indigo carmine to settle into the mucosal contours; methylene blue takes approximately 60 seconds to be absorbed. Once that segment has been examined, the next segment is sprayed and so on until the anal margin is reached. On average, 60 to 100 mL of solution is required to spray the entire colorectal mucosa.

Dye spraying greatly aids in the detection of intraepithelial neoplasia (see Box 1, augmented detection with dyes). Areas of villiform (velvet-like) mucosa with clear borders (circumscript lesions) are of particular concern. Areas of nodularity or friable mucosa may also indicate intraepithelial neoplasia (see Fig. 1). Sessile (polypoid) lesions are easier to detect, but careful delineation of the edge of the lesion is required (aided by dye spraying), and if the lesion is endoscopically resectable, it is essential to take additional biopsies from the surrounding mucosa to ensure that there is no residual neoplastic tissue and to tattoo the site to permit reinspection later.

The combination of chromoendoscopy and new-generation magnifying colonoscopes enables detailed mucosal analysis (see Box 1, crypt architecture analysis). Neoplastic changes are characterized by an irregular, tubular, or villous crypt architecture staining pattern. Nonneoplastic changes are characterized by stellar or regular round pits. The different staining patterns are categorized using the pit-pattern classification [10].

By targeting biopsies toward mucosal abnormalities (see Box 1, endoscopic targeted biopsies), the specificity of each biopsy for dysplasia is increased and the total number of biopsies taken per colonoscopic examination can be reduced in comparison to random biopsies with standard colonoscopy [11–14].

Efficiency of Chromoendoscopy

The first randomized controlled trial was published in 2003 to test whether chromoendoscopy and magnifying endoscopy might facilitate early detection of intraepithelial neoplasia in patients with UC by using magnifying chromoendoscopy [11]. One hundred sixty-five patients with long-standing UC were randomized at a 1:1 ratio to undergo conventional colonoscopy or colonoscopy with chromoendoscopy using 0.1% methylene blue. Circumscript lesions in the colon were evaluated according to a modified pit-pattern classification. In the chromoendoscopy group, there was significantly better correlation between the endoscopic assessment of degree and extent of colonic inflammation and the histopathologic findings compared with the conventional colonoscopy group. More targeted biopsies were possible and significantly more intraepithelial neoplasia was detected in the chromoendoscopy group (32 versus 10 cases). Using the modified pit-pattern classification, the sensitivity and specificity for differentiation between nonneoplastic and neoplastic lesions were 93%. The overall sensitivity of magnifying chromoendoscopy to predict neoplasia was 97%, with a specificity of 93%. The ability of the dye technique to differentiate neoplastic from nonneoplastic lesions so as to enhance detection of more dysplastic lesions in flat mucosa is a potential major advance in dysplasia surveillance. These first promising data about chromoendoscopy in UC were confirmed by Hurlstone [12]. In a prospective study, 162 patients with long-standing UC and established pancolitis underwent total colonoscopy by a single endoscopist using a magnifying colonoscope. After detection of subtle mucosal changes, such as fold convergence, air-induced deformation, interruption of innominate grooves, or focal discrete color change, targeted intravital staining with indigo carmine was used. The macroscopic type and the staining pattern were defined. The control group consisted of 162 disease-matched patients undergoing conventional colonoscopy. Chromoendoscopy with targeted biopsy significantly increased the diagnostic yield for intraepithelial neoplasia and the number of flat neoplastic changes as opposed to conventional colonoscopy. Intraepithelial neoplasia in flat mucosal change was observed in 37 lesions, of which 31 were detected using chromoendoscopy.

In a follow-up trial by Hurlstone and colleagues [13], a total of 350 patients with long-standing UC underwent surveillance colonoscopy using high-magnification chromoscopic colonoscopy. Quadrantic biopsies at 10-cm intervals were taken on extubation in addition to targeted biopsies of abnormal mucosal areas. Defined lesions were further evaluated using modified Kudo crypt pattern analysis. These data were compared with data from 350 disease duration– and disease extent–matched control patients who had undergone conventional colonoscopic surveillance between January 2001 and April 2005. Significantly more intraepithelial neoplastic lesions were detected in the magnification chromoscopy group compared with controls (69 versus 24 patients; $P < .0001$). Intraepithelial neoplasia was observed in 67 lesions, of which 53 (79%) were detected using magnification chromoscopy alone. Chromoscopy increased the number of flat lesions with intraepithelial neoplasia detected compared with controls ($P < .001$).

Rutter and coworkers [14] performed the third prospective trial in UC on 100 patients with back-to-back colonoscopies, starting with random and targeted biopsies, followed by indigo carmine–aided panchromoendoscopy with targeted biopsies only. The diagnostic yield of dysplastic changes was increased in this study by the use of chromoendoscopy from 2 to 7 patients (3.5-fold increase) and from two to nine dysplastic lesions (4.5-fold increase).

Based on these trials, chromoendoscopy is now incorporated into the US guidelines for surveillance in patients with long-standing UC [15]. The committee (Crohn's and Colitis Foundation of America Colon Cancer in IBD Study Group) endorses the incorporation of chromoendoscopy into surveillance colonoscopy for appropriately trained endoscopists. Additionally, it was stated that the development of newer techniques may further refine the current surveillance recommendations and the understanding of the natural history of dysplasia. It is important to point out that chromoendoscopy requires appropriate training of the endoscopist and should be performed according to well-accepted criteria.

It has to be noted that chromoendoscopy helps to unmask lesions in patients with long-standing UC. Magnifying or high-resolution endoscopy is necessary to characterize the plethora of lesions further after staining according to the classification of Kudo and colleagues [10] so as to reduce the number of lesions that should be biopsied.

In conclusion, magnifying chromoendoscopy is a new valid tool for improving endoscopic detection of intraepithelial neoplasia in patients with long-standing UC. Chromoendoscopy increased the diagnostic yield of intraepithelial neoplasia as compared with conventional colonoscopy and biopsy techniques 3- to 4.5-fold, which further suggests that more patients with UC could be considered as candidates for colectomy. Differentiation of nonneoplastic from neoplastic lesions is possible with high overall sensitivity and specificity [17].

Limitations of Chromoendoscopy and Magnifying Endoscopy

Until now, there were no severe side effects reported regarding the local use of indigo carmine. Olliver and colleagues [18] recently raised some concerns about the intravital dye methylene blue, however, despite a harmless transient discoloration of stool and urine. They found oxidative DNA damage after chromoendoscopy (as measured by single-cell gel electrophoresis) in patients with Barrett's esophagus and argued that methylene blue, together with white light, during endoscopy could also be a risk for patients to drive carcinogenesis. Therefore, the question arises as to whether methylene blue–aided chromoendoscopy may contribute to the carcinogenic process in other diseases, such as UC, and lead to an increase in intraepithelial neoplasias in follow-up. Nevertheless, in a follow-up report (median follow-up of 23 months) examining the safety of methylene blue staining, patients with previous chromoendoscopies showed fewer intraepithelial neoplastic lesions as compared with patients who were screened by colonoscopy [19]. These data suggest that chromoendoscopy with methylene blue is a safe and highly effective approach for the detection of flat colonic lesions in UC. The reported increase in DNA lesions on methylene blue–light treatment is unlikely to have biologic significance in vivo, and unwanted side effects seem to be negligible in view of the advantages of the method.

The visual evaluation of minute detail allowed by magnification endoscopy is promising, but some points of criticism must be discussed. Inflammation can cause significant disturbance of the image seen when magnifying endoscopy is used to look for the minute changes indicative of neoplasia, and there is a danger of false-positive results. Inflamed epithelium should be treated before final endoscopic evaluation whenever possible. It is not useful or practical to use the zoom mode permanently when screening the lower gastrointestinal tract. The initial evaluation is performed in the conventional mode and depends strictly on the knowledge and experience of the endoscopist. After the initial detection of discrete lesions, chromoendoscopy and magnification endoscopy are the tools used to enhance surface mucosal patterns. These techniques disclose a plethora of mucosal detail, the evaluation of which increases the procedure time, at least when the endoscopist is learning the technique.

The proposed classification for colorectal lesions is too complex relative to their practical clinical value. Simplification is recommended. We are facing the same dilemma as our pathologist colleagues when evaluating dysplasia, with the difference that histologic preparation is widely standardized, whereas standardized procedure recommendations are lacking for chromoendoscopy and magnification endoscopy. Another difficulty in the use of magnifying endoscopes is the high magnification levels. The newly developed systems allow enlargement of up to 150 times. A sharp image is focused by manually adjusting the movable lens. Close examination can be difficult because of peristalsis and respiratory movements.

NARROW BAND IMAGING

Narrow band imaging (NBI) is an innovative optical technology that can clearly visualize the microvascular structure of the mucosal layer [20]. NBI illuminates the tissue surface using special filters that narrow the respective red-green-blue bands while simultaneously increasing the relative intensity of the blue band. This enhances the tissue microvasculature, mainly as a result of the differential optical absorption of light by hemoglobin in the mucosa associated with initiation and progression of dysplasia, particularly in the blue range. The resulting images look like "chromoendoscopy without dye" focusing on capillaries. Gono and colleagues [20] found that by using narrow band illumination of 415 ± 30 nm, the contrast of the capillary pattern in the superficial layer of the human tongue was markedly improved. They suggested that this approach was optimal for visualizing the capillary pattern in vivo and was complementary to conventional magnification classification. In their study, Machida and coworkers [21] used a newly developed NBI technique in which modified optical filters were used in the light source of a videoendoscope system and could be applied during colonoscopy in a clinical setting. This pilot study evaluated the clinical feasibility of the NBI system for colonoscopy. A total of 34 colorectal lesions in 34 patients were included. Differentiation between neoplastic and nonneoplastic lesions using the NBI system was evaluated in comparison with results from conventional colonoscopy and chromoendoscopy.

NBI and chromoendoscopy showed the same sensitivity (each 100%) and specificity (each 75%) to differentiate neoplastic from nonneoplastic lesions. In addition, both techniques were superior to conventional endoscopy (83% sensitivity and 44% specificity). NBI achieved a better visualization of vascular network, however, whereas chromoendoscopy was more precise in characterization of the surface pit pattern.

The value of NBI in face of UC is not yet determined. It can be speculated that focusing on capillary structures might be difficult because of background inflammation in patients with UC.

OPTICAL COHERENCE TOMOGRAPHY

Optical coherence tomography (OCT) is an optical analogue of ultrasound, providing 10-μm resolution and real-time cross-sectional images of the luminal gastrointestinal tract [22]. Thus, OCT allows real-time high-resolution in analogy to B-scan ultrasonography, which detects back-scattered sound waves. OCT images are formed by detecting light that is reflected back from subsurface tissue microstructure, based on optical interferometry. OCT has a more limited imaging depth (~2 mm) compared with high-frequency ultrasonography probes; however, it may offer the possibility to predict malignant infiltration into the submucosa precisely because of its higher resolution. This would be of crucial clinical importance, because mucosal resection could be limited to adenomas or early cancers with malignant infiltration into the upper third of the submucosal layer.

Shen and colleagues [23] investigated the clinical value of OCT for differentiating between Crohn's disease and UC. Crohn's disease is characterized by transmural chronic inflammation, whereas UC is typically limited to the mucosal layer. OCT was performed in 40 patients with Crohn's disease (309 images) and 30 patients with UC (292 images). Thirty-six patients with Crohn's disease

(90.0%) had a disrupted layered structure as compared with only 5 patients with UC (16.7%). This difference was highly significant ($P < .001$). The disrupted layered structure on OCT indicative of transmural inflammation has had diagnostic sensitivity and specificity of 90.0% and 83.3%, respectively. Resolution of the current available OCT probes is still unsatisfactory, however. Improvements in axial and lateral resolutions are needed to refine the diagnostic possibilities further, especially to assess the submucosal layer accurately on a subcellular level.

FLUORESCENCE ENDOSCOPY

Light-induced fluorescence endoscopic imaging can be used to unmask neoplastic lesions by autofluorescence or induced fluorescence by contrast agents. Messmann and coworkers [24] used orally (20 mg/kg) or locally administered 5-aminolevulinic acid (5-ALA) in 37 patients with long-standing UC. This leads to differential endogenous production of the fluorophore protoporphyrin IX. The sensitivity of fluorescence for dysplastic lesions was high, ranging from 87% to 100% after local sensitization. The value decreased to only 43% after systemic administration of 5-ALA, however.

The value of fluorescence endoscopy has been studied in combination with fiber endoscopes. Currently, a system has been developed that combines autofluorescence with videoendoscopy (Prototype Olympus, Tokyo, Japan). Initial data are available from the upper gastrointestinal tract [25]. It can be speculated that this technologic breakthrough may significantly improve the diagnostic yield of fluorescence endoscopy, enabling one to image neoplastic tissue selectively.

PERSPECTIVES AND FUTURE TRENDS

The limits and concerns of magnifying chromoendoscopy are few and can be overcome by training and increased knowledge of the endoscopists. Nevertheless, the dream and goal of ideal colonoscopy is virtual histology, or "on-line" in vivo histology. The endoscopists can decide which is the area of interest and can remove the lesion in a targeted fashion without prior biopsy. Chromoendoscopy can illustrate the surface structure. Of more interest, however, is the cellular structure. Many new optical developments try to advance early diagnosis of colorectal cancer. Raman spectroscopy, OCT, light-scattering spectroscopy, confocal fluorescence endoscopy, and immunofluorescence endoscopy are some of the new methods, each with advantages and disadvantages. The closest step toward virtual histology is confocal laser endoscopy, however [26].

CONFOCAL LASER ENDOMICROSCOPY

Confocal laser endomicroscopy allows subsurface analysis of the intestinal mucosa and in vivo histologic examination during ongoing endoscopy. The components of a confocal laser endoscope are based on integration of a confocal laser microscope in the distal tip of a conventional videoendoscope (Fig. 3). During laser endoscopy, a single-line laser delivers an excitation wavelength of 488 nm and the maximum laser power output is 1 mW or less at the surface of the tissue. Confocal image data are collected at a scan rate of 0.8 frames per second (1024 × 512 pixels) or 1.6 frames per second (1024 × 1024 pixels). The optical slice thickness is 7 µm, with a lateral resolution of 0.7 µm. The field of view is 500 µm × 500 µm. The range of the z-axis was 0 to 200 µm below the surface layer. Confocal images can be generated simultaneously with endoscopic images (Fig. 4).

Technique of Confocal Laser Endomicroscopy

A fluorescent contrast agent is used to achieve high-contrast images using confocal endomicroscopy. Potentially suitable agents are fluorescein, acriflavine, tetracycline, or cresyl violet. The contrast agents can be applied systemically (fluorescein) or topically (all others) by using a spraying catheter. The most common dye used so far is fluorescein. The confocal endoscope can be handled similar to a standard endoscope. After the systemic application of a contrast dye (eg, fluorescein), the distal tip of the endoscope is placed in gentle contact with the mucosa and the position of the focal plane within the specimen is adjusted using the buttons on the endoscope control body. In every region of interest, images from the surface to deeper parts of the mucosal layer can be obtained and stored digitally in a specific folder associated with the site of collection. Targeted biopsies are possible because of the proximity of the working channel and the endomicroscopic window at the distal tip of the endoscope,

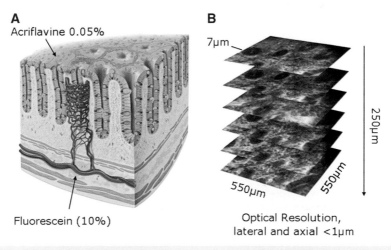

A
Acriflavine 0.05%

Fluorescein (10%)

B
7µm

250µm

550µm

550µm

Optical Resolution,
lateral and axial <1µm

Fig. 3. Scheme of endomicroscopy. (A) Microarchitecture of the colonic wall. Topical acriflavine or systemic application of fluorescein is mandatory for confocal endomicroscopy. (B) Confocal images are orientated in a horizontal fashion. The optical slice thickness is 7 µm with a lateral resolution of 0.7 µm. The field of view is 500 µm × 500 µm. The range of the z-axis is 0 to 250 µm below the surface layer.

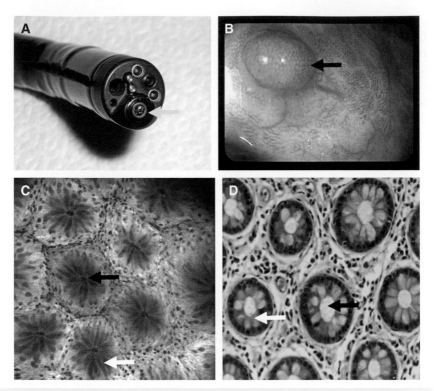

Fig. 4. Endomicroscopy in UC: nonneoplastic lesion. (*A*) Confocal laser colonoscope. The confocal microscope is integrated in the distal tip. An additional microscopic window (*arrow*) enables the emission of blue laser light facilitating in vivo histologic examination. (*B*) Small polypoid lesion with a regular staining pattern is clearly visible after methylene blue–aided chromoendoscopy. (*C*) Targeted endomicroscopic imaging shows a normal contribution of crypts and crypt openings (*black arrow*). The goblet cells within the crypts are displayed in black (*white arrow*). Connective tissue is arranged regularly in a hexagonal fashion. (*D*) Corresponding histologic examination confirms the endomicroscopic diagnosis. Normal crypts and round openings (*black arrow*) are visible. In addition, mucin is visible in the goblet cells (*white arrow*). Note that because of shrinking artifacts, the spaces between the tissue are wider in conventional histologic findings as compared with in vivo histologic findings.

which allows the position of the confocal scanner on the tissue to be seen via the conventional videoendoscopic view.

Clinical Data

The confocal laser endoscope can be used routinely for screening and surveillance. Suspected lesions can be examined in a targeted fashion by placing the endomicroscopic window onto the lesion. Confocal images can be graduated according to cellular and vascular changes. The images correlated well with conventional histologic findings after targeted biopsies. In the first prospective trial, 13,020 confocal images from 390 different locations (256 inconspicuous areas and 134 circumscript lesions) were compared with histologic data from 1038 biopsies. Subsurface analysis during confocal laser endoscopy allowed detailed analysis of cellular structures. The presence of neoplastic changes could be predicted by using the newly developed confocal pattern classification (see Fig. 3; Fig. 5) with high accuracy (97.4% sensitivity, 99.4% specificity, and 99.2% accuracy) [26]. In addition, the combination of chromoendoscopy and confocal laser endoscopy facilitates surveillance in UC. Chromoendoscopy unmasks circumscript lesions, and confocal laser endomicroscopy can be used to predict intraepithelial neoplasia with high accuracy.

In the first randomized trial using endomicroscopy, 153 patients with long-term UC in clinical remission (SURFACE guidelines) were randomized at a 1:1 ratio to undergo conventional colonoscopy or panchromoendoscopy using 0.1% methylene blue in conjunction with endomicroscopy to detect intraepithelial neoplasia or colorectal cancer. Circumscript lesions in the colonic mucosa detected by chromoendoscopy were evaluated with endomicroscopy for cellular and vascular changes according to the confocal pattern classification so

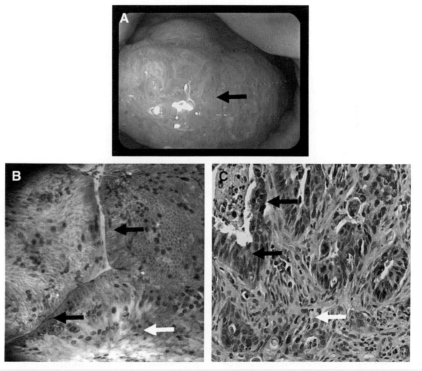

Fig. 5. Endomicroscopy in UC: neoplastic lesion. (A) Large polypoid lesion is visible in the sigmoid. Chromoendoscopy is not necessary to recognize the lesion. (B) Endomicroscopy shows neoplasia with tubular arranged epithelium with loss of goblet cells (*black arrows*). In some parts, vessel and cell architecture is totally irregular (*white arrow*). (C) Corresponding histologic examination shows high-grade intraepithelial neoplasia with similar architecture.

as to predict neoplasia. Targeted biopsies of the examined areas were performed and histologically graduated according to the new Vienna classification [7].

In the standard colonoscopy group, randomized biopsies every 10 cm between the anus and cecum and targeted biopsies of visible mucosal changes were performed. Primary outcome analysis was the histologic diagnosis of neoplasia. Using chromoendoscopy in conjunction with endomicroscopy (80 patients, average examination time of 42 minutes), significantly more intraepithelial neoplasia could be detected (19 versus 4 cases; $P = .007$) as with standard colonoscopy (73 patients, average examination time of 31 minutes). Endomicroscopy revealed different cellular structures (epithelial and blood cells), capillaries, and connective tissue limited to the mucosal layer. A total of 5580 confocal images from 134 circumscript lesions were compared with histologic results from 311 biopsies. The presence of neoplastic changes could be predicted with high accuracy (94.7% sensitivity, 98.3% specificity, and 97.8% accuracy) (see Figs. 3 and 5) [27].

SUMMARY

The newly developed high-resolution and magnification endoscopes offer features that allow more and new mucosal details to be seen. They are commonly used in conjunction with chromoendoscopy. The analysis of mucosal surface details is beginning to resemble histologic examination. More accurate recognition of small flat and depressed neoplastic lesions is possible. Endoscopic prediction of neoplastic and nonneoplastic tissue is possible by analysis of surface architecture of the mucosa, which influences the endoscopic management. For the diagnosis of flat adenomas, chromoendoscopy should be a part of the endoscopist's armamentarium. In inflammatory bowel disease, chromoendoscopy can be used for patients with long-standing UC to unmask flat intraepithelial neoplasia and is likely to become the new standard method for surveillance colonoscopy in the near future. The new detailed images seen with magnifying chromoendoscopy are the beginning of a new era in which advances in optical development, such as confocal endomicroscopy, allow a unique look at detailed cellular structures.

References

[1] Gilat T, Fireman Z, Grossman A, et al. Colorectal cancer in patients with ulcerative colitis. Gastroenterology 1988;94:870–7.

[2] Winawer S, et al. Colorectal cancer screening and surveillance: clinical guidelines and rationale—update based on new evidence. Gastroenterology 2003;124(2):544–60.

[3] Odze RD, Farraye FA, Hecht JL, et al. Long-term follow-up after polypectomy treatment for adenoma-like dysplastic lesions in ulcerative colitis. Clin Gastroenterol Hepatol 2004;2(7):534–41.

[4] Sinicrope FA, Wang K. Treating polyps in ulcerative colitis: adenoma-like lesions and dysplasia-associated mass lesions. Clin Gastroenterol Hepatol 2004;2(7):531–3.

[5] Itzkowitz SH, Harpaz N. Diagnosis and management of dysplasia in patients with inflammatory bowel diseases. Gastroenterology 2004;126(6):1634–48.

[6] Suzuki K, Muto T, Shinozaki M, et al. Differential diagnosis of dysplasia-associated lesion or mass and coincidental adenoma in ulcerative colitis. Dis Colon Rectum 1998;41(3):322–7.

[7] Schlemper RJ, Riddell RH, Kato Y, et al. The Vienna classification of gastrointestinal epithelial neoplasia. Gut 2000;47:251–5.

[8] Jung M, Kiesslich R. Chromoendoscopy and intravital staining techniques. Baillieres Best Pract Res Clin Gastroenterol 1999;13(1):11–9.

[9] Rutter M, Bernstein C, Matsumoto T, et al. Endoscopic appearance of dysplasia in ulcerative colitis and the role of staining. Endoscopy 2004;36(12):1109–14.

[10] Kudo S, Tamura S, Nakajima T, et al. Diagnosis of colorectal tumorous lesions by magnifying endoscopy. Gastrointest Endosc 1996;44:8–14.

[11] Kiesslich R, Fritsch J, Hottmann M, et al. Methylene blue-aided chromoendoscopy for the detection of intraepithelial neoplasia and colon cancer in ulcerative colitis. Gastroenterology 2003;124(4):880–8.

[12] Hurlstone DP. Further validation of high-magnification-chromoscopic colonoscopy for the detection of intraepithelial neoplasia and colon cancer in ulcerative colitis. Gastroenterology 2004;126:376–8.

[13] Hurlstone DP, Sanders DS, Lobo AJ, et al. Indigo carmine-assisted high-magnification chromoscopic colonoscopy for the detection and characterisation of intraepithelial neoplasia in ulcerative colitis: a prospective evaluation. Endoscopy 2005;37(12):1186–92.

[14] Rutter MD, Saunders BP, Schofield G, et al. Pancolonic indigo carmine dye spraying for the detection of dysplasia in ulcerative colitis. Gut 2004;53:256–60.

[15] Itzkowitz SH, Present DH. Consensus conference: colorectal cancer screening and surveillance in inflammatory bowel disease. Inflamm Bowel Dis 2005;11(3):314–21.

[16] Rutter M, Saunders B, Wilkinson K, et al. Severity of inflammation is a risk factor for colorectal neoplasia in ulcerative colitis. Gastroenterology 2004;126:451–9.

[17] Kiesslich R, Neurath MF. Chromoendoscopy: an evolving standard in surveillance for ulcerative colitis. Inflamm Bowel Dis 2004;10:695–6.

[18] Olliver JR, Wild CP, Sahay P, et al. Chromoendoscopy with methylene blue and associated DNA damage in Barrett's oesophagus. Lancet 2003;362:373–4.

[19] Kiesslich R, Burg J, Kaina B, et al. Safety and efficacy of methylene blue aided chromoendoscopy in ulcerative colitis: a prospective pilot study upon previous chromoendoscopies. Gastrointest Endosc 2004;59:AB97.

[20] Gono K, Obi T, Yamaguchi M, et al. Appearance of enhanced tissue features in narrowband endoscopic imaging. J Biomed Opt 2004;9(3):568–77.

[21] Machida H, Sano Y, Hamamoto Y, et al. Narrow-band imaging in the diagnosis of colorectal mucosal lesions: a pilot study. Endoscopy 2004;36(12):1094–8.

[22] Dacosta RS, Wilson BC, Marcon NE. New optical technologies for earlier endoscopic diagnosis of premalignant gastrointestinal lesions. J Gastroenterol Hepatol 2002;17:85–104.

[23] Shen B, Zuccaro G, Gramlich TL, et al. In vivo colonoscopic optical coherence tomography for transmural inflammation in inflammatory bowel disease. Clin Gastroenterol Hepatol 2004;2(12):1080–7.

[24] Messmann H, Endlicher E, Freunek G, et al. Fluorescence endoscopy for the detection of low and high grade dysplasia in ulcerative colitis using systemic or local 5-aminolaevulinic acid sensitization. Gut 2003;52(7):1003–7.

[25] Kara MA, Peters FP, Ten Kate FJ, et al. Endoscopic video autofluorescence imaging may improve the detection of early neoplasia in patients with Barrett's esophagus. Gastrointest Endosc 2005;61(6):679–85.

[26] Kiesslich R, Burg J, Vieth M, et al. Confocal laser endoscopy for diagnosing intraepithelial neoplasias and colorectal cancer in vivo. Gastroenterology 2004;127:706–13.

[27] Kiesslich R, Goetz M, Schneider C, et al. Confocal endomicroscopy as a novel method to diagnose colitis associated neoplasias in ulcerative colitis: a prospective randomized trial. [abstract]. Gastroenterology 2005;4(Suppl 2):28.

Gastroenterol Clin N Am 35 (2006) 621–639

GASTROENTEROLOGY CLINICS
OF NORTH AMERICA

Cancer in Crohn's Disease

Sonia Friedman, MD[a,b,*]

[a]Department of Medicine, Harvard Medical School, 25 Shattuck Street, Boston, MA 02115, USA
[b]Division of Gastroenterology, Brigham and Women's Hospital, 75 Francis Street, Boston, MA 02115, USA

C rohn's disease (CD) is a chronic inflammatory disease that can affect the entire gastrointestinal tract from the mouth to the anus. There has been a multitude of case reports, population studies, and studies from inflammatory bowel disease referral centers that links CD to intestinal and extraintestinal cancers. There is good evidence to support a link between CD and small and large bowel cancer. There is less evidence to support a link between CD and lymphomas, leukemias, and carcinoids. For the cancers of the colon, small intestine, and of chronic perianal fistulas, vigilance on the part of the physician is required. For lymphomas, leukemias, and carcinoids, more population- and hospital-based studies are needed to better define their incidence and prevalence.

HISTORY OF COLORECTAL CANCER IN CROHN'S DISEASE

The first description of colorectal cancer (CRC) in Crohn's colitis was reported in 1948 [1]. Since then, there have been hundreds of reports of CRC complicating Crohn's colitis [2–13]. In a 1983 National Foundation for Ileitis and Colitis survey that was sent out to physicians with a specific interest in inflammatory bowel disease (IBD), there was a sixfold greater risk for the development of CRC in patients who had CD [14]. The main observations of this study were (1) the multicentricity of the carcinoma in 18 cases, (2) the occurrence of carcinoma in at least 3 cases at the site of a fistula, and (3) the occurrence of the carcinoma at the site of an otherwise benign CD stricture. Although this study was conducted 23 years ago, these three observations have held true.

POPULATION- AND HOSPITAL-BASED STUDIES

Population- [15–22] and hospital-based [6,7,23–31] studies that span at least 35 years support an increased risk for CRC in CD. Many of these papers, however, did not study the patients who are specifically at risk—those who have Crohn's colitis. One cannot compare the risk for CRC in CD with that of

*Division of Gastroenterology, Brigham and Women's Hospital, 75 Francis Street, Boston, MA 02115. E-mail address: sfriedman1@partners.org

0889-8553/06/$ – see front matter
doi:10.1016/j.gtc.2006.07.008 © 2006 Elsevier Inc. All rights reserved.
gastro.theclinics.com

ulcerative colitis (UC) unless patients with equal extent and duration of disease are studied. Most likely, patients who have only ileal or upper gastrointestinal tract CD do not have an increased risk for CRC. In addition, these papers report standardized incidence ratios and only rarely cumulative incidence rates. Thus, caution must be used when comparing results between studies. Table 1 compares the results of all of the hospital- and population-based studies of CRC in CD. Many of these studies looked at all patients who had CD, not just those who had Crohn's colitis. Only a few studies looked specifically at the relative risk for CRC in patients who had colitis [7,17,20,24,30,31]. All except one [31] showed a much-increased risk for CRC, particularly in the setting of macroscopic colonic disease. In addition, all of these studies looked at patient data that were decades old in a treatment era in which surgery was probably more commonplace and there were few effective medicines for CD. Although increased intestinal inflammation probably increased the risk for cancer in these populations, surgical resection certainly decreased the risk for cancer by decreasing the length of the colon at risk. The results of a more current study might be different.

RISK FACTORS: COLONIC DISEASE

A few studies specifically have addressed the risk for CRC in colonic CD. Gyde and colleagues [7] reported a relative risk of 23.8 ($P < .001$) in patients who had Crohn's colitis compared with 4.3 ($P < .001$) in the general Crohn's population. Greenstein and colleagues [24] reported a relative risk of 6.9 ($P < .001$) in patients who had Crohn's colitis. Ekbom and colleagues [17] found a relative risk of 5.6 (95% CI, 2.1–12.2) for CRC in Crohn's colitis alone and a relative risk of 3.2 (95% CI, 0.7–9.2) in Crohn's ileitis and colitis. Gillen and colleagues [30] found an 18.2 (7.8–35.8) excess risk in patients who had extensive colitis. One conflicting study that was done by Jess and colleagues [32] found an overall increased risk for CRC (1.9; 95% CI, 1.4–2.7) in patients who had CD, but disease location and extent did not impact upon the result; however, this was a meta-analysis of 6 population-based studies and 2 studies did not separate out patients who had colonic disease. Another more recent study by Jess and colleagues [31] also gave conflicting results; the risk for CRC in patients who had colonic involvement only was 0.8 (95% CI, 0.02–4.7). The extent of colonic involvement was not reported, however, and many patients may not have had extensive colitis. In a recent meta-analysis of 12 hospital- and population-based studies, Canavan and colleagues [33] estimated an overall relative risk for CRC in CD of 2.5 (95% CI, 1.3–4.7). The relative risk was 4.5 (95% CI, 1.3–14.9) when patients who had colonic disease were studied [33]. This meta-analysis did not include the last study by Jess and colleagues [31].

RISK FACTORS: YOUNG AGE OF ONSET

Young age of onset of disease also may increase the risk for colon cancer in CD. Weedon and colleagues [27] reported the highest relative risk for CRC

Table 1
Risk for colorectal cancer in hospital-and population-based studies

Study	Type of study	N	# Subjects who had colonic disease	Cases of CRC	SIR or RR (95% CI)	SIR or RR in Patients who had colonic disease
Farmer et al, 1971 [6]	(H)	466	NR	1	NR	NR
Fielding et al, 1972 [23]	(H)	295	NR	3	NR	NR
Weedon et al, 1973 [27]	(H)	449	356	8	26.6 (8.6–34.4)	NR
Gyde et al, 1980 [7]	(H)	513	381a	9	4.3 (P < .001)	23.8 (P < .001)
Greenstein et al, 1981 [24]	(H)	579	327	7	NR	6.9 (P < .001)
Kvist et al, 1986 [25]	(H)	473	350	3	NR	NR
Gollop et al, 1987 [19]	(P)	103	67	1	2.0 (0.1–1.1)	NR
Fireman et al, 1989 [18]	(P)	365	207	1	1.14 (NR)	NR
Ekbom et al, 1990 [17]	(P)	1655	830	12	2.5 (1.3–4.3)	5.6 (2.1–12.2)
Munkholm et al, 1993 [28]	(H)	373	208	2	1.1 (0.04–5.8)	NR
Persson et al, 1994 [22]	(P)	1251	790	5	0.89 (0.29–2.07)	NR
Connell et al, 1994 [29]	(H)	2480	NR	15	NR	NR
Gillen et al, 1994 [30]	(H)	281	214a	8	3.4 (1.47–6.71)	18.2 (7.8–35.8)
Mellemkjaer et al, 2000 [21]	(P)	2645	NR	15	1.1 (0.6–1.9)	NR
Bernstein et al, 2001 [15]	(P)	2857	NR	29	2.64 (1.69–4.12)	NR
Friedman et al, 2001 [26]	(H)	259	259b	8	NR	NR
Jess et al, 2004 [20]	(P)	374	250	4	1.14 (0.31–2.92)	1.64 (0.2–5.92)
Jess et al, 2006 [31]	(P)	314	223	6	1.9 (0.7–4.1)	0.8 (0.02–4.7)

Abbreviations: H, hospital based; NR, not reported; P, population based; SIR, standardized incidence ratio.

aLimited to patients who had extensive colitis.

b90% of patients had extensive colitis.

of 26.6 (95% CI, 8.6–34.4). This study was limited to patients who were younger than 21 years old at presentation to the Mayo Clinic with CD. Because the incidence of CRC in the general population is low before the age of 50, the presence of eight cases of CRC in this study resulted in a large estimate of the relative risk. Ekbom and colleagues [17] did a subgroup analysis of patients who had Crohn's colitis who had been diagnosed before the age of 30 years and also found a much increased relative risk for CRC: 20.9 (95% CI, 6.8–48.7) compared with 2.2 (95% CI, 0.6–5.7) in those who were 30 years of age or older. Gillen and colleagues [30] looked at patients who had CD who were younger than 25 years of age at diagnosis and found a 13.3 (95% CI, 3.6–34.1) excess risk for CRC. It is unclear whether this effect is due to the young age itself or to the long duration of disease. When this subset of patients was restricted to only those who had extensive colitis, the excess risk increased to 57.2 (95% CI, 15.4–146.3). The relative risk for this series as a whole was 3.4 (95% CI, 1.47–6.71). In the most recent study by Jess and colleagues [31], men who were younger than 30 years at diagnosis had a 22-fold increased risk for CRC, yet the confidence interval was wide (95% CI, 2.7–80.3).

RISK FACTORS: EXTENT OF DISEASE

In addition, it seems that the extent of Crohn's colitis affects the risk for CRC, and patients who have extensive colitis have the highest risk for CRC. Of the hundreds of patients from published series and case reports of CRC, almost all had macroscopic colitis. Among the patients for whom extent of disease was reported, most had extensive or pancolitis. When looking at extent of disease, it is most helpful to look at the studies that compare extent of Crohn's colitis with the extent of UC and then calculate the risk for CRC. Gillen and colleagues [34] studied 125 patients who had extensive Crohn's colitis. "Extensive" was defined as disease involving the whole colon as far proximally as the hepatic flexure. These patients were compared with 486 patients who had extensive UC. The absolute cumulative frequency of risk for developing CRC in extensive colitis was 8% at 22 years from onset of symptoms in the group that had CD and 7% at 20 years from onset in the group that had UC. The second study that compared the risk for CRC in CD and UC is that by Greenstein and colleagues [24]. This study grouped together patients who had ileocolitis and colitis, and did not separate out patients who had extensive or total Crohn's colitis; however the seven cases of CRC were found only in patients whose CD involved the colon, including 327 patients who had Crohn's colitis and ileocolitis. The relative risk was 6.9 ($P <$ .001), similar to that found in left-sided UC (8.6; $P <$ .001) in this study, but less than that found in total UC (26.5; $P <$ .001) in this study. This result makes sense because many of the patients who had CD may have had resections or did not have extensive colitis.

RISK FACTORS: DURATION OF DISEASE

There are only a few studies that looked specifically at the influence of disease duration on the risk for colon cancer. Weedon and colleagues [27] reported a CRC risk of 0.3% at 10 years and 2.8% at 20 years from the onset of symptoms of CD. In the series that was reported by Ekbom and colleagues [17], the duration of the underlying CD did not influence the CRC risk (<10 years, 2.5-fold increased risk [95% CI, 1.0–5.1]; 10–19 years, twofold increased risk [95% CI, 0.4–6.0]; >20 years 3.2-fold increased risk [95% CI, 0.4–11.4]). The series was not analyzed by extent of colitis. In the study by Gillen and colleagues [30], the cumulative risk among patients who had extensive colitis increased to around 30% at 25 years (95% CI, 3.5–43.8) from onset of their CD, but because of the comparatively small numbers, the confidence intervals are wide. Jess and colleagues [31] reported a cumulative incidence of CRC of 0.3% at 5 years (95% CI, 0.0%–1.1%), 1.6% at 15 years (95% CI, 0.0%–3.6%), and 2.4% at 25 years (95% CI, 0.0%–5.8%) after CD diagnosis. This series also was not analyzed by extent of colitis. Canavan and colleagues [33] reported the cumulative risk for CRC at 10 years following a diagnosis of CD as 2.9% (95% CI, 1.5%–5.3%).

Many case reports and series of patients who had CRC complicating CD support a relation between duration of underlying CD and the risk for developing CRC. In the series of 25 patients that was reported by Stahl and colleagues [35], the mean interval from diagnosis of CD to the diagnosis of cancer was 18.5 years (range, 0–32 years). In the series of 30 patients that was reported by Ribeiro and colleagues [11], 87% had a disease duration greater than 20 years (range, 0–44 years). A prospective surveillance program would clarify greatly the risk for CRC as related to disease duration but most likely, as in UC, the risk for CRC increases with the duration of Crohn's colitis.

SCREENING AND SURVEILLANCE IN CHRONIC CROHN'S COLITIS

In 1967, Morson and Pang [36] demonstrated an association between mucosal dysplasia and CRC in patients who had chronic UC. A similar relationship seems to exist in Crohn's colitis. The theory in Crohn's colitis is the same as that in UC; dysplasia represents a half-way point on the continuum from colitis to cancer. As with UC, dysplasia has been demonstrated to exist adjacent to and distant from the CRC. These findings support the colitis-dysplasia-carcinoma sequence in Crohn's colitis. The percentage of distant dysplasia varies with the particular study, however, with estimates ranging from 27% to 100% (Table 2) [39].

There is only one single-center study that reports the experience of a surveillance program in chronic Crohn's colitis. Given the increased risk for CRC in UC and the above evidence of a comparable risk for CRC in Crohn's colitis, especially in patients with long duration and extensive disease, Friedman and colleagues [26] reported on a surveillance program that had been in place for 20 years at a single tertiary-referral practice in New York City. Since 1980, all patients who have had CD of at least 8 years' duration and at least one third of the colon involved were offered the opportunity to undergo colonoscopic screening (first examination) and surveillance (subsequent examinations).

Table 2
Distant dysplasia in colorectal cancer

Study	# Patients who had CRC	# Patients who had distant dysplasia
Craft et al, 1981 [3]	2	2 (100%)
Simpson et al, 1981 [37]	3	1 (33%)
Petras et al, 1987 [10]	6	4 (67%)
Cooper et al, 1984 [2]	2	1 (50%)
Hamilton et al, 1985 [8]	10	6 (60%)
Richards et al, 1989 [12]	5	5 (100%)
Stahl et al, 1992 [35]	22	6 (27%)
Sigel et al, 1999 [38]	19	9 (41%)

Adapted from Ullman TA. Dysplasia and colorectal cancer in Crohn's disease. J Clin Gastroenterol 2003;(36):S76.

Colonoscopic technique was the same as that used for patients who had chronic UC, namely four circumferential biopsies performed at approximately 10-cm intervals and additional biopsies if strictures or suspicious polypoid lesions were observed.

A total of 663 examinations was performed on 259 patients, 90% of whom had extensive colitis. The median disease duration was 19 years (range, 8–49 years). Thirty-four percent of patients had undergone a previous partial colon resection. Most likely, this would most decrease the risk for cancer because it decreases the extent of disease. On screening or surveillance examinations, the highest degree of dysplasia found was indefinite in 10 patients, low grade in 23 patients, high grade in 4 patients, and cancer in 5 patients. Six patients who had low-grade dysplasia had surgical resections and one additional case of cancer was found. All four patients who had high-grade dysplasia had surgical resections and one additional case of cancer was found. On continued surveillance, another case of cancer was found in a patient who previously had indefinite dysplasia. Therefore, a total of eight cases of cancers was found in this study. The finding of neoplasia (low grade, high grade, cancer) was associated with age greater than 45 years and increased symptoms. By life table analysis, the probability of detecting dysplasia or cancer after a negative screening colonoscopy was 22% by the fourth surveillance examination (Fig. 1). Although this was not strictly a prospective study, it certainly makes the argument for colonoscopic screening and surveillance in extensive Crohn's colitis. The American Gastroenterological Association and the American Society for Gastrointestinal Endoscopy recommend colonoscopic screening and surveillance in Crohn's colitis just as in UC. These same screening and surveillance recommendations for Crohn's colitis are supported further by the Consensus Conference of Colorectal Cancer Screening and Surveillance in Inflammatory Bowel Disease [40].

RISK FACTORS: COLONIC STRICTURES

Strictures of the colon have been reported to occur in 4% to 16% of patients who have Crohn's colitis. Many patients with refractory strictures that are

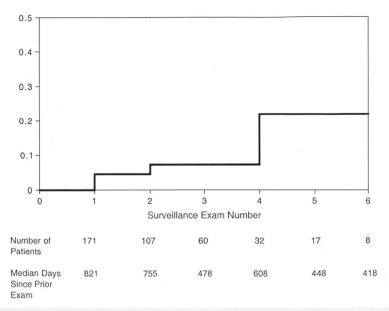

Number of Patients	171	107	60	32	17	8
Median Days Since Prior Exam	821	755	478	608	448	418

Fig. 1. Probability of finding definite dysplasia or carcinoma on surveillance examinations. (*From* Friedman S, Rubin PH, Bodian C, et al. Screening and surveillance colonoscopy in crotis colitis. Gastroenterology 2001;120:823; with permission.)

treated surgically to relieve obstruction are found to have malignancies arising in these Crohn's strictures. Yamazaki and colleagues [41] found 10 malignancies in 132 colonic strictures in 980 patients (13.5%) who had Crohn's ileocolitis or colitis; they concluded that the risk for developing colon cancer with stricture was ten times greater than without stricture (6.8% versus 0.7%; $P > .001$). The risk for cancer was increased especially in short strictures ($P > .0001$). The recommendations of the Consensus Conference of Colorectal Cancer Screening and Surveillance in Inflammatory Bowel Disease are that if the endoscopist is able to traverse a stricture in Crohn's colitis, repeat endoscopic examination within 1 year is appropriate. If the endoscopist is unable to pass the stricture and perform surveillance with a standard pediatric endoscope (11 mm), a barium enema or CT colonography should be considered to evaluate the proximal colon, with possible referral to an expert center. If there is more than 20 years of disease, the rate of concomitant CRC (~12%) warrants consideration of surgery (total colectomy or segmental resection) if the endoscopist is unable to evaluate the colon proximal to the stricture. Endoscopic balloon dilation works best for de novo and anastomotic Crohn's strictures that are short (<6 cm). Dilation of long, narrow strictures increases the risk for perforation. If the patient is having symptoms of chronic obstruction, surgical resection should be done for relief of symptoms [40].

In the study by Friedman and colleagues [26], a pediatric colonoscope allowed the investigators to improve their percentage of complete screening examinations by 16% and surveillance examinations by 33%, which brought total colonic visualization to 88% (screening) and 93% (surveillance). In five patients, the first positive finding of dysplasia or cancer was achieved only by the use of a pediatric colonoscope.

RISK FACTORS: BYPASSED SEGMENTS

A bypass procedure that left the inflamed segment behind was acceptable and favored by some surgeons in the early days of surgical management of CD. Although the relative risk for developing a cancer in a bypassed segment of small or large bowel has not been studied specifically, almost every case series of intestinal cancer in CD reports cancer in diverted segments, some in ileum and some in colon. Greenstein and colleagues [42] reported on seven patients who developed cancer in diverted segments, three in colon and four in ileum. Six cases of the cancer occurred at sites of previous active inflammatory disease and one case occurred in a mostly normal "skipped" area of cecum. Four of the cancers were associated with fistulas; two with enterovesical fistula, one with enterocutaneous fistula, and one with both. A tumor mass was palpable in only one patient. All seven patients underwent operation and all showed metastatic spread to liver, lymph nodes, or adjacent organs. All patients died within 2 years of the diagnostic laparotomy. All patients had had a long duration of CD (range, 17–44 years) before the development of cancer. Patients with bypassed segments of colon are at increased risk for cancer in the bypassed segment because there is ongoing inflammation, the bypassed area cannot be surveyed by periodic colonoscopy, and medications often do not reach the bypassed area. This operation is now used infrequently, but there are some patients who have long-standing CD and have bypassed loops. CT colonography may be helpful in assessing disease activity and mass lesions, but it is not adequate in assessing flat dysplasia or cancer. As such, clinicians should consider revising or removing such segments from their patients, especially because diagnosis of cancer in a bypassed loop is difficult to make and it often is advanced when discovered.

COMPARISON OF COLORECTAL CANCER IN CROHN'S DISEASE WITH ULCERATIVE COLITIS

CRC is the most common malignant complication that is found in patients who have both UC and CD. From the studies by Gillen and colleagues [34] and Greenstein and colleagues [24], it is known that the risk for developing cancer is similar given the same duration and extent of disease. In another study, Choi and Zelig [43] looked at the clinicopathologic features of colon cancer in patients who have UC and CD. Using the computerized medical records system at the Lahey Clinic Medical Center in Massachusetts, the investigators found 6217 patients who had IBD, 3124 patients who had CD, and 3093 patients who had UC. Among these patients, 80 had concomitant CRC (28 CD, 52 UC). These cases were compared with 5266 patients who had CRC but no IBD. The median age at diagnosis of CRC in patients who had CD was

54.5 years (range, 32–76 years), older than that in patients who had UC (43 years, range 17–75 years; $P = .005$). The median duration of disease to the time of the diagnosis of cancer was 15 years for patients who had CD and 18 years for patients who had UC. The median age at diagnosis of sporadic CRC was 65 years (range, 7–99 years) for patients who did not have IBD. Thus, cancer developed at a younger age in the patients who had CD ($P < .001$) and UC ($P < .001$). CRC was diagnosed in 7 (25%) of the patients who had CD and 5 (10%) of the patients who had UC within the first 8 years of disease. Multiple tumors were seen at the time of diagnosis in CD (11% of patients) and UC (12% of patients). In the patients who had CD, no instance of CRC was found without concomitant colonic disease, and CRC was found inside the area of macroscopic disease 85% of the time. All patients who had UC had CRC within the area of macroscopic disease. Mucinous and signet ring carcinomas were equally common (CD 29%, UC 21%) and greater than the reported frequencies (7%–11% and 1%–2%, respectively) in sporadic CRC. Forty-two percent of the cases of CRC in patients who had CD were right-sided as compared with 16% of the cases in patients who had UC. Dysplasia was present with similar frequency in both diseases (CD 73%; UC 50%). The 5-year survival rates were similar between the groups that had CD and UC (10.1% and 9.7%, respectively). These results are similar to the previously reported survival data in patients who had sporadic CRC [44,45].

SUMMARY: COLORECTAL CANCER IN CROHN'S COLITIS

Risk factors for developing CRC are long duration and extensive macroscopic disease. Patients with bypassed segments and colonic strictures also are at increased risk. Probable risk factors for developing CRC in CD (as in UC) are young age at diagnosis, family history of CRC [46], and primary sclerosing cholangitis [47]. In patients who have both CD and UC, there is a higher proportion of mucinous and signet ring histology and a greater proportion of synchronous lesions compared with sporadic CRC. There is a greater proportion of right-sided lesions in patients who only have CD only. In addition, dysplasia frequently is present adjacent to and distant from the tumor, demonstrating a field effect. The survival rates of CRC in CD, UC, and sporadic CRC are similar after detection. There has not been a prospective randomized trial of colonoscopic surveillance in CD or UC.

SMALL BOWEL CANCER IN CROHN'S DISEASE

Primary adenocarcinoma of the small intestine is an extremely rare disease. Patients who have CD have been identified as having an increased risk, with results varying between a 3-fold and 91-fold excess risk. There are eight population-based studies that show an increased risk (Table 3) [15,17,20–22,28,31,48] as well as several hospital-based studies [7,23,24,49] and multiple case reports [2,10,12,23,25,36,50,51]. The estimates have been based on only a few cases in each series. In addition, the hospital study that reported the lowest risk combined all cancers that occurred from the buccal cavity to the terminal

Table 3
Risk for small bowel cancer in population-based studies

Study	# patients who had CD of small bowel	Observed cases	Excepted cases	SIR or RR (95% CI)
Fireman et al, 1989 [18]	196	0	NR	0
Ekbom et al, 1990 [17]	1040	1	0.3	3.4 (0.1–18.6)
Munkolm et al, 1993 [28]	230	2	0.04	50 (37.1–65.9)
Persson et al, 1994 [22]	1019	4	0.26	15.6 (4.3–40)
Mellemkjaer et al, 2000 [21]	NR	5	0.3	17.9 (5.8–4.2)
Bernstein et al, 2001 [15]	NR	5	0.29	17.4 (4.2–73)
Jess et al, 2004 [20]	244	4	0.06	66.7 (18.1–171)
Palascak-Juif et al, 2005 [48]	1935	a		
Jess et al, 2006 [31]	221	3	0.07	40.6 (8.4–118)

Abbreviations: NR, not reported; RR, relative risk.
    acumulative risk: 0.2% 10 years (0–0.8); 2.2% 25 years of disease (0.7–6.4)

ileum [7], whereas all other studies limited their analyses to the small intestine. Only one Israeli population-based study did not show an increased risk, possibly because of the overall rarity of the disease, difference in therapy in different locations, and difference in biology in different locations [18]. Jess and colleagues [32] reported the pooled standardized incidence ratio (SIR) from 5 of the population-based studies as 21.7 (95% CI, 10.4–45.1). One hospital-based study by Greenstein and colleagues [24] looked at 507 patients who had regional enteritis and ileocolitis, and found the relative risk for small bowel adenocarcinoma (SBA) to be 85.8 ($P < .001$). If only the patients who had regional enteritis are studied, the relative risk increased to 114.5 ($P < .001$). Jess and colleagues [31] found an increased risk for developing small bowel cancer of 40.6 (95% CI, 8.4–118) in patients who had small bowel involvement. Of three cases of cancers reported, only one was adenocarcinoma; there also was one case each of leiomyosarcoma and lymphoma. Canavan and colleagues [33] did a meta-analysis of eight population and hospital-based studies that were done before 2005, and reported the relative risk for small bowel cancer in CD as 33.2 (95% CI, 15.9–60.9). The types of small bowel cancer were not specified in this paper, but an examination of the individual studies [15,17,20–24,30] determined that most were adenocarcinomas.

There have been several studies that looked at the risk factors, presentation, and prognosis of SBA in CD. The earliest, a case-control study by Lasher [52], reported that jejunal inflammatory disease; occupational exposure to halogenated aromatic compounds with aliphatic amines, asbestos, and solvents; and 6-mercaptopurine (6-MP) were risk factors. Further case-control studies need to be done to substantiate this reported risk for 6-MP, especially because its use is so widespread. Another case-control study looked at the presenting symptoms and prognosis of CD-associated SBA. The investigators identified nine cases of SBA, and found that patients frequently presented with abdominal pain (89%), obstruction (89%), and weight loss. Medications, fistulas, excluded loops, strictures, and personal history of malignancy did not increase risk. All patients but one had lymph node involvement or metastasis. The mortality at 1 and 2 years were 42% and 61%, respectively [53].

A recent study compared sporadic SBA with CD-associated small bowel cancer, and found that long-standing ileal inflammation is a risk factor [48]. In this study, small bowel cancer was difficult to diagnose and was made preoperatively in only 1 of 20 patients who had CD as compared with 22 of 40 patients who had sporadic adenocarcinoma. Signet ring cells were found in 35% of patients who had CD but not in patients who had SBA de novo. Relative survival was not different in these two categories of patients (54% versus 37% and 35% versus 30% in patients who did and did not have CD at 2 and 5 years, respectively). This is the only study that reported cumulative risk for developing small bowel cancer in patients who had small bowel involvement at diagnosis. At 10 years, the cumulative risk is 0.2% (95% CI, 0–0.8); but at 25 years it is 2.2% (95% CI, 0.7–6.4). It has been stated that given the extremely low incidence of SBA in the general population, even a large relative risk for SBA associated with CD does not result in a high rate of small bowel cancers. The one cumulative incidence of 2.2% should give us pause, however, and it might be prudent to consider screening for cancers, possibly with CT enterography, in patients who have long-standing small bowel disease.

CANCERS ASSOCIATED WITH PERIANAL FISTULAE

Severe chronic complicated perianal disease in patients who have CD seems to be associated with an increased risk for cancer in the lower rectum and anal canal. Among 2480 patients who had CD who were seen between 1940 and 1992 at St. Mark's hospital, follow-up information regarding rectal and anal malignancy could be obtained in approximately half of the patients [29]. Fifteen patients were known to have developed carcinoma of the lower gastrointestinal tract. The carcinomas were located in the anus (5 cases), lower third of the rectum (7 cases), upper two thirds of the rectum (1 case), and the colon (2 cases). The 12 patients who had cancer of the lower rectum and anus had severe anorectal CD with strictures, fistulae, abscesses, proctitis, and large skin tags. The association between complicated perianal CD and cancer of the rectum and anus also was reported by other investigators. Ky's [54] series demonstrated carcinoma related to fistulae eight times in 7 patients who were seen during a 14-year time period. This represents a prevalence of approximately 0.7% in patients who had CD. Greenstein and colleagues [24,55,56] reported a relative risk of 30 (P < .005) for developing squamous cell cancers of the anus in patients who had CD and a relative risk of 14.2 ($P < .005$) for developing vulvar cancers in female patients who had CD. Most of these cases of cancers were associated with severe perianal disease. In addition, there are multiple case reports of cancers arising in perianal or rectovaginal fistulae in patients who have CD [57–69].

There are no formal guidelines for screening and surveillance of cancers associated with perianal CD. Clinical practice has been to send patients who have perianal disease or rectovaginal fistulae to an experienced colorectal surgeon for yearly examination and biopsy if necessary. Most patients who have active perianal disease already are under the care of a colorectal surgeon for drainage of perirectal abscesses or Seton placement that should be done before or concurrently with medical therapy. Patients with an ileostomy and a rectal remnant should have their rectum surveyed endoscopically or removed.

LYMPHOMA AND LEUKEMIA IN CROHN'S DISEASE

J. Arnold Bargen [70] first described lymphoma occurring in the setting of IBD in 1928. Since then, there have been multiple case reports and case series linking IBD with lymphoma. Population- and hospital-based studies have yielded conflicting results. Patient cohorts in these studies range from inpatient and hospital referral IBD databases to national practitioner databases. The most reassuring results have come from large population-based studies and multicenter databases that suggest that earlier reported cases of lymphoma risk from single centers might have reflected a referral bias. There are 17 population- and hospital-based studies that have analyzed the risk for lymphoma in IBD; most failed to identify a significant association [71–80]. One of the most convincing studies, using the General Practice Research Database in the United Kingdom, screened the database of 8 million patients and comparable age- and gender-matched controls [78]. The study included 6605 patients who had CD, 10,931 patients who had UC, and 60,506 controls who were followed for an average of 3.7, 3.9, and 4.4 years, respectively. Patients who developed lymphoma within 1 year of IBD diagnosis were excluded, and all patients who were included in the trial had at least 1 year of follow-up. There were 18 cases of lymphoma with a calculated relative risk of 1.20 (95% CI, 0.67–2.06). Patients who had CD demonstrated a relative risk of 1.39 (95% CI, 0.50–3.40), whereas patients who had UC demonstrated a relative risk of 1.11 (95% CI, 0.51–2.19). Because azathioprine (AZA) and 6-MP may be associated with lymphoma, the investigators performed additional analyses to examine this subgroup of patients. Eight hundred and thirty-seven patients who had CD and 628 patients who had UC had received at least one prescription for AZA or 6-MP. None of the 837 patients who had CD were diagnosed with lymphoma following AZA/6-MP therapy, and a single patient who had UC was diagnosed with Hodgkin's lymphoma. Compared with patients who had IBD who did not receive therapy with AZA/6-MP, the relative risk for lymphoma in treated patients was not increased significantly (1.27; 95% CI, 0.03–8.20).

A more recent study, because of its large size and conflicting results, also deserves discussion. Askling and colleagues [72] performed a population-based cohort study using three Swedish population cohorts and an inpatient register. There were 27,559 patients who had UC and 20,120 patients who had CD. There was no increased risk for lymphoma in patients who had UC; however, in patients who had CD there was a borderline significant increased lymphoma risk (SIR, 1.3; 95% CI, 1.0–1.6) that was confined to the first 5 years of disease. The cumulative incidence of malignant lymphomas after 3 decades was 1.1% and 0.7% for patients who had UC and CD, respectively. Thus, although the population-based studies may disagree regarding the statistical significance of the relative risk for lymphoma in CD, the data indicate that the absolute risk is extremely low. The increased risk, if any, with the addition of immunomodulators and biologics that are used for treatment of CD has been reviewed elsewhere [81–91].

There is much less data on the risk for leukemia in CD, with only several case reports and hospital series identifying a possible link [56,71,92]. The only population-based data were included in the aforementioned study by Askling and colleagues [72]. In this study, the SIR of myeloid leukemia was 1.8 (95% CI, 1.2–2.6) in patients who had UC and 1.2 (95% CI, 0.6–2.0) in patients who had CD. Although this shows a slightly increased risk for myeloid leukemia in UC, more population-based studies need to be done.

One population-based study and several case reports have suggested a link between myclodysplastic syndromes (MDSs) and CD [93–97]. The MDSs encompass a heterogeneous group of bone marrow stem cell disorders that are characterized by normo- or hypercellular dysplastic bone marrows and peripheral cytopenias. Many of the patients in these series had chromosome 20 abnormalities in bone marrow cells; however, the relation of this cytogenic abnormality to CD is unknown. In the only population-based study from Olmsted County, Minnesota, the investigators found an MDS prevalence of 0.17% in patients who had IBD. This is significantly higher than in the general population (0.01%–0.025%). Therefore, MDSs should be a consideration in patients who have CD with refractory anemia.

SQUAMOUS CELL CANCERS AND CARCINOIDS

An increased risk for squamous cell cancers was found in two large studies; one was hospital based and the other was population based. In the first study, Greenstein and colleagues [24,56] found an increased risk for squamous cell cancers in patients who had CD; however, they were all anal cancers in patients who had anorectal CD. In the second study, Ekbom [74] found an SIR of 5.5 (95% CI, 2.0–11.9) for squamous skin cancers in patients who had CD; however, the location of these cancers was not provided and they could have been anal cancers in patients who had perianal disease. The association of squamous cell cancers and adenocarcinomas with perianal fistulizing CD has been documented fairly well, and it is likely that most CD-associated squamous cell cancers are in this category.

The possibility of an increased risk for carcinoids in CD comes from case reports and case series [98–102]. There are no hospital- or population-based data to support this claim. Carcinoids are found at approximately 0.33% of appendectomies, which matches the incidence of carcinoids that were found at surgery for CD (0.3%) in one case series [100]. Autopsy studies of noninflamed appendixes reported an incidence of approximately 0.03% [102]. In a series from Mount Sinai Hospital, 11 cases of carcinoid tumor in patients who had CD (six patients) and UC (five patients) were analyzed [101]. All carcinoids were found incidentally after surgery for IBD; none of the patients had metastases or carcinoid syndrome. The investigators concluded that there is no evidence to substantiate a direct association between IBD and carcinoid tumor because the frequencies are equivalent in operated patients who do and do not have IBD.

SUMMARY

There has been a multitude of case reports, case series, hospital-based, and population-based studies that link CD to various types of cancers. When each of these studies is scrutinized, however, there is only enough evidence to support a link between colorectal adenocarcinoma, SBA, and squamous and adenocarcinomas that are associated with perianal fistulizing disease. All of the studies of large bowel adenocarcinoma or SBA follow patients in an era during which there were far fewer effective medicines to treat CD and surgery was more commonplace. The only surveillance study of patients who had extensive, long-duration Crohn's colitis showed a 22% risk for developing neoplasia (low grade, high grade, or cancer) after four surveillance examinations. Overall results from this study and the multitude of other studies show that the risk for cancer in Crohn's colitis is equal to that in UC given equal extent and duration of disease. Patients who have Crohn's colitis that affects at least one third of the colon and with at least 8 years of disease should undergo screening and surveillance, just as in UC. Although the absolute risk for SBA in CD is low (2.2% at 25 years in one study), we should not rule out screening and surveying for this complication that is associated with significant morbidity and mortality in patients who have long-standing, extensive, small bowel disease. The risk for lymphoma and leukemia in CD is low, but immunomodulators and biologics may increase this risk. The evidence that links carcinoid tumors to CD is weak, and population-based studies need to be done. The study of cancers that are associated with CD is an evolving field that surely will change given that immunomodulators and biologics are being used with greater frequency.

References
  [1] Warren S, Sommers SC. Cicatrizing enteritis as a pathological entity. Am J Pathol 1948;24:475–501.
  [2] Cooper DJ, Weinstein MA, Korelitz BI. Complications of Crohn's disease predisposing to dysplasia and cancer of the intestinal tract: considerations of a surveillance program. J Clin Gastroenterol 1984;6(3):217–24.

[3] Craft CF, Mendelsohn G, Cooper HS, et al. Colonic "precancer" in Crohn's disease. Gastroenterology 1981;80(3):578–84.

[4] Darke SG, Parks AG, Grogono JL, et al. Adenoma, carcinoma and Crohn's disease. A report of two cases and analysis of the literature. Br J Surg 1973;60(3):169–75.

[5] Dobbins WO III. Dysplasia and malignancy in inflammatory bowel disease. Annu Rev Med 1984;35:33–48.

[6] Farmer RG, Hawk WA, Turnbull RB Jr. Carcinoma associated with mucosal ulcerative colitis, and with transmural colitis and enteritis (Crohn's disease). Cancer 1971;28(2):289–92.

[7] Gyde SN, Prior P, Macartney JC, et al. Malignancy in Crohn's disease. Gut 1980;21(12): 1024–9.

[8] Hamilton SR. Colorectal carcinoma in patients with Crohn's disease. Gastroenterology 1985;89(2):398–407.

[9] Kraft SC. Crohn's disease and digestive tract cancer. Gastroenterology 1981;81(3): 626–7.

[10] Petras RE, Mir-Madjlessi SH, Farmer RG. Crohn's disease and intestinal carcinoma. A report of 11 cases with emphasis on associated epithelial dysplasia. Gastroenterology 1987;93(6):1307–14.

[11] Ribeiro MB, Greenstein AJ, Sachar DB, et al. Colorectal adenocarcinoma in Crohn's disease. Ann Surg 1996;223(2):186–93.

[12] Richards ME, Rickert RR, Nance FC. Crohn's disease-associated carcinoma. A poorly recognized complication of inflammatory bowel disease. Ann Surg 1989;209(6): 764–73.

[13] Warren R, Barwick W. Crohn's colitis with carcinoma and dysplasia. Report of a case and review of 100 small and large bowel resections for Crohn's disease to detect incidence of dysplasia. Am J Surg 1983;7:151–9.

[14] Korelitz BI. Carcinoma of the intestinal tract in Crohn's disease: results of a survey conducted by the National Foundation for Ileitis and Colitis. Am J Gastroenterol 1983;78(1):44–6.

[15] Bernstein CN, Blanchard JF, Kliewer E, et al. Cancer risk in patients with inflammatory bowel disease: a population-based study. Cancer 2001;91(4):854–62.

[16] Bernstein D, Rogers A. Malignancy in Crohn's disease. Am J Gastroenterol 1996;91(3): 434–40.

[17] Ekbom A, Helmick C, Zack M, et al. Increased risk of large-bowel cancer in Crohn's disease with colonic involvement. Lancet 1990;336(8711):357–9.

[18] Fireman Z, Grossman A, Lilos P, et al. Intestinal cancer in patients with Crohn's disease. A population study in central Israel. Scand J Gastroenterol 1989;24(3):346–50.

[19] Gollop JH, Phillips SF, Melton LJ III, et al. Epidemiologic aspects of Crohn's disease: a population based study in Olmsted County, Minnesota, 1943–1982. Gut 1988;29(1): 49–56.

[20] Jess T, Winther KV, Munkholm P, et al. Intestinal and extra-intestinal cancer in Crohn's disease: follow-up of a population-based cohort in Copenhagen County, Denmark. Aliment Pharmacol Ther 2004;19(3):287–93.

[21] Mellemkjaer L, Johansen C, Gridley G, et al. Crohn's disease and cancer risk (Denmark). Cancer Causes Control 2000;11(2):145–50.

[22] Persson PG, Karlen P, Bernell O, et al. Crohn's disease and cancer: a population-based cohort study. Gastroenterology 1994;107(6):1675–9.

[23] Fielding JF, Prior P, Waterhouse JA, et al. Malignancy in Crohn's disease. Scand J Gastroenterol 1972;7(1):3–7.

[24] Greenstein AJ, Sachar DB, Smith H, et al. A comparison of cancer risk in Crohn's disease and ulcerative colitis. Cancer 1981;48(12):2742–5.

[25] Kvist N, Jacobsen O, Norgaard P, et al. Malignancy in Crohn's disease. Scand J Gastroenterol 1986;21(1):82–6.

[26] Friedman S, Rubin PH, Bodian C, et al. Screening and surveillance colonoscopy on chronic Crohn's colitis. Gastroenterology 2001;120:820–6.

[27] Weedon DD, Shorter RG, Ilstrup DM, et al. Crohn's disease and cancer. N Engl J Med 1973;289(21):1099–102.

[28] Munkholm P, Langholz E, Davidsen M, et al. Intestinal cancer risk and mortality in patients with Crohn's disease. Gastroenterology 1993;105:1716–23.

[29] Connell WR, Sheffield JP, Kamm MA, et al. Lower gastrointestinal malignancy in Crohn's disease. Gut 1994;35(3):347–52.

[30] Gillen CD, Andrews HA, Prior P, et al. Crohn's disease and colorectal cancer. Gut 1994;35(5):651–5.

[31] Jess T, Loftus E, Velayos F, et al. Risk of intestinal cancer in inflammatory bowel disease: a population-based study from Olmsted, Minnesota. Gastroenterology 2006;130: 1039–46.

[32] Jess T, Gamborg M, Matzen P, et al. Increased risk of intestinal cancer in Crohn's disease: a meta-analysis of population-based cohort studies. Am J Gastroenterol 2005;100(12): 2724–9.

[33] Canavan C, Abrams KR, Mayberry J. Meta-analysis: colorectal and small bowel cancer risk in patients with Crohn's disease. Aliment Pharmacol Ther 2006;23: 1097–104.

[34] Gillen CD, Walmsley RS, Prior P, et al. Ulcerative colitis and Crohn's disease: a comparison of the colorectal cancer risk in extensive colitis. Gut 1994;35(11):1590–2.

[35] Stahl TJ, Schoetz DJ, Roberts PL, et al. Crohn's disease and carcinoma: increasing justification for surveillance? Dis Colon Rectum 1992;35:850–6.

[36] Morson BC, Pang LA. Rectal biopsy as an aid to cancer control in ulcerative colitis. Gut 1967;8:423–34.

[37] Simpson S, Traube J, Riddell RH. The histologic appearance of dysplasia (precarcinomatous change) in Crohn's disease of the small and large intestine. Gastroenterology 1981;81(3):492–501.

[38] Sigel JE, Petras RE, Lashner BA, et al. Intestinal adenocarcinoma in Crohn's disease: a report of 30 cases with a focus on coexisting dysplasia. Am J Surg Pathol 1999;23(6): 651–5.

[39] Ullman TA. Dysplasia and colorectal cancer in Crohn's disease. J Clin Gastroenterol 2003;36(5 Suppl):S75–8 [discussion S94–6].

[40] Itzkowitz SH, Present DH. Consensus conference: Colorectal Cancer Screening and Surveillance in Inflammatory Bowel Disease. Inflamm Bowel Dis 2005;11(3):314–21.

[41] Yamazaki Y, Ribeiro MB, Sachar DB, et al. Malignant colorectal strictures in Crohn's disease. Am J Gastroenterol 1991;86:882–5.

[42] Greenstein AJ, Sachar D, Pucillo A, et al. Cancer in Crohn's disease after diversionary surgery. A report of seven carcinomas occurring in excluded bowel. Am J Surg 1978;135(1): 86–90.

[43] Choi PM, Zelig MP. Similarity of colorectal cancer in Crohn's disease and ulcerative colitis: implications for carcinogenesis and prevention. Gut 1994;35(7):950–4.

[44] Corman ML, Veidenheimer MC, Coller JA. Colorectal carcinoma: a decade of experience at the Lahey Clinic. Dis Colon Rectum 1979;22:477–9.

[45] DeLeon ML, Schoetz DJ Jr, Coller JA, et al. Colorectal cancer: Lahey Clinic Experience, 1972–1976. An analysis of prognostic indicators. Dis Colon Rectum 1987;30:237–42.

[46] Askling J, Dickman PW, Karlen P, et al. Family history as a risk factor for colorectal cancer in inflammatory bowel disease. Gastroenterology 2001;120(6):1356–62.

[47] Lewis JD, Deren JJ, Lichtenstein GR. Cancer risk in patients with inflammatory bowel disease. Gastroenterol Clin North Am 1999;28(2):459–77.

[48] Palascak-Juif V, Bouvier AM, Cosnes J, et al. Small bowel adenocarcinoma in patients with Crohn's disease compared with small bowel adenocarcinoma de novo. Inflamm Bowel Dis 2005;11(9):828–32.

[49] Greenstein AJ, Sachar DB, Smith H, et al. Patterns of neoplasia in Crohn's disease and ulcerative colitis. Cancer 1980;46(2):403–7.

[50] Abrahams NA, Halverson A, Fazio VW, et al. Adenocarcinoma of the small bowel: a study of 37 cases with emphasis on histologic prognostic factors. Dis Colon Rectum 2002;45(11):1496–502.

[51] Collier PE, Turowski P, Diamond DL. Small intestinal adenocarcinoma complicating regional enteritis. Cancer 1985;55(3):516–21.

[52] Lashner B. Risk factors for small bowel cancer in Crohn's disease. Dig Dis Sci 1992;37:1179–84.

[53] Solem CA, Harmsen WS, Zinsmeister AR, et al. Small intestinal adenocarcinoma in Crohn's disease: a case-control study. Inflamm Bowel Dis 2004;10(1):32–5.

[54] Ky A. Carcinomas arising in anorectal fistulas of Crohn's disease. Dis Colon Rectum 1998;41:992–6.

[55] Greenstein AJ. Cancer in inflammatory bowel disease. Mt Sinai J Med 2000;67(3):227–40.

[56] Greenstein AJ, Gennuso R, Sachar D, et al. Extraintestinal cancers in inflammatory bowel disease. Cancer 1985;56:2914–21.

[57] Bahadursingh AM, Longo WE. Malignant transformation of chronic perianal Crohn's fistula. Am J Surg 2005;189(1):61–2.

[58] Buchman P, Allan RN, Thompson H, et al. Carcinoma in a rectovaginal fistula in a patient with Crohn's disease. Am J Surg 1980;140:462–3.

[59] Buchman AL, Ament ME, Doty J. Development of squamous cell carcinoma in chronic perineal sinus and wounds in Crohn's disease. Am J Gastroenterol 1991;86:1829–32.

[60] Church JM, Weakley FL, Fazio VW, et al. The relationship between fistulas in Crohn's disease and associated carcinoma: report of four cases and review of the literature. Dis Colon Rectum 1985;28:361–6.

[61] Devroe H, Coene L, Mortelmans LJ, et al. Colloid carcinoma arising in an anorectal fistula in Crohn's disease: a case report. Acta Chir Belg 2005;105(1):110–1.

[62] Ficari F, Fazi M, Garcea A, et al. Anal carcinoma occurring in Crohn's disease patients with chronic anal fistula. Suppl Tumori 2005;4(3):S31.

[63] Fox LP, Pasternack FR, Geyer AS, et al. Perineal squamous cell cancer in a patient with fistulizing and ulcerating Crohn's disease. Clin Exp Dermatol 2005;30(6):718–9.

[64] Laurent S, Barneaux A, Detroz B, et al. Development of adenocarcinoma in chronic fistula in Crohn's disease. Acta Gastroenterol Belg 2005;68(1):98–100.

[65] Moore-Maxwell CA, Robboy SJ. Mucinous adenocarcinoma arising in rectovaginal fistulas associated with Crohn's disease. Gynecol Oncol 2004;93(1):266–8.

[66] Nikias G, Eisner T, Katz S, et al. Crohn's disease and colorectal carcinoma: rectal cancer complicating long-standing perianal disease. Am J Gastroenterol 1995;90:216–9.

[67] Preston DM, Fowler EF, Lennard-Jones JE, et al. Carcinoma of the anus in Crohn's disease. Br J Surg 1983;70:346–7.

[68] Sjodahl RI, Myrelid P, Soderholm JD. Anal and rectal cancer in Crohn's disease. Colorectal Dis 2003;5(5):490–5.

[69] Zagoni T, Peter Z, Sipos F, et al. Carcinoma arising in enterocutaneous fistulae of Crohn's disease patients: description of two cases. Int J Colorectal Dis 2005;18:1–4.

[70] Bargen J. Chronic ulcerative colitis associated with malignant disease. Arch Surg 1928;93:1307–11.

[71] Arseneau KO, Stukenborg GJ, Connors AF Jr, et al. The incidence of lymphoid and myeloid malignancies among hospitalized Crohn's disease patients. Inflamm Bowel Dis 2001;7(2):106–12.

[72] Askling J, Brandt L, Lapidus A, et al. Risk of haematopoietic cancer in patients with inflammatory bowel disease. Gut 2005;54(5):617–22.

[73] Collins WJ. Malignant lymphoma complicating regional enteritis: case report and review of the literature. Am J Gastroenterol 1977;68(2):177–81.

[74] Ekbom A. Extracolonic malignancies in Crohn's disease. Cancer 1991;67:2015–9.

[75] Freeman HJ. Tabulation of myeloid, lymphoid and intestinal malignancies in Crohn's disease. Can J Gastroenterol 2002;16(11):779–84.
[76] Greenstein AJ, Mullen GE, Strauchen JA, et al. Lymphoma in inflammatory bowel disease. Cancer 1992;69:1119–23.
[77] Kwon JH, Farrell RJ. The risk of lymphoma in the treatment of inflammatory bowel disease with immunosuppressive agents. Crit Rev Oncol Hematol 2005;56(1):169–78.
[78] Lewis JD, Bilker WB, Brensinger C, et al. Inflammatory bowel disease is not associated with an increased risk of lymphoma. Gastroenterology 2001;121(5):1080–7.
[79] Loftus EV Jr, Tremaine WJ, Habermann TM, et al. Risk of lymphoma in inflammatory bowel disease. Am J Gastroenterol 2000;95(9):2308–12.
[80] Losco A, Gianelli U, Cassani B, et al. Epstein-Barr virus-associated lymphoma in Crohn's disease. Inflamm Bowel Dis 2004;10(4):425–9.
[81] Aithal GP, Mansfield JC. Review article: the risk of lymphoma associated with inflammatory bowel disease and immunosuppressive treatment. Aliment Pharmacol Ther 2001;15(8):1101–8.
[82] Biancone L, Orlando A, Kohn A, et al. Infliximab and newly diagnosed neoplasia in Crohn's disease: a multicentre matched pair study. Gut 2006;55(2):228–33.
[83] Bickston SJ, Lichtenstein GR, Arseneau KO, et al. The relationship between infliximab treatment and lymphoma in Crohn's disease. Gastroenterology 1999;117(6):1433–7.
[84] Brown SL, Greene MH, Gershon SK, et al. Tumor necrosis factor antagonist therapy and lymphoma development: twenty-six cases reported to the Food and Drug Administration. Arthritis Rheum 2002;46(12):3151–8.
[85] Connell WR, Kamm MA, Dickson M, et al. Long-term neoplasia risk after azathioprine treatment in inflammatory bowel disease. Lancet 1994;343(8908):1249–52.
[86] Dayharsh GA, Loftus EV Jr, Sandborn WJ, et al. Epstein-Barr virus-positive lymphoma in patients with inflammatory bowel disease treated with azathioprine or 6-mercaptopurine. Gastroenterology 2002;122(1):72–7.
[87] Fraser AG, Orchard TR, Robinson EM, et al. Long-term risk of malignancy after treatment of inflammatory bowel disease with azathioprine. Aliment Pharmacol Ther 2002;16(7):1225–32.
[88] Kandiel A, Fraser AG, Korelitz BI, et al. Increased risk of lymphoma among inflammatory bowel disease patients treated with azathioprine and 6-mercaptopurine. Gut 2005;54(8):1121–5.
[89] Korelitz BI, Mirsky FJ, Fleisher MR, et al. Malignant neoplasms subsequent to treatment of inflammatory bowel disease with 6-mercaptopurine. Am J Gastroenterol 1999;94(11):3248–53.
[90] Lewis JD, Schwartz JS, Lichtenstein GR. Azathioprine for maintenance of remission in Crohn's disease: benefits outweigh the risk of lymphoma. Gastroenterology 2000;118(6):1018–24.
[91] Present DH, Meltzer SJ, Krumholz MP, et al. 6-Mercaptopurine in the management of inflammatory bowel disease: short- and long-term toxicity. Ann Intern Med 1989;111(8):641–9.
[92] Makarem JA, Otrock ZK, Sharara AI, et al. Crohn's disease in leukemia: report of a case, with a review of the literature. Dig Dis Sci 2005;50(10):1950.
[93] Hebbar M, Kozlowski D, Wattel E, et al. Association between myelodysplastic syndromes and inflammatory bowel diseases. Report of seven new cases and review of the literature. Leukemia 1997;11:2188–91.
[94] Casellote J, Porta F, Tuset E, et al. Crohn's disease and the myelodysplastic syndrome. J Clin Gastroenterol 1997;24(4):286–7.
[95] Eng C, Farraye F, Shulman LN, et al. The association between the myelodysplastic syndromes and Crohn's disease. Ann Intern Med 1992;117:661–2.
[96] Bosch X, Bernadich O, Vera M. The association between Crohn's disease and the myelodysplastic syndromes: report of 3 cases and review of the literature. Medicine 1998;77(6):371–7.

[97] Harewood GC, Loftus EV, Tefferi A, et al. Concurrent inflammatory bowel disease and mye-lodysplastic syndromes. Inflamm Bowel Dis 1999;5(2):98–103.
[98] Brown GA, Kollin J, Rajan RK. The coexistence of carcinoid tumor and Crohn's disease. J Clin Gastroenterol 1986;82:286–9.
[99] Cioffi U, De Simone M, Ferrero S, et al. Synchronous adenocarcinoma and carcinoid tumor of the terminal ileum in a Crohn's disease patient. BMC Cancer 2005;5:157.
[100] Freeman HJ. Appendiceal carcinoids in Crohn's disease. Can J Gastroenterol 2003; 17(1):43–6.
[101] Greenstein AJ, Balasubramanian S, Harpaz N, et al. Carcinoid tumor and inflammatory bowel disease: a study of eleven cases and review of the literature. Am J Gastroenterol 1997;92(4):682–5.
[102] Moertel CG, Dockerty MB, Judd ES. Carcinoid tumors of the vermiform appendix. Cancer 1968;21:270–8.

Gastroenterol Clin N Am 35 (2006) 641–673

GASTROENTEROLOGY CLINICS
OF NORTH AMERICA

ELSEVIER
SAUNDERS

Surgical Approaches to Cancer in Patients Who Have Inflammatory Bowel Disease

Arthur F. Stucchi, PhD[a], Cary B. Aarons, MD[b],
James M. Becker, MD[c],*

[a]Departments of Surgery, Pathology, and Laboratory Medicine, Boston University School of Medicine, 700 Albany Street W402, Boston, MA 02118, USA
[b]Department of Surgery, Boston University School of Medicine, 700 Albany Street W402, Boston, MA 02118, USA
[c]Department of Surgery, Boston University Medical Center, 88 East Newton Street C-500, Boston, MA 02118, USA

I t is estimated that nearly 150,000 Americans will be diagnosed with colorectal cancer (CRC) this year [1], and despite the underlying cause, approximately 75% to 90% are candidates for surgical resection at presentation. Although most patients undergo curative resection, nearly half will experience a recurrence of their disease [2]. CRC is a serious and life-threatening complication of inflammatory bowel disease (IBD). Patients who have long-standing Crohn's disease (CD) or ulcerative colitis (UC) are at a substantially increased risk for developing gastrointestinal (GI) cancers, especially CRC [3–5]. Because the prevalence of IBD in the general population is low, the cumulative risk for developing dysplasia or CRC has been difficult to quantify; however, it is estimated that patients who have extensive, long-standing UC have up to a 30-fold increased risk for developing CRC, whereas CD is associated with up to a 20-fold increase in the incidence of CRC [5]. Although the relative risk of colorectal and small bowel cancers is increased significantly in patients who have CD, a recent meta-analysis [6] indicated that the cumulative risk of CRC at 10 years is reduced to less than 3%, which suggests a potential benefit from routine screening. This same study showed that the relative risk for small bowel cancer in CD is still substantially greater than in the general population, which indicates the need for better small bowel screening methods for these patients. This increase also accounts, in part, for the increase in the number of patients who had CD that required small bowel resection for adenocarcinoma over the last decade [7,8].

Although IBD-associated CRC accounts for only approximately 1% to 2% of all cases of CRC in the general population, the mortality in this subset of

*Corresponding author. *E-mail address*: james.becker@bmc.org (J.M. Becker).

0889-8553/06/$ – see front matter
doi:10.1016/j.gtc.2006.07.009
© 2006 Elsevier Inc. All rights reserved.
gastro.theclinics.com

patients that has CRC is higher than for those who are afflicted with sporadic CRC [9]; it accounts for approximately 15% of all deaths in patients who have IBD [10]. Early age at diagnosis, extensive colonic involvement, and duration of the disease are significant risk factors [11]. The incidence of CRC in IBD, especially in patients who have UC, begins to increase substantially 8 to 10 years after the initial diagnosis, after which the risk for CRC increases by approximately 0.5% to1.0% annually [3]. Thus, by the time the patient has had extensive colitis for 20 years, the risk for CRC may be as high as 20%, and increases to nearly 40% in patients who have had even quiescent disease for longer than 25 to 30 years [12,13]. Subsets of patients who have IBD, especially those with comorbid conditions, such as primary sclerosing cholangitis, can be at a significantly greater risk [13,14].

Although this increased risk clearly emphasizes the importance of regular screening and surveillance programs, standardized guidelines have been lacking for some time. The Crohn's and Colitis Foundation of America recently convened a consensus conference during which a panel of international experts developed recommendations for standardized surveillance guidelines [15]. These guidelines are discussed elsewhere in this issue; however, the cornerstone of surveillance is regular colonoscopies with numerous biopsies from the entire colon and rectum to detect mucosal dysplasia or CRC early enough so that patients can benefit from surgical intervention [16]. Because the length of time between the onset of IBD and the development of CRC can be substantial, establishing an optimal strategy for surveillance early in the course of the patient's disease is a key to reducing the risk for CRC [17].

INDICATIONS FOR SURGERY

Until primary chemoprevention for sporadic and IBD-related CRC is understood better [18], surgical intervention with the addition of neoadjuvant or adjuvant therapy in more advanced disease remains the only effective treatment for these high-risk patients. Endoscopic surveillance remains the gold standard in the early detection of patients who have long-standing colitis who are at an increased risk for dysplasia and the development of CRC, and in identifying patients who are likely to benefit from surgical intervention [15,19,20]. Although the surgical options for GI cancers can be different depending on whether the patient is diagnosed with UC or CD, the indications for surgical intervention are similar for all patients who have IBD-associated CRC and follow similar oncologic guidelines. In patients who have IBD-associated CRC, total proctocolectomy remains the only surgical modality for cancer prophylaxis; however, because of the low absolute risk for cancer, this option is recommended rarely as the first-line treatment [7].

There are several indications for which surgical intervention clearly is the only therapeutic option (Box 1); however, some controversy still remains. For example, the presence of flat low-grade dysplasia is a difficult clinical issue for which an ideal management strategy has not been established clearly (see the article by Bernstein elsewhere in this issue). Although dysplasia of any

Box 1: Indications for surgery

Prophylaxis after long-standing disease

Flat low-grade dysplasia

Flat high-grade dysplasia

Unresectable DALM

Obstructive strictures

Documented adenocarcinoma

Adapted from Greenstein AJ. Cancer in inflammatory bowel disease. Mt Sinai J Med 2000;67(3):236.

grade increases the probability of coexistent cancer [21], the presence of low-grade dysplasia is a powerful predictor of synchronous and future adenocarcinoma [22]. Although many clinicians would recommend increasing the frequency of surveillance colonoscopies rather than surgery, it has been the authors' experience (J.M.B.) that any degree of flat dysplasia should be viewed with a high degree of suspicion. Many surgeons now believe that any grade of flat mucosal dysplasia that is verified by an experienced GI pathologist, regardless of the patient's age, diagnosis, duration, or extent of disease, is a potential indication for surgery, and the patient should be referred to a surgeon for further evaluation [7]. At this point, a thorough discussion with the patient regarding the risks and benefits of colectomy versus continued surveillance should be undertaken, stressing that a colectomy should be considered seriously. If the patient refuses surgery at this time, repeat endoscopy and biopsies should be performed on a more frequent basis within 3 to 6 months. Because patients who have IBD are clearly at an increased risk for CRC and developing synchronous lesions [10], most surgeons also agree that surgical intervention is indicated for biopsies that are positive for dysplasia in flat mucosa not associated with excised polyps, high-grade dysplasia in flat mucosa, unresectable dysplasia-associated lesion or mass (DALM), obstructive strictures, or malignancy [7,22].

Strictures of the colon are common in patients who have IBD, and they are associated with an overall 10-fold risk for colon cancer: 30-fold for UC and 6-fold for CD [23]. Many surgeons believe that any colonic stricture that is significant enough to cause obstructive symptoms, even if it appears benign on endoscopy, may be harboring a malignancy [24] and should be treated surgically [25].

Because of the increased risks for developing cancer in the near future and having synchronous lesions, surgery is indicated, especially when any of the indications discussed above are confirmed by an experienced GI pathologist. In some situations, patients who have chronic or long-standing UC are choosing to undergo elective proctocolectomy much earlier in the course of their disease [26], especially now that there are restorative procedures that offer low complication rates and excellent outcomes [27].

Patients who have primary colorectal carcinomas also may have more than one malignant lesion within the colon or rectum at the time of initial presentation. The incidence of synchronous colorectal carcinomas has been as high as 12.4% [28]. Preoperative or intraoperative screening for the presence of synchronous colorectal carcinomas is important because if they go undetected, they can present postoperatively with advanced stages and usually require re-operation. If synchronous carcinomas are detected intraoperatively, the surgical procedure occasionally needs to be altered [28].

PREOPERATIVE EVALUATION AND STAGING

Surgery is the only effective treatment for patients who have any type of CRC; however, before any patient who is diagnosed with CRC undergoes surgical therapy, a thorough preoperative evaluation is necessary to assess the patient's risk and optimize outcome [29]. Although preoperative evaluation is important in the staging process, it also is critical in deciding which surgical option will be the most beneficial to the patient. When considering the options, careful attention must be given to the most effective treatment of the patient's potentially life-threatening CRC; however, the optimal surgical management of one's IBD also is an important consideration with long-term implications. For this reason, patients who have IBD-associated GI cancers should be referred to a surgeon who is experienced in treating these comorbidities.

Patients who have IBD and present with colon or rectal cancer or both may require different preoperative assessments (Table 1); however, the foundation

Table 1
Preoperative assessment of patients who have colorectal cancer

Evaluation	Presentation	
	Colon	Rectal
History & physical examination	Yes	Yes
Digital rectal examination	Yes	Yes
Family history	Yes	Yes
Colonoscopy	Yes	Yes
Proctoscopy or sigmoidoscopy	No	Yes
Basic laboratory tests	Yes	Yes
Liver function tests	Select pts	Select Pts
CEA	Yes	Yes
Chest radiograph	Yes	Yes
Abdominal/pelvic CT scan	Select pts	Yes
Endoscopic ultrasound	No	Yes
MRI	No	Select Pts
PET scan	No	No

Abbreviations: CEA, carcinoembryonic antigen; PET, positron emission tomography; pts, patients.
Adapted from McCormick JT, Gregorcyk S.G. Preoperative evaluation of colorectal cancer. Surg Oncol Clin N Am 2006;15(1):39–49.

of the assessment for any presentation is the history and physical examination. The surgeon must obtain a detailed history of the patient's symptoms, family history, and a thorough physical examination. The patient's overall health and current physical status is important in assuring that the patient is able to undergo major surgery successfully. In addition, depending on the presentation and any previous work-up, a comprehensive imaging assessment must be undertaken preoperatively to ascertain as much information about the stage of the tumor as possible. Accurate tumor staging is an absolute prerequisite for effective surgical therapy, whether the patient suffers from IBD-related or sporadic CRC. Anatomic features of the tumor, lymph node status, and presence of metastatic disease are key elements that the surgeon must consider in deciding which operation is best for the patient, and if preoperative adjuvant therapy will be of benefit, especially for rectal cancer.

Based on the history and physical examination findings, several imaging and laboratory tests may be appropriate. Conventional optical colonoscopy is useful for tumor detection, tissue sampling, and to detect synchronous lesions; however, it generally is most effective when performed in conjunction with several noninvasive imaging techniques. Preoperative contrast enhanced CT has emerged as one of the more effective imaging tools for staging CRC [30], and along with ultrasound, has been the mainstay in detecting local and metastatic spread of malignancy. To enable the use of new surgical techniques and more effective use of neoadjuvant therapies, even more accurate preoperative tumor staging has become necessary. Although MRI for the detection of local tumor extension is particularly useful for rectal tumors, F-18 fluorodeoxyglucose positron emission tomography (FDG-PET) is becoming used more widely for the detection of metastatic nodal and soft tissue disease and as an adjunct to preoperative staging [31]. Radioimmunoscintigraphic imaging or carcinoembryonic antigen (CEA) scintigraphy after administration of radiolabeled CEA antibodies also is becoming an important radionuclide technique that can add clinically significant information in assessing the extent and location of disease [32]. Deciding on the appropriate surgical therapy for patients who have IBD-related GI malignancies also may require tumor staging with whole-body coverage. More recently, a whole-body PET/CT protocol for tumor staging and a protocol for PET/CT colonography were integrated into one comprehensive examination that was found to be a particularly accurate staging modality in patients who had CRC, especially patients with incomplete optical colonoscopy or questionable synchronous lesions [33].

For patients who present with sporadic or IBD-associated rectal cancer, accurate preoperative staging is crucial for developing an optimal surgical plan and determining the need for adjuvant therapy. Although CT and MRI are useful in detecting metastatic disease, they are too insensitive for use in the local staging of rectal cancers. Endorectal or endoscopic ultrasound (EUS) has become a powerful imaging modality and the most accurate technique for staging rectal cancer preoperatively [34]. Further improvements to this technology, such as three-dimensional EUS, high-frequency miniprobes for color Doppler imaging, and transrectal ultrasound-guided biopsy techniques, are widening the role of EUS in the staging of rectal carcinomas significantly [35]. As an adjunct to EUS in determining which patients may benefit the most from preoperative adjuvant therapy, recent studies suggest that patients who respond favorably to preoperative chemoradiation tend to have a better prognosis following surgery. Patients who had rectal cancer that had a poor response to preoperative chemoradiation had elevated serum CEA levels before chemoradiation, which suggests that serum CEA levels also may provide useful information about tumor responsiveness to preoperative adjuvant therapy [36]. After a comprehensive preoperative assessment is complete, the surgeon can discuss the surgical options and expected outcomes confidently with the patient.

SURGICAL TREATMENT
Surgical Principles
When there is a suspected or confirmed IBD-associated GI cancer, the surgical approach is based primarily on oncologic principles that adhere to the currently accepted standards of cancer surgery. As is the case for surgery in sporadic CRC, unless a total proctocolectomy is being performed, this involves wide excision of the involved segment of colon or small bowel with appropriate margins and an adequate lymphadenectomy. In conjunction with the appropriate surgery for CRC, however, the operative selection must include a consideration of the IBD diagnosis, especially if indeterminate, the extent and severity of colonic and small bowel involvement, previous surgical resections, and the presence of rectal or perineal disease [23].

Surgical Options
Although the surgical options for CRC can be different, depending on whether the patient is diagnosed with UC or CD, there are four broad surgical options for these patients: (1) segmental resection, (2) total proctocolectomy with end ileostomy or ileal pouch–anal anastomosis (IPAA), (3) subtotal colectomy with ileostomy or ileorectal anastomosis (IRA), and (4) various palliative procedures, including diverting colostomy or ileostomy (Fig. 1). Stage for stage, the prognosis for patients who have IBD-related GI malignancies generally is similar to that of patients who have sporadic GI malignancies [37]; however, IBD-associated GI cancers usually are detected at a later stage, especially small bowel adenocarcinomas [38]. Patients who have IBD who have undergone surgical treatment tolerate chemotherapy quite well, and, as a general rule, if oncologic principles are not compromised, a surgical procedure can be performed without any deleterious impact on oncologic outcome.

Surgical Approaches
As with most GI cancers that arise sporadically, surgical therapy is the only definitive treatment for patients who are diagnosed with IBD-associated CRC. Although the molecular pathogenesis and clinical, endoscopic, and histologic features of IBD-associated CRC can differ from CRC that arises

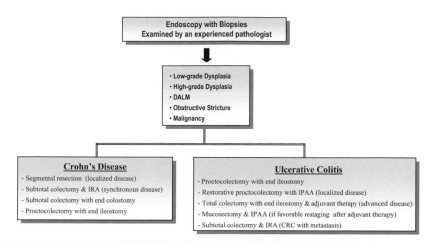

Fig. 1. Surgical approaches to dysplasia and invasive colon cancer in ulcerative colitis & Crohn's disease. (*Adapted from* Greenstein AJ. Cancer in inflammatory bowel disease. Mt Sinai J Med 2000;67(3):237; and Kaiser AM, Beart RW. Surgical management of ulcerative colitis. Swiss Med Wkly 2001;131;327.)

sporadically [39], the surgical paradigms and oncologic principles that govern the management of these patients are essentially the same.

Ulcerative Colitis

Surgery continues to play a central role in the overall management of patients who have UC. Surgery will be required in up to 40% of these patients at some stage of their disease for several indications, including CRC [40,41]. Although the risk for CRC is substantial in these patients in general, subsets of patients who have UC and primary sclerosing cholangitis are at an even higher risk; a significant fraction of these patients develops CRC that tends to have a poorer prognosis [42]. Therefore, patients who have this extraintestinal manifestation require careful and more frequent surveillance (see article by Rubin and Kavitt elsewhere in this issue). Significant advances in the surgical management of UC have been made in the past 50 years, and these same surgical paradigms are applicable to the treatment of CRC in these patients. Although restorative proctocolectomy has evolved as the procedure of choice (see later discussion), there are several surgical approaches, depending on the patient's presentation and preference as well as the surgeon's experience (Table 2).

In patients who are diagnosed with UC, the presence of flat low- or high-grade dysplasia, unresectable DALM, or suspected carcinoma of the colon or rectum is not a contraindication to restorative proctocolectomy with mucosal proctectomy and IPAA [43], unless the tumor is of an advanced stage or is located within the distal rectum. Mucosal proctectomy with IPAA is contraindicated for rectal tumors that are located in the middle and lower thirds of the rectum. In these patients, a standard proctocolectomy with permanent Brooke ileostomy is indicated. Because low rectal tumors are prone to local recurrence,

Table 2
Surgical approaches to common presentations of ulcerative colitis–associated colorectal cancer

Presentation	Surgical approach
Localized colon cancer	Restorative proctocolectomy, mucosal proctectomy with IPAA
Colon cancer of uncertain stage	Staged colectomy with ileostomy and Hartmann closure of the rectum. If favorable pathology, then IPAA. If unfavorable pathology, permanent ileostomy.
Metastatic or advanced colon cancer requiring chemotherapy	Colectomy with permanent ileostomy and Hartmann closure of the rectum
Proximal or high rectal cancer (early stage)	Restorative proctocolectomy, mucosal proctectomy with IPAA
Proximal or high rectal cancer (advanced stage)	Subtotal proctocolectomy with permanent ileostomy and low Hartmann closure of the rectum
Distal (low) rectal cancer	Proctocolectomy with permanent ileostomy and Hartmann closure of the rectum
Obstructive stricture	Restorative proctocolectomy, mucosal proctectomy with IPAA

Adapted from Greenstein AJ. Cancer in inflammatory bowel disease. Mt Sinai J Med 2000;67(3):227–40; with permission; and Ullman TA. Cancer in inflammatory bowel disease. Curr Treat Options Gastroenterol 2002;5:163–71; with permission.

postoperative radiation therapy may be required; however, it can compromise sphincter tone and contribute to poor long-term function. In contrast, patients who have tumors that are located in the proximal one third of the rectum may undergo distal mucosal proctectomy with IPAA safely after neoadjuvant therapy, except in cases where the tumor is large or advanced; in these cases, proctocolectomy with Brooke ileostomy is a safer option. If there is uncertainty about the stage of the tumor at the time of the initial operation, a staged subtotal colectomy with ileostomy and Hartmann closure of the rectum is indicated until the pathologic stage is confirmed. If the pathology is favorable and the patient remains disease-free, a subsequent conversion to an IPAA is recommended, especially if the patient desires restoration of continence. If the pathology is unfavorable, a permanent ileostomy is recommended. Colon cancers that have metastasized to the liver should be treated with colectomy or proctocolectomy with Brooke ileostomy, which is a safer option than is mucosal proctectomy with IPAA. Although there is some degree of morbidity associated with every surgical option, functional results generally are good and patient satisfaction is high.

Total proctocolectomy and ileostomy
A single-stage total proctocolectomy with permanent Brooke ileostomy (Fig. 2) historically has been the procedure of choice for UC-associated CRC [44]. This

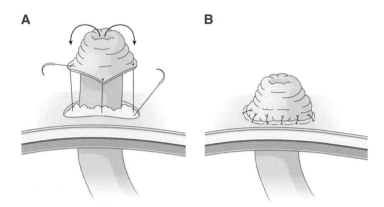

Fig. 2. Construction of an end ileostomy. (A) The terminal ileum is brought 5 cm through an abdominal wall defect, everted, and (B) sutured to the more proximal ileal seromuscularis and the dermis to mature the ileostomy. (*From* Becker, JM, Stucchi, AF. Inflammatory bowel disease. In: Becker JM, Stucchi AF, editors. Essentials of surgery. Philadelphia: Saunders; 2006. p. 240–56; with permission.)

procedure removes the entire colon and ablates the rectum, anus, and anal sphincters. Although this procedure eliminates all diseased tissue and the malignancy, requires a single operation, and provides patients with a predictable functional result, it remains poorly accepted primarily because of patient aversion to the permanent ileostomy. Although a Brooke ileostomy facilitates the rapid maturation of the stoma and eliminates many of the functional problems that previously were associated with a permanent ileostomy, patients who receive even the most carefully constructed ileostomies are incontinent and must contend with external collecting devices.

This procedure also is associated with not insignificant postoperative complications. In addition to a 30% overall morbidity, patients risk hemorrhage, contamination, sepsis, and neural injury to the genitourinary tract. Up to 25% of patients requires stoma revision and experience perineal wound problems after a standard abdominal perineal proctectomy. Fifteen to 20% of patients experience small bowel obstruction at some point in the postoperative period. Of major concern are bladder and sexual dysfunction that are associated with parasympathetic nerve injury.

Despite the fact that most patients with a Brooke ileostomy eventually adjust to the stoma, nearly 50% experience some level of appliance-related problems, including skin irritation or excoriation, discomfort, leakage and odor, or just the time, effort, and financial burden of caring for an ileostomy. Perhaps more central than these problems are the significant psychologic and psychosocial implications of a permanent ileostomy, particularly for young and physically active patients. Unless there are overriding oncologic concerns that preclude other options, surgeons generally suggest alternatives to a total proctocolectomy and ileostomy. In addition, patient dissatisfaction that is due to mechanical and functional problems with the ileostomy and the associated incontinence motivated surgeons to seek alternatives to preserving continence.

Continent ileostomy

Although used rarely as an alternative to a permanent ileostomy in patients who have UC with low rectal cancers or metastatic disease, this article would not be complete without mention of the continent ileostomy or Kock pouch [45]. The significance of this operation for its time was that patients could be offered an operation that cured their malignancy, allowed them to remain continent, and did not require the use of an external appliance. Constructed entirely of ileum, the intestinal pouch serves as a reservoir for stool, with an ileal conduit connecting the pouch to a cutaneous stoma. The operation was modified by the addition of an intestinal nipple valve between the pouch and the stoma to facilitate evacuation with a soft plastic tube passed through the valve by way of the stoma. Although this procedure had clear theoretic advantages over the Brooke ileostomy, its high rate of functional complications restricted its clinical usefulness. The continent ileostomy may be useful in patients who already have undergone total proctocolectomy and ileostomy for CRC, and, after careful counseling, wish to undergo a continence-restoring procedure. This operation also remains an option for patients who wish to remain continent but are not candidates for, or have failed, restorative proctocolectomy or who for other reasons, prefer a permanent ileostomy [46]. In major centers that offer all surgical alternatives to patients who have UC-associated CRC, the Kock pouch has limited clinical usefulness. Few such pouches are being constructed, despite recent reports of satisfactory long-term function in more than two thirds of patients for up to 30 years [47]. Although surgical revisions may be needed to restore proper function, the continent ileostomy seems to have good durability. In a more recent study, patients reported adequate function, high satisfaction, and a health-related quality of life that was similar to the general population [48]. A Kock pouch is contraindicated in patients who have CD-associated CRC.

Total proctocolectomy with ileal pouch–anal anastomosis

Until about 25 years ago, proctocolectomy with a permanent Brooke ileostomy essentially was the only viable option that surgeons could offer patients who had UC-associated CRC that required a total colectomy. Although this procedure eliminated all diseased and malignant tissue, patients were averse to this option because it required a permanent abdominal ileostomy. It is for this reason that surgeons sought to develop more innovative, functional, and acceptable procedures.

More than half a century ago, the pioneering efforts of two surgeons, Mark Ravitch and David Sabiston Jr, introduced the concept of restorative proctocolectomy with anal sphincter preservation [49]. Instead of ablating the entire rectum, anus, and anal sphincter during a standard proctocolectomy, they purported that because UC is a mucosal disease, the disease-bearing rectal mucosa could be dissected completely down to the dentate line (Fig. 3). This

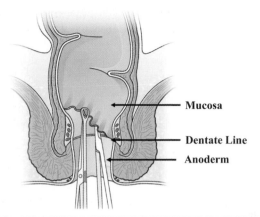

Fig. 3. Transanal mucosal proctectomy. A circumferential incision is made at the dentate line, and the rectal mucosa is dissected away from the anal sphincter and the rectal muscularis carefully. (*From* Becker JM, Stucchi AF. Inflammatory bowel disease. In: Becker JM, Stucchi AF, editors. Essentials of surgery. Philadelphia: Saunders; 2006. p. 240–56; with permission.)

would allow for the preservation of the rectal muscular cuff and the anal sphincter apparatus. The subsequent extension of the terminal ileum into the pelvis endorectally, and suturing it circumferentially to the anus in an end-to-end fashion, would reestablish the continuity of the intestinal tract. This novel surgical advance incorporated several potential advantages, including preservation of parasympathetic innervation to the bladder and genitalia, elimination of the abdominal perineal proctectomy, and, if performed carefully, preservation of the anorectal sphincter. Most importantly, the permanent abdominal ileostomy was eliminated and continence was maintained. This original operation essentially was abandoned shortly thereafter because of poor functional results that were due, in part, to an inadequate understanding of pelvic floor anatomy and anal sphincter physiology. The pioneering efforts of these surgeons set the stage for what has become the definitive procedure for patients who are seeking surgical intervention for UC-associated CRC.

It was not until some 30 years later that Parks and Nicholls [50] and Utsunomiya and colleagues [51] independently initiated the resurgence of the modern IPAA procedure. Because ileal compliance was shown to be correlated inversely with stool frequency in patients after the end-to-end ileoanal anastomosis [52], it was suggested that ileal adaptation might be facilitated by the surgical construction of an ileal pouch or reservoir proximal to the ileoanal anastomosis. These surgeons were among the first to use an ileal reservoir or pelvic pouch successfully to improve the functional outcome following total colectomy and mucosal proctectomy. Several variations of ileal reservoirs were proposed and constructed, including the S-pouch, W-pouch, the lateral side-to-side isoperistaltic pouch [53], and the J-pouch, which is used the most commonly in major centers that perform this operation, including the authors'

(Fig. 4) [27]. Studies that compared the functional results after ileoanal anastomosis with and without an ileal reservoir demonstrated that stool frequency was reduced significantly in patients in whom an ileal pouch was constructed. Using a temporary loop ileostomy, which allows fecal diversion during the early weeks following surgery to allow for ileal pouch and ileoanal anastomotic healing, the incidence of postoperative complications, such as pelvic sepsis and anastomotic dehiscence, can be reduced significantly [27]. Since the addition of the ileal pouch, there has been a dramatic increase in the use of restorative proctocolectomy, especially as surgeons became more familiar with the technical aspects of the procedure. Despite the controversies surrounding methodologic issues (eg, mucosectomy, stapled versus hand-sewn anastomoses, diverting loop ileostomy, pouch configurations, staged procedures), most surgeons agree that restorative proctocolectomy with IPAA is the definitive operation for the surgical treatment of patients who have UC and UC-associated CRC. This procedure also is the choice for patients who have inherited CRC syndromes (eg, familial adenomatous polyposis [FAP]), and, more recently, in select patients who have hereditary nonpolyposis CRC (HNPCC) [54]. Although this procedure generally is contraindicated for patients who have CD, there are reports of acceptable long-term outcomes in select patients [55].

CRC can present at any time during the course of a patient's UC, and at any age; therefore, some guidelines for patient selection must be considered. Although strict adherence to careful patient selection always has been a guiding principle for success with IPAA, the selection process has become less stringent as surgeons have become more familiar with the technical aspects of the

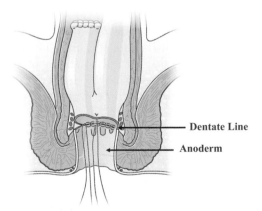

Fig. 4. Creating the ileal J-pouch–anal anastomosis. The ileal J-pouch is secured to the sphincter in each quadrant with a suture. The purse string stitch closing the enterotomy is cut to allow the apex of the pouch to open. An anastomosis is then created between the apex of the pouch and the anoderm with interrupted absorbable sutures. (*From* Becker JM, Stucchi AF. Inflammatory bowel disease. In: Becker JM, Stucchi AF, editors. Essentials of surgery. Philadelphia: Saunders; 2006. p. 240–56; with permisson).

operation. There still remain established factors associated with improved outcomes, however.

Until recently, age was not a significant consideration because most patients who had UC and required surgery for any indication, including dysplasia or CRC, were young. It was believed previously that long-term functional outcomes after IPAA were poor in patients who were older than 45 years at the time of surgery, and IPAA was not recommended for elderly patients [56]. Because older and even elderly patients presented with UC that was unresponsive to medical therapy or with UC-associated CRC, surgeons needed to evaluate the impact of age on long-term functional outcome. Tan and colleagues [57] evaluated the outcomes in patients from 50 years of age to beyond 70 years; they found no significant differences in major complications or functional outcomes when patients older than 65 years were compared with younger patients. Thus, as the authors and others have shown, IPAA is not a contraindication in healthy older patients, as long as anal sphincter tone is good.

Preoperative sphincter function may be one of the more important predictors of postoperative functional outcome. Anorectal manometry is used routinely at the authors' center to establish preoperative sphincter tone. IPAA generally is contraindicated in patients who have poor preoperative resting or squeeze pressures; however, the authors find that most patients, even into their sixth and seventh decades, meet the minimum acceptable criteria. This raises the confidence of the patient and surgeon that the outcome will be acceptable. When proposing IPAA, it also is imperative that the patient fully understands the physiology as well as the operative procedure, and has reasonable expectations regarding the long-term outcome.

One final consideration in patient selection pertains to offering IPPA to women of child-bearing age who present with CRC. Although young women who have undergone proctocolectomy with Brooke or continent ileostomy can anticipate a normal pregnancy and delivery, IPPA seems to reduce fertility [41,58]. Women who do become pregnant are at no increased risk for complications during pregnancy or after delivery [41]. Furthermore, ileal pouch function and the incidence of long-term complications following pregnancy seem to be unaffected [59]. Thus, until more definitive studies evaluate fertility in women who are considering IPAA, surgeons should inform their patients of decreased fertility.

Surgical controversies of ileal pouch–anal anastomosis

Since IPAA became the most common surgical option offered to patients who require colectomy for chronic UC or UC-associated CRC, controversy has surrounded several aspects of the operation. Although several small procedural issues are debated often, perhaps the foremost controversies regarding the procedure are those most relevant to CRC recurrence: the rectal mucosectomy and the choice of ileoanal anastomotic technique [41].

For some time, mucosal proctectomy (see Fig. 3) and hand-sewn IPAA (see Fig. 4) versus a double-stapled IPAA (Fig. 5) to the intact anal transition zone [60] has been an ongoing technical controversy amongst surgeons who perform

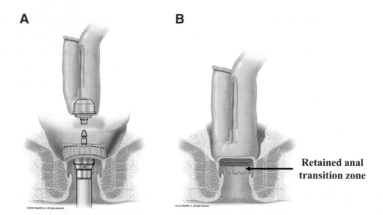

Fig. 5. Double-staple technique for IPAA using an end-to-end anastomosing (EEA) stapler. After the ileal pouch is constructed, (A) the head of an EEA stapler is secured in the apex of the pouch and connected to the pin of the stapler, which is placed upward through the anus, and, (B) the anastomosis to the anal transition zone is completed. (*From* Cima RR, Young-Fadok T, Pemberton JH. Procedure of ulcerative colitis: Gastrointestinal tract and abdomen. In: Souba WW, Fink MJ, Jurkovich GJ, et al, editors. ACS surgery. WebMD; New York: 2004; with permission.)

this procedure. The disagreement arises over two main issues. Although the increased risk for recurrent proctitis is of concern, perhaps of more importance to the patient who has CRC is the increased risk for recurrent rectal cancer if a mucosal proctectomy is not performed. Although the patient's clinical condition and mitigating complications may play some role, the choice of anastomotic technique generally depends on the surgeon's preference and experience. Because mucosal proctectomy removes the columnar epithelial layer from the anal transition zone, the subsequent risk for recurrent inflammation, dysplasia, or cancer is eliminated; however, dissection of the rectal mucosa can be technically demanding and cause damage to underlying smooth muscle layers of the anal sphincter that can compromise function [61]. Mucosectomy is indicated absolutely in patients who have UC who present with dysplasia or cancer in the rectum, or in patients who undergo IPAA for FAP or HNPCC [54].

Several major centers that perform IPAA now advocate an alternative approach to the pouch–anal anastomosis that eliminates the mucosal proctectomy. In this alternative, the distal rectum is stapled and divided near the pelvic floor, leaving 1 to 4 cm of the anal transition zone largely intact. The ileal pouch is then stapled to the top of the anal canal with a transanally placed circular stapler (see Fig. 5). The obvious objective of surgical therapy for CRC is to remove all or as much of the disease and potentially disease-bearing mucosa as possible, thereby eliminating the subsequent risk for rectal cancer. Because the double-stapled technique does not involve a mucosal proctectomy, this raises concerns regarding the risk for developing dysplasia or cancer in the retained mucosa of the anal transitional zone. IPAA is a technically difficult and demanding procedure with the mucosal proctectomy and the pouch–anal anastomosis perhaps requiring the most experience. The ease of use has made the double-stapled anastomosis a widely used technique, especially in light of a recent study that showed that it was significantly faster and easier to learn than was the hand-sewn technique [62]. In addition, pundits claim that preserving the distal internal anal sphincter muscle and anal transitional zone contributes to significant functional advantages over the mucosectomy [63]. Although most studies demonstrate that both anastomotic techniques are safe and result in rapid and profound improvement in quality of life, the obvious concern is that by leaving disease-bearing mucosa in the anal canal, patients are exposed to a lifelong risk for malignant transformation that will require careful annual postoperative surveillance [64]. In addition, recurrent inflammation of the retained mucosa in the anal transition zone, sometimes referred to as "cuffitis," can mimic other postoperative complications, such as pouchitis [65]. Therefore, the best available evidence suggests that there are risks and benefits to both pouch–anal anastomotic techniques; these must be weighed carefully by the surgeon given each patient's presentation, the stage of the CRC, whether the rectum is involved, and the ability to comply with careful follow-up.

Outcomes and complications after ileal pouch–anal anastomosis

Most large series now conclude that restorative proctocolectomy with IPAA is a viable, safe, and effective therapeutic option for select patients who have UC with associated CRC. In one author's (JMB) experience with more than 750 patients in whom IPAA was performed using mucosal proctectomy and a hand-sewn ileoanal anastomosis over a 25 year period at three major institutions, long-term follow-up has shown that good functional results are durable for more than 15 years and patient satisfaction remains high [66]. In patients who present with low-grade dysplasia, there has been a trend toward earlier surgical intervention as gastroenterologists and surgeons realize the substantial benefits and reduced risk to the patient. Most patients who have UC report a significant improvement in their quality of life after undergoing IPAA [67–69], which further supports the notion for surgical treatment as soon as evidence of dysplasia is verified by an experienced GI pathologist. In addition, the authors and other investigators [70] have had excellent results in older patients who present with UC-related CRC, and now feel confident in offering the operation to patients who are older than 65 years of age as long as they meet the preoperative anal manometric standards and the lower rectum is not compromised by cancer.

The use of preoperative and postoperative radiation therapy for patients who have UC and rectal cancer alone, who otherwise are candidates for restorative proctocolectomy, is not established; however, post-IPAA radiation may compromise pouch integrity [71]. Long-term functional results for patients who have cancer are similar to those seen in patients who have UC but do not have cancer [72].

In the authors' series, as in most, poor stool consistency, increased stool frequency, and nocturnal leakage are some of the more common postoperative complaints. Data from the larger series, including the authors', demonstrated an overall mean of five or six bowel movements per 24 hours and 0.5 bowel movements at night 1 year after closure of the ileostomy. Although the severity and frequency of short- and long-term complications that are related to IPAA have decreased significantly since its inception—especially as surgeons become more technically adept with the operation—significant morbidity can be associated with IPAA. Short-term complications or those that occur within 30 days of surgery include pelvic sepsis and abscesses that primarily are due to anastomotic or pouch leakage. Long-term complications include small bowel obstruction, anastomotic strictures, fistulas, sexual dysfunction, pouchitis, and adhesions [27,66]. These reports also demonstrated that, despite the fact that patients experience between four and seven bowel movements per day and episodes of pouchitis, the patient satisfaction rate and quality of life indices were high. In the authors' series [27], the morbidity and complication rate after IPAA are lower than reported from other major centers [69,70]. The pouch failure rate in the authors' series, which necessitated conversion to permanent Brooke ileostomy, is approximately 2%, as compared with the pooled estimate of 6.2% found in a survey of the literature [66]. Single-surgeon experience with IPAA contributes significantly to the absence of mortality and low morbidity that can be achieved with this operation if it is performed frequently, carefully, and with a standard operative technique. No operative deaths have occurred in the authors' series, and the overall operative morbidity after IPAA is about 10%. The authors' major operative morbidity is small bowel obstruction, and although it is lower than the reported incidence, is likely is due to the high rate of adhesion formation that is associated with IPAA [73]; this clearly suggests the need for more effective adhesion prevention measures.

Of the long-term complications after IPAA, pouchitis may be the most problematic. This nonspecific, idiopathic inflammation of the ileal pouch remains the most common and significant late, long-term complication that, in some cases, overshadows the benefits of IPAA. In some series, pouchitis occurred in more than 50% of patients who had UC [74]; therefore, surgeons and gastroenterologists should be familiar with its diagnosis and treatment. Patients who have pouchitis can present with any number of colitis-like symptoms, including increased stool frequency, watery diarrhea, fecal urgency, incontinence, rectal bleeding, abdominal cramping, fever, and malaise. A review of the literature indicates that the incidence of pouchitis can vary from just 6% [75] to upwards of 58% [74] and 59% [76], depending on the diagnostic criteria used. In the authors' series, the overall incidence of pouchitis is approximately 22%, although most patients experience only acute episodes with few chronic or refractory cases. Broad-spectrum antibiotics continue to be the mainstay of medical management, especially for patients with acute or episodic flare-ups. In the authors' experience [77], rapid relief often is achieved with a

10-day combination course of ciprofloxacin (250 mg, twice a day) and metronidazole (250 mg, four times a day).

Perhaps one of the more infrequent complications that is reported in patients with IPAA is dysplasia and carcinoma of the ileal pouch. The authors reported that although the ileal pouch mucosa goes through morphologic changes that is called "colonic metaplasia" by some investigators, these represent adaptive responses to inflammation and do not precede dysplasia or adenocarcinoma [78]. In addition to the authors' series, others also showed that dysplastic transformations within the ileal pouch mucosa are rare, even after a long follow-up [79]. Although these findings can be reassuring for patients and surgeons, the authors advocate routine surveillance with endoscopic biopsy every 5 years.

The development of primary or recurrent rectal cancer essentially has been nonexistent in the authors' series; however, they are encountering more patients who have high-grade dysplasia and adenocarcinomas of the anal canal who had undergone a double-stapled IPAA elsewhere. Some surgeons believe that preservation of the mucosa in the anal transition zone significantly improves function. Resting pressures do tend to be higher following stapled IPAA [80]; however, this does not necessarily translate into significantly better long-term function. Thus, to alleviate further and unwarranted risk, the authors advocate that mucosectomy should be recommended in all patients who undergo IPAA for UC and especially for UC-related CRC [81].

Indeterminate Colitis

Indeterminate colitis (IC) refers to the approximately 10% of patients who have IBD in whom a definitive diagnosis of UC or CD cannot be made at colonoscopy or in colonic biopsies. Typically, these patients present with clinical, pathologic, and histologic features of UC and CD [82]. This lack of a definitive diagnosis can be a particular challenge for the surgeon when these patients present with CRC, particularly with regards to the surgical option offered. From a surgical standpoint, every attempt to differentiate UC from CD should be made preoperatively, because this can play a significant role in the options that are presented to the patient. The gastroenterologist, pathologist, and surgeon should review all clinical, endoscopic, radiographic, and pathologic records carefully. The final diagnosis may be aided by serologic markers, such as perinuclear antineutrophil cytoplasmic antibodies and anti-*Saccharomyces cerevisiae* mannan antibodies for UC and CD, respectively [83]; however, these serology tests are not diagnostic by themselves. If the diagnosis is seriously in question, the first concern is to remove all CRC-bearing tissue. In most of these patients, a colectomy with a Hartmann's closure of the rectum and a Brooke ileostomy is a safe and definitive choice that will leave the surgical option for future restorative surgery. Some surgeons believe that if there is any evidence that is suggestive of CD or if there is dysplasia or cancer in the lower rectum, then a proctocolectomy with permanent Brooke ileostomy should be performed. Several recent series showed that most patients who have IC and undergo IPAA for CRC experience functional outcomes and failure rates similar to those of patients who have UC [84]. Because it was shown recently that most patients who have IC most likely have UC [82], many surgeons believe that they can safely offer patients who have IC who present with uncomplicated CRC IPAA, with the expectation of a reasonably good outcome [85].

Crohn's Disease

Surgery also plays a significant role in the management of patients who have CD. More than three quarters of patients who have CD eventually require surgery for several indications, including small bowel and colorectal carcinoma [41]. The disease almost always recurs postoperatively with a median time to second operation of about 10 years [86]. It was shown recently that by 1 year after a first resection, up to 80% of patients show endoscopic recurrence, 10% to 20% have clinical relapse, and 5% have surgical recurrence [87]. Hence, when a patient who has CD presents with dysplasia or cancer anywhere in the GI tract, careful consideration must be given to the surgical approach so as to conserve as much bowel as possible without compromising oncologic principles.

Small Bowel

Small bowel adenocarcinomas are uncommon and represent less than 5% of all GI tract malignancies; however, in patients who have CD, the risk for small bowel cancer is substantially higher, reportedly up to 60-fold greater than in the general population [3,7,8]. Much like UC, the cumulative risk for developing small bowel adenocarcinomas increases significantly after 8 to 10 years of small bowel inflammation, even if quiescent [88]. Risk factors for small bowel adenocarcinomas in CD are long-standing, complicated disease, especially those associated with strictures or fistulas; onset of disease before the age of 30 years; male gender; and smoking [89]. The preoperative diagnosis continues to present challenges, and patients often present in later stages of cancer; thus the long-term prognosis remains poor.

Segmental resection

Segmental resection is used commonly to treat CD-related adenocarcinomas of the small intestine. Because ileocecal disease is the most common presentation of CD, it is not surprising that ileal adenocarcinomas are the most frequent of all small bowel malignancies that are associated with CD [90]. Most frequently, CD-related ileal adenocarcinomas are located in strictures and often are diagnosed postoperatively [91]. In general, CD-related small bowel adenocarcinomas are difficult to diagnose, and usually are discovered from evaluation of symptoms or incidentally. Patients may present with recurrent low-grade fever and repeated episodes of abdominal pain, but usually no diarrhea.

Surgical therapy for CD-associated small bowel adenocarcinomas is guided by standard oncologic principles, while keeping in mind that there is a high risk that CD or adenocarcinoma may recur and require subsequent surgery. Studies have identified metaplastic changes, adenomas, and epithelial dysplasia adjacent to resected sections of small bowel that increase the likelihood of disease recurrence and emphasize the importance of postoperative surveillance [92,93]. Palliation of unresectable disease can be of benefit to patients who have late-stage or advanced tumors. Chemotherapy and radiation play a limited role in the management of these tumors, because they often are of advanced stage at the time of presentation [94]. Some extraintestinal cancers also have been noted to occur at increased rates in these patients.

Although strictureplasty is a well-established bowel-sparing alternative for surgical treatment of complicated CD [95], many surgeons are now questioning the long-term safety of this procedure because of the risk for occult adenocarcinomas in strictures [23]. Diagnosis of occult tumors and small bowel adenocarcinomas, in general, poses a challenge because conventional diagnostic modalities (eg, small bowel series, upper and lower endoscopy) reveal little, if any, information. Until recently, screening methods for detecting small bowel adenocarcinomas has been limited; however, multidetector-row and three-dimensional CT imaging of small bowel neoplasms have been effective noninvasive imaging modalities [96]. Abdominal MRI also can be used as a diagnostic tool for evaluation of the small bowel in patients who have CD; it may provide more useful information than conventional enteroclysis [97]. Although push-and-pull enteroscopy allows a complete visualization of the entire small bowel with biopsy capabilities in patients who have CD, the invasiveness of this procedure often limits its use [98]. Perhaps the more promising new diagnostic tool for imaging the small bowel directly is video capsule endoscopy, which allows for direct endoscopic visualization of the entire small intestine in patients who have CD [99]. Several studies have revealed significant improvement in detection results with capsule endoscopy [100]. This technology is emerging rapidly as a safe and relatively noninvasive imaging device for detecting small bowel tumors [101,102]. Capsule endoscopy recently was shown to be a highly accurate technique for the detection of small bowel polyps in patients who had hereditary GI polyposis syndromes, and it represents a valuable alternative to barium contrast series [103]. This technique likely will become a standard pre- and postoperative surveillance tool for patients who have long-standing small bowel CD that undoubtedly will reduce the risk of these rare, but often fatal, cancers.

In general, no matter what the underlying cause, the prognosis for patients who have small bowel adenocarcinoma is poor, perhaps because of the nonspecific symptoms and delay in diagnosis; however, surgical resection may be possible in patients who have tumors that are detected at an early stage [104]. The mortality can be as high as 60%, depending on the stage at presentation [105]. Other factors that affect prognosis are based on histologic findings, such as positive surgical margins, poor differentiation, depth of tumor invasion, and positive lymph nodes [104].

Surgical complications after segmental resection of the small bowel include hemorrhage, sepsis, and anastomotic leak. The recurrence of CD is always an overshadowing risk of any surgical procedure in these patients. In addition, metachronous cancer in the remaining small bowel is a continuing risk that requires careful postoperative surveillance.

Colon

There are several options that surgeons can offer to patients who have CD who present with pathologically confirmed low- or high-grade dysplasia, early-stage cancer, or frank malignancy in the colon, depending on the location of the disease (Table 3). Although a total proctocolectomy with IPAA generally is contraindicated because of the high risk for developing CD of the ileal pouch, there are reports of patients who have undergone this procedure and report good long-term function [55]. Because most patients who have CD are at risk for subsequent surgeries, segmental resections or a subtotal colectomy with IRA is a safer approach, unless the tumor is found to be of an advanced stage or is located within the rectum. For these patients, a standard proctocolectomy and permanent Brooke ileostomy is indicated.

Segmental resection

Although segmental colonic resection or hemicolectomy is performed commonly in patients who have CD-associated colon cancer, this option remains controversial because of the high rate of disease recurrence. Compared with subtotal colectomy with IRA, segmental resection of the colon, even for colon cancer, is reported to be associated with a higher rate of reoperation [106]. Other investigators showed that segmental colonic resection and subtotal colectomy were equally effective as treatment options for colonic CD; however, patients in the group that underwent segmental resection exhibited

Table 3
Surgical approaches to common presentations of crohn's disease-associated colorectal and small bowel cancer.

Presentation	Surgical approach
Localized colon cancer	Hemicolectomy or segmental resection with reanastomosis
Colon cancer of uncertain stage	Staged colectomy with ileostomy and Hartmann closure of the rectum. If favorable pathology, then IRA. If unfavorable pathology, permanent ileostomy.
Metastatic or advanced colon cancer requiring chemotherapy	Colectomy with permanent ileostomy and Hartmann closure of the rectum
Proximal (high) rectal cancer	Subtotal colectomy with IRA
Distal (low) rectal cancer	Proctocolectomy with permanent ileostomy and Hartmann closure of the rectum
Obstructive stricture	Segmental resection with reanastomosis
Small bowel	Segmental resection with reanastomosis

Adapted from Greenstein AJ. Cancer in inflammatory bowel disease. Mt Sinai J Med 2000;67(3):227–40; with permission; and Ullman TA. Cancer in inflammatory bowel disease. Curr Treat Options Gastroenterol 2002;5:163–71; with permission.

recurrence earlier than did those who underwent IRA [107]. Whether this is the case following segmental resection for CD-associated CRC remains to be tested by a prospective, randomized study. Hence, at the time of resection of the colon cancer, if there is any evidence of coexisting CD in the colon, a subtotal colectomy may be a better option for the patient.

Surgical complications after segmental resection of the colon include hemorrhage, sepsis, neural injury, and anastomotic leak. The recurrence of CD is always an overshadowing risk of any surgical procedure in these patients. In addition, metachronous cancer in the remaining small bowel or colon is a continuing risk that requires careful postoperative surveillance (see later discussion).

Subtotal colectomy and ileorectal anastomosis

Subtotal colectomy and IRA (Fig. 6) has been used in the surgical treatment of IBD and related CRC for more than 50 years [108]. An ileorectal anastomosis eliminates the need for an abdominal stoma and because the pelvic autonomic nerves are not disturbed, the risk for impotence and bladder dysfunction are low. Abdominal colectomy with IRA is a less extensive operation that avoids the pelvic floor, and, as a result, usually leaves the patient with full continence. Although it removes the malignancy, it is not curative for the original disease itself. Inflammation can recur in the retained rectum and there is still an ongoing risk for malignancy that increases with time. Even in the absence of malignancy, function in the early postoperative period can be poor, averaging four or five stools per 24 hours. IRA also is associated with several postoperative complications, including small bowel obstruction and leakage of the anastomosis between the ileum and the rectum. Subtotal colectomy with IRA is

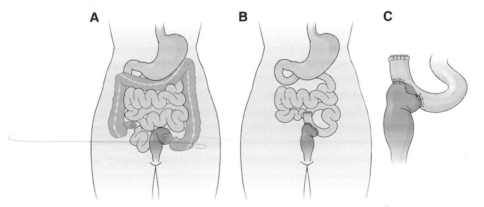

Fig. 6. Ileorectal anastomosis. (*A*) After an abdominal subtotal colectomy is performed, (*B*) the rectum is anastomosed to the terminal ileum (*C*) using an end to side anastomosis. This operation is used primary in patients who have CD and represents a nondefinitive operation for patients who have UC. (*From* Becker JM, Stucchi AF. Inflammatory bowel disease. In: Becker JM, Stucchi AF, editors. Essentials of surgery. Philadelphia: Saunders; 2006. p. 240–56; with permission.)

contraindicated in patients who have anal sphincter dysfunction, rectal disease, dysplasia, or malignancy.

If there is uncertainty about the stage of a colonic tumor at the time of the initial operation, a staged subtotal colectomy with ileostomy and Hartmann closure of the rectum is indicated until the pathology is confirmed. If the pathology is favorable and the patient remains disease-free, conversion to an IRA is recommended, especially if the patient desires continence. If the pathology is unfavorable, a permanent ileostomy is recommended. CD-associated colon cancers that have metastasized to the liver should be treated with a subtotal colectomy or total proctocolectomy with a Brooke ileostomy, which is a safer option, especially in patients who present with lymph node–positive tumors.

Laparoscopy and Minimally Invasive Techniques

The use of minimally invasive surgery and other laparoscopic techniques is emerging rapidly in the treatment of small bowel, colon, and rectal cancers that are due to any cause [109]. Laparoscopic colorectal surgery is associated with decreased postoperative pain, reduced ileus, shorter hospital stays, and improved cosmesis when compared with a laparotomy for the same indication [110]. Although laparoscopic approaches provide significant benefits for colorectal resection, there were initial concerns regarding their ability to meet oncologic standards. The Clinical Outcomes of Surgical Therapy trial, which compared the outcomes of laparoscopic and open colectomy for cancer, recently validated the efficacy of laparoscopy for colon cancer [111]. This multicenter, randomized study definitively demonstrated that the rates of recurrent cancer were similar between laparoscopically-assisted colectomy and open colectomy, which suggested that the laparoscopic approach is an acceptable, oncologically safe alternative to open surgery for colon cancer.

Laparoscopic techniques were used first to perform total proctocolectomy with ileostomy in patients who had UC in the early 1990s [112]. Since then, this area has advanced rapidly, and restorative proctocolectomy with IPAA is being performed increasingly using laparoscopic-assisted and minimally invasive techniques at most major centers [113,114]. In the hands of a skilled surgeon, laparoscopic restorative proctocolectomy is a technically feasible, safe, and durable alternative [115]. Function and quality of life for patients who undergo laparoscopic-assisted IPAA is equivalent to patients who undergo an open procedure [116]. Laparoscopic techniques for the treatment of rectal cancers also are used widely and result in an earlier postoperative recovery and a resected specimen that is oncologically comparable to open surgery [117]. Minimally invasive techniques also are ideally suited for patients who have CD who undergo segmental resections for disease-related complications, including cancers, with excellent results [118].

Metastatic Disease

Approximately one in five patients who are diagnosed with CRC, whether sporadic or IBD-related, presents with stage IV metastatic disease at diagnosis [119]. This additional complication presents a challenge for the surgeon, because it most certainly affects the outcome of the primary surgery. The liver is the most common site of metastatic disease from CRC. Although hepatic resection is the most effective therapy, only a minority of patients that has metastatic disease has resectable tumors. Among patients who present with apparent localized disease and undergo curative resection, more than 50% experience a metastatic recurrence [120]. Up to 30% of these patients who are candidates for resection of liver metastases can have prolonged survival, with a median survival of between 24 and 40 months [121]. The overall 5-year survival rate for patients who have metastatic CRC is less than 10% [122].

Novel and more effective systemic therapies for metastatic colon cancer in the adjuvant setting are emerging rapidly [123,124], and often can optimize the outcome of surgery [125]. Although randomized studies showed a survival benefit for patients who received adjuvant chemotherapy [126], whether radiation therapy for resectable colon cancer adds any survival benefit depends largely on the presentation. Adjuvant radiation therapy may be of benefit in patients with a high risk for local recurrence [124]. Although adjuvant chemotherapy is important as an independent prognostic factor in terms of disease-free survival, recent studies suggest that select patients also may benefit from aggressive surgical therapy alone. The 5-year overall survival was 74% in patients who underwent multiple metastasectomies versus 42% for those who underwent a single metastasectomy; this suggests that, in selected patients, this aggressive approach is safe and results in excellent long-term survival [127].

POSTOPERATIVE SURVEILLANCE

Nearly 150,000 Americans were diagnosed with CRC last year. Of the approximately 75% to 90% that was treated surgically, nearly half experienced a recurrence of their disease [2]. It was estimated recently that about 500,000 patients in the United States return to their gastroenterologist or surgeon every year for postoperative surveillance following curative resection for CRC [128]. Given the high risk for locoregional recurrence or distant metastasis, for which the greatest risk exists within the first 3 to 5 years after resection [129], a comprehensive postoperative surveillance program is a prerequisite to providing optimal patient care, early detection of treatable recurrences, and, above all, improving long-term survival [128,130]. Despite this large patient population that requires surveillance, there is little consensus with respect to the most effective screening strategy. Although there have been a few recent randomized trials that have attempted to address this issue, none has proposed a definitive surveillance strategy that improves survival [131–133]. Several organizations, including the American Society of Clinical Oncology [134] and the American Society of Colon and Rectal Surgeons [133], recently convened expert panels to develop algorithms that can be used as general surveillance guidelines for these patients. These recommendations concur with a recent multicenter, randomized, controlled trial that showed that more intensive surveillance strategies significantly improved prognosis, especially in patients who had stage II CRC [135]. Although the risk is substantially higher, after a patient who has a resectable IBD-related cancer undergoes surgery, standard oncologic principles for the specific presentation generally guide the postoperative surveillance protocol.

The obvious goal of postoperative surveillance is to identify resectable recurrences as early as possible. Many gastroenterologists and surgeons believe that the cornerstone of these surveillance programs is a thorough history and physical examination every 3 to 6 months. Depending on the circumstances, the surgical option, and the stage of the disease at resection, a combination of comprehensive endoscopic examinations and serum tumor marker testing is undertaken over the next 5 years (Fig. 7). If there is clinical suspicion of recurrence or CEA levels are elevated—and especially if CT scans are equivocal—adjunct imaging modalities are recommended to establish evidence of metastasis [129,135]. Although MRI is particularly sensitive in detecting hepatic metastases [136], FDG-PET and CEA scintigraphy can be useful in detecting occult metastases. FDG-PET and PET/CT also have emerged as powerful imaging tools in the restaging of established disease, and, clinically, to evaluate the response to adjuvant therapy [137].

Obviously, the surveillance guidelines are different in patients who have undergone a colectomy for IBD-related CRC. In patients who have UC with IPAA, there are no clear guidelines for postoperative survey of the ileal pouch for dysplasia. Although rare [78], there are isolated accounts of neoplastic transformation within the ileal pouch; therefore, pouchoscopy with biopsies should be performed at least every 5 years [20,27].

A significant controversy that surrounds total proctocolectomy with IPAA in UC is a technical one that relates to the debate over stapled anastomosis of the ileal pouch to the upper anal canal or mucosectomy and hand-sewn anastomosis. Although the long-term risk for dysplasia may be low, the stapled

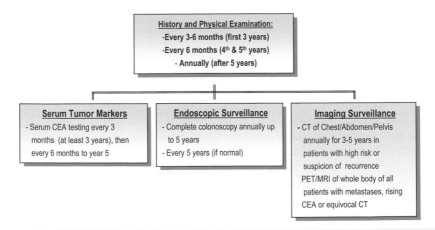

Fig. 7. Postoperative surveillance guidelines after curative resection of colorectal cancer. (*Data from* Refs. [128–130].)

anastomosis does leave up to 4 cm of distal mucosa in the anal transition zone that is at risk for dysplasia, cancer, and recurrent inflammation. Thus, long-term, regular monitoring of the retained rectal mucosa in the anal transition zone for the presence of dysplasia is advisable in patients with a stapled anastomosis [27]. Therefore, it is recommended that patients who have UC who have rectal dysplasia, rectal cancer in the mid or lower third of the rectum, or diffuse colonic dysplasia, and patients who have FAP or HNPCC undergo a complete mucosectomy.

PROGNOSIS AND LONG-TERM OUTCOMES

Although much of the variability in outcomes depends on the stage of the disease and other tumor characteristics, it is becoming more apparent to surgeons that other variables can affect recurrence and patient survival. Operative techniques, such as laparoscopic and other minimally invasive procedures, and surgical decisions that involve the choice of procedure and treatment of metastatic disease can affect outcomes significantly [2].

It is generally believed that sporadic CRC and IBD-related CRC arise from dysplastic precursors; however, there are notable differences with respect to morphology, location, molecular pathogenesis, and clinicopathologic features [23,39]. IBD-related CRCs typically occur in younger patients and often are multiple, broadly infiltrating, and uniformly distributed throughout the colon [138]. These differences seem to suggest that although similar, sporadic CRC and IBD-related CRC are two distinct disease entities, with potentially different implications for prognosis. In general, long-term survival following surgical resection for CRC is better than in small bowel cancers associated with CD. Although early reports suggested a poorer long-term prognosis in IBD-related CRC, more recent studies indicate that the overall 5-year survival rates are similar to sporadic CRC [23,139].

In CRC, the pathologic stage at resection is considered to be a strong prognostic indicator of outcome and survival; however, several serum tumor markers have been reported to be of prognostic value as well. Recent reports suggested that serum CEA, CA 19-9, CA 242, CA 72-4, and the free β subunit of human chorionic gonadotropin (hCG β) are independent prognostic factors. Elevated serum values of all of these markers correlated with poor outcome and worse survival in CRC; however, independent prognostic significance was observed with hCG β, CA 72-4, and CEA [140]. More recent studies indicated that after the location of the primary tumor, only CEA provided significant diagnostic information. CEA had the highest diagnostic accuracy in detecting recurrent CRC, especially to the liver [141]. Thus, CEA seems to be the surveillance marker of choice for patients who are treated surgically for CRC [142].

CEA is produced by 90% of CRCs, and reportedly contributes to the malignant characteristics of a tumor [141]. Because CEA lacks sensitivity in the early stages of CRC, it is an unsuitable risk marker for population screening; however, an elevated preoperative serum CEA level is a poor prognostic indication and correlates with reduced overall survival after surgical resection of CRC [143]. The subsequent failure of the CEA to return to normal levels after surgical resection can be indicative of inadequate resection or of occult metastatic disease. Many surgeons believe, as do the authors, that frequent monitoring of CEA levels postoperatively may identify patients who have metastatic disease for whom surgical resection or other adjuvant therapy might be beneficial [32]. Other studies are ongoing to stratify prognostically distinct groups of CRC further, and have identified new independent indicators of prognosis [144].

SUMMARY

IBD clearly increases the risk for GI malignancies, especially CRC. The absolute number of patients that develops such malignancies is low compared with the overall cancer rate; however, younger age of onset, higher relative risk, unique clinical presentations, and problems with early diagnosis make this a serious complication of IBD. With the exception of patients with comorbid complications, such as primary sclerosing cholangitis, the prognosis is no worse for CRCs that arise as the result of IBD compared with those that arise sporadically. The prognosis remains poor for small bowel adenocarcinomas in patients who have CD, primarily because of their advanced stage at detection. Diligent surveillance is essential for early detection and treatment of IBD-related CRCs in patients with unresected colons, long-standing or extensive disease, and in those who have early-onset CD, although pundits still question whether it significantly affects prognosis and survival. Better surveillance techniques for small bowel dysplasia or malignancy in patients who have CD is needed, especially given the poor prognosis of these patients when advanced cancers are detected. Depending on the presentation and disease diagnosis, patients have several surgical treatment options and can expect good outcomes for all. When the appropriate surgical technique is used in patients who have colon or rectal cancer, along with adjuvant chemotherapy when appropriate, prognosis and function is good; however, the experience of the surgeon can affect the prognosis for IBD-related GI cancers. Surgical therapy is based not only on general oncologic principles, but also on the surgery that is appropriate for the IBD diagnosis. Resection of the mesentery and lymphadenectomy should be performed according to oncologic principles. Postoperative survival for IBD-related CRC is good, and diligent surveillance and follow-up are critical to the patient's overall prognosis.

References

[1] Jemal A, Siegel R, Ward E, et al. Cancer statistics, 2006. CA Cancer J Clin 2006;56(2): 106–30.

[2] Rossi H, Rothenberger DA. Surgical treatment of colon cancer. Surg Oncol Clin N Am 2006;15(1):109–27.

[3] Bernstein CN, Blanchard JF, Kliewer E, et al. Cancer risk in patients with inflammatory bowel disease: a population-based study. Cancer 2001;91(4):854–62.

[4] Judge TA, Lewis JD, Lichtenstein GR. Colonic dysplasia and cancer in inflammatory bowel disease. Gastrointest Endosc Clin N Am 2002;12(3):495–523.

[5] Hill LB, O'Connell JB, Ko CY. Colorectal cancer: epidemiology and health services research. Surg Oncol Clin N Am 2006;15(1):21–37.

[6] Canavan C, Abrams KR, Mayberry J. Meta-analysis: colorectal and small bowel cancer risk in patients with Crohn's disease. Aliment Pharmacol Ther 2006;23(8): 1097–104.

[7] Ullman TA. Cancer in inflammatory bowel disease. Curr Treat Options Gastroenterol 2002;5(3):163–71.

[8] Solem CA, Harmsen WS, Zinsmeister AR, et al. Small intestinal adenocarcinoma in Crohn's disease: a case-control study. Inflamm Bowel Dis 2004;10(1):32–5.

[9] Vagefi PA, Longo WE. Colorectal cancer in patients with inflammatory bowel disease. Clin Colorectal Cancer 2005;4(5):313–9.

[10] Munkholm P. Review article: the incidence and prevalence of colorectal cancer in inflammatory bowel disease. Aliment Pharmacol Ther 2003;18(Suppl 2):1–5.

[11] Itzkowitz SH, Harpaz N. Diagnosis and management of dysplasia in patients with inflammatory bowel diseases. Gastroenterology 2004;126(6):1634–48.

[12] Sharan R, Schoen RE. Cancer in inflammatory bowel disease. An evidence-based analysis and guide for physicians and patients. Gastroenterol Clin North Am 2002;31(1):237–54.

[13] Harford WV. Colorectal cancer screening and surveillance. Surg Oncol Clin N Am 2006;15(1):1–20.

[14] Shetty K, Rybicki L, Brzezinski A, et al. The risk for cancer or dysplasia in ulcerative colitis patients with primary sclerosing cholangitis. Am J Gastroenterol 1999;94(6):1643–9.

[15] Itzkowitz SH, Present DH. Consensus conference: colorectal cancer screening and surveillance in inflammatory bowel disease. Inflamm Bowel Dis 2005;11(3):314–21.

[16] Sjoqvist U. Dysplasia in ulcerative colitis–clinical consequences? Langenbecks Arch Surg 2004;389(5):354–60.

[17] Lichtenstein GR. Reduction of colorectal cancer risk in patients with Crohn's disease. Rev Gastroenterol Disord 2002;2(Suppl 2):S16–24.

[18] Shanahan F. Review article: colitis-associated cancer—time for new strategies. Aliment Pharmacol Ther 2003;18(Suppl 2):6–9.

[19] Toruner M, Harewood GC, Loftus EV Jr, et al. Endoscopic factors in the diagnosis of colorectal dysplasia in chronic inflammatory bowel disease. Inflamm Bowel Dis 2005;11(5): 428–34.

[20] Fefferman DS, Farrell RJ. Endoscopy in inflammatory bowel disease: indications, surveillance, and use in clinical practice. Clin Gastroenterol Hepatol 2005;3(1):11–24.

[21] Gorfine SR, Bauer JJ, Harris MT, et al. Dysplasia complicating chronic ulcerative colitis: is immediate colectomy warranted? Dis Colon Rectum 2000;43(11):1575–81.

[22] Odze R. Diagnostic problems and advances in inflammatory bowel disease. Mod Pathol 2003;16(4):347–58.

[23] Greenstein AJ. Cancer in inflammatory bowel disease. Mt Sinai J Med 2000;67(3): 227–40.

[24] Reiser JR, Waye JD, Janowitz HD, et al. Adenocarcinoma in strictures of ulcerative colitis without antecedent dysplasia by colonoscopy. Am J Gastroenterol 1994;89(1):119–22.

[25] Cima RR, Pemberton JH. Surgical indications and procedures in ulcerative colitis. Curr Treat Options Gastroenterol 2004;7(3):181–90.

[26] Cima RR, Pemberton JH. Protagonist: early surgical intervention in ulcerative colitis. Gut 2004;53(2):306–7.

[27] Becker JM, Stucchi AF. Proctocolectomy with ileoanal anastomosis. J Gastrointest Surg 2004;8(4):376–86.

[28] Kimura T, Iwagaki H, Fuchimoto S, et al. Synchronous colorectal carcinomas. Hepatogastroenterology 1994;41(5):409–12.

[29] McCormick JT, Gregorcyk SG. Preoperative evaluation of colorectal cancer. Surg Oncol Clin N Am 2006;15(1):39–49.

[30] Sosna J, Morrin MM, Kruskal JB, et al. Colorectal neoplasms: role of intravenous contrast-enhanced CT colonography. Radiology 2003;228(1):152–6.

[31] Saunders TH, Mendes Ribeiro HK, Gleeson FV. New techniques for imaging colorectal cancer: the use of MRI, PET and radioimmunoscintigraphy for primary staging and follow-up. Br Med Bull 2002;64:81–99.

[32] Goldstein MJ, Mitchell EP. Carcinoembryonic antigen in the staging and follow-up of patients with colorectal cancer. Cancer Invest 2005;23(4):338–51.

[33] Veit P, Kuhle C, Beyer T, et al. Whole body positron emission tomography/computed tomography (PET/CT) tumour staging with integrated PET/CT colonography: technical feasibility and first experiences in patients with colorectal cancer. Gut 2006;55(1): 68–73.

[34] Akbari RP, Wong WD. Endorectal ultrasound and the preoperative staging of rectal cancer. Scand J Surg 2003;92(1):25–33.

[35] Giovannini M, Ardizzone S. Anorectal ultrasound for neoplastic and inflammatory lesions. Best Pract Res Clin Gastroenterol 2006;20(1):113–35.

[36] Park YA, Sohn SK, Seong J, et al. Serum CEA as a predictor for the response to preoperative chemoradiation in rectal cancer. J Surg Oncol 2006;93(2):145–50.

[37] Delaunoit T, Limburg PJ, Goldberg RM, et al. Colorectal cancer prognosis among patients with inflammatory bowel disease. Clin Gastroenterol Hepatol 2006;4(3): 335–42.

[38] Delaunoit T, Neczyporenko F, Limburg PJ, et al. Pathogenesis and risk factors of small bowel adenocarcinoma: a colorectal cancer sibling? Am J Gastroenterol 2005;100(3): 703–10.

[39] Itzkowitz SH, Yio X. Inflammation and cancer IV. Colorectal cancer in inflammatory bowel disease: the role of inflammation. Am J Physiol Gastrointest Liver Physiol 2004;287(1): G7–G17.

[40] McLeod R. Surgery for ulcerative colitis. World Gastrenterology News 2002;6(3):35–6.

[41] Larson DW, Pemberton JH. Current concepts and controversies in surgery for IBD. Gastroenterology 2004;126(6):1611–9.

[42] Loftus EV Jr, Harewood GC, Loftus CG, et al. PSC-IBD: a unique form of inflammatory bowel disease associated with primary sclerosing cholangitis. Gut 2005;54(1):91–6.

[43] Remzi FH, Preen M. Rectal cancer and ulcerative colitis: does it change the therapeutic approach? Colorectal Dis 2003;5(5):483–5.

[44] Meagher AP, Farouk R, Dozois RR, et al. J ileal pouch-anal anastomosis for chronic ulcerative colitis: complications and long-term outcome in 1310 patients. Br J Surg 1998;85(6): 800–3.

[45] Kock NG. Intra-abdominal "reservoir" in patients with permanent ileostomy. Preliminary observations on a procedure resulting in fecal "continence" in five ileostomy patients. Arch Surg 1969;99(2):223–31.

[46] Borjesson L, Oresland T, Hulten L. The failed pelvic pouch: conversion to a continent ileostomy. Tech Coloproctol 2004;8(2):102–5.

[47] Lepisto AH, Jarvinen HJ. Durability of Kock continent ileostomy. Dis Colon Rectum 2003;46(7):925–8.

[48] Berndtsson IE, Lindholm E, Oresland T, et al. Health-related quality of life and pouch function in continent ileostomy patients: a 30-year perspective. Dis Colon Rectum 2004;47(12):2131–7.

[49] Ravitch MM, Sabiston DL Jr. Anal ileostomy with preservation of the sphincter: a proposed operation in patients requiring total colectomy for benign lesions. Surg Gynecol Obstet 1947;84:1095–9.

[50] Parks AG, Nicholls RJ. Proctocolectomy without ileostomy for ulcerative colitis. BMJ 1978;2(6130):85–8.

[51] Utsunomiya J, Iwama T, Imajo M, et al. Total colectomy, mucosal proctectomy, and ileoanal anastomosis. Dis Colon Rectum 1980;23(7):459–66.

[52] Heppell J, Kelly KA, Phillips SF, et al. Physiologic aspects of continence after colectomy, mucosal proctectomy, and endorectal ileo-anal anastomosis. Ann Surg 1982;195(4): 435–43.

[53] Becker JM, Stucchi AF. Ulcerative colitis. In: Greenfield LJ, editor. Surgery: scientific principles and practice. 3rd edition. Philadelphia: Lippincott, Williams and Wilkins; 2001. p. 1070–89.

[54] Becker JM, Stucchi AF. Inherited colorectal polyposis syndromes. In: Cameron JL, editor. Current surgical therapy. 8th edition. Philadelphia: Elsevier Mosby; 2004. p. 200–11.

[55] Panis Y. Is there a place for ileal pouch-anal anastomosis in patients with Crohn's colitis? Neth J Med 1998;53(6):S47–51.

[56] Farouk R, Pemberton JH, Wolff BG, et al. Functional outcomes after ileal pouch-anal anastomosis for chronic ulcerative colitis. Ann Surg 2000;231(6):919–26.

[57] Tan HT, Connolly AB, Morton D, et al. Results of restorative proctocolectomy in the elderly. Int J Colorectal Dis 1997;12(6):319–22.

[58] Gorgun E, Remzi FH, Goldberg JM, et al. Fertility is reduced after restorative proctocolectomy with ileal pouch anal anastomosis: a study of 300 patients. Surgery 2004;136(4): 795–803.

[59] Hahnloser D, Pemberton JH, Wolff BG, et al. Pregnancy and delivery before and after ileal pouch-anal anastomosis for inflammatory bowel disease: immediate and long-term consequences and outcomes. Dis Colon Rectum 2004;47(7):1127–35.

[60] Knight CD, Griffen FD. An improved technique for low anterior resection of the rectum using the EEA stapler. Surgery 1980;88(5):710–4.

[61] Becker JM, LaMorte W, St. Marie G, et al. Extent of smooth muscle resection during mucosectomy and ileal pouch-anal anastomosis affects anorectal physiology and functional outcome. Dis Colon Rectum 1997;40(6):653–60.

[62] Tekkis PP, Fazio VW, Lavery IC, et al. Evaluation of the learning curve in ileal pouch-anal anastomosis surgery. Ann Surg 2005;241(2):262–8.

[63] Ziv Y, Fazio VW, Church JM, et al. Stapled ileal pouch anal anastomoses are safer than handsewn anastomoses in patients with ulcerative colitis. Am J Surg 1996;171(3):320–3.

[64] Fazio VW, Ziv Y, Church JM, et al. Ileal pouch-anal anastomoses complications and function in 1005 patients. Ann Surg 1995;222(2):120–7.

[65] Shen B, Lashner BA, Bennett AE, et al. Treatment of rectal cuff inflammation (cuffitis) in patients with ulcerative colitis following restorative proctocolectomy and ileal pouch-anal anastomosis. Am J Gastroenterol 2004;99(8):1527–31.

[66] Lehrmann J, Stucchi AF, LaMorte WW, et al. Complications and outcomes after ileal pouch-anal anastomosis (IPAA): a meta-analysis of more than 8300 patients. Gastroenterology 2003;124(4):A814.

[67] Muir AJ, Edwards LJ, Sanders LL, et al. A prospective evaluation of health-related quality of life after ileal pouch anal anastomosis for ulcerative colitis. Am J Gastroenterol 2001;96(5):1480–5.

[68] Michelassi F, Lee J, Rubin M, et al. Long-term functional results after ileal pouch anal restorative proctocolectomy for ulcerative colitis: a prospective observational study. Ann Surg 2003;238(3):433–41.

[69] Hahnloser D, Pemberton JH, Wolff BG, et al. The effect of ageing on function and quality of life in ileal pouch patients: a single cohort experience of 409 patients with chronic ulcerative colitis. Ann Surg 2004;240(4):615–21. [discussion 621–3].

[70] Delaney CP, Fazio VW, Remzi FH, et al. Prospective, age-related analysis of surgical results, functional outcome, and quality of life after ileal pouch-anal anastomosis. Ann Surg 2003;238(2):221–8.

[71] Kaiser AM, Beart RW Jr. Surgical management of ulcerative colitis. Swiss Med Wkly 2001;131(23–24):323–37.

[72] Gorfine SR, Harris MT, Bub DS, et al. Restorative proctocolectomy for ulcerative colitis complicated by colorectal cancer. Dis Colon Rectum 2004;47(8):1377–85.

[73] Becker JM, Dayton MT, Fazio VW, et al. Prevention of postoperative abdominal adhesions by a sodium hyaluronate-based bioresorbable membrane: a prospective, randomized, double-blind multicenter study. J Am Coll Surg 1996;183(4):297–306.

[74] Kuisma J, Jarvinen H, Kahri A, et al. Factors associated with disease activity of pouchitis after surgery for ulcerative colitis. Scand J Gastroenterol 2004;39(6):544–8.

[75] Reissman P, Piccirillo M, Ulrich A, et al. Functional results of the double-stapled ileoanal reservoir. J Am Coll Surg 1995;181(5):444–50.

[76] Simchuk EJ, Thirlby RC. Risk factors and true incidence of pouchitis in patients after ileal pouch-anal anastomoses. World J Surg 2000;24(7):851–6.

[77] Becker JM, Stucchi AF, Bryant DE. How do you treat refractory pouchitis and when do you decide to remove the pouch? Inflamm Bowel Dis 1998;4(2):167–9 [discussion 170–1].

[78] Fruin AB, El-Zammer O, Stucchi AF, et al. Colonic metaplasia in the ileal pouch is associated with inflammation and is not the result of long-term adaptation. J Gastrointest Surg 2003;7(2):246–54.

[79] Borjesson L, Willen R, Haboubi N, et al. The risk of dysplasia and cancer in the ileal pouch mucosa after restorative proctocolectomy for ulcerative proctocolitis is low: a long-term term follow-up study. Colorectal Dis 2004;6(6):494–8.

[80] Reilly WT, Pemberton JH, Wolff BG, et al. Randomized prospective trial comparing ileal pouch-anal anastomosis performed by excising the anal mucosa to ileal pouch-anal anastomosis performed by preserving the anal mucosa. Ann Surg 1997;225(6):666–76.

[81] Becker JM. What is the better surgical technique in ileal-pouch-anal anastomosis? Mucosectomy. Inflamm Bowel Dis 1996;2:151–4.

[82] Odze RD. Pathology of indeterminate colitis. J Clin Gastroenterol 2004;38(5 Suppl): S36–40.

[83] Vernier G, Sendid B, Poulain D, et al. Relevance of serologic studies in inflammatory bowel disease. Curr Gastroenterol Rep 2004;6(6):482–7.

[84] Dayton MT, Larsen KR, Christiansen DD. Similar functional results and complications after ileal pouch-anal anastomosis in patients with indeterminate vs ulcerative colitis. Arch Surg 2002;137(6):690–4 [discussion 694–5].

[85] Delaney CP, Remzi FH, Gramlich T, et al. Equivalent function, quality of life and pouch survival rates after ileal pouch-anal anastomosis for indeterminate and ulcerative colitis. Ann Surg 2002;236(1):43–8.

[86] Penner RM, Madsen KL, Fedorak RN. Postoperative Crohn's disease. Inflamm Bowel Dis 2005;11(8):765–77.

[87] Froehlich F, Juillerat P, Felley C, et al. Treatment of postoperative Crohn's disease. Digestion 2005;71(1):49–53.

[88] Palascak-Juif V, Bouvier AM, Cosnes J, et al. Small bowel adenocarcinoma in patients with Crohn's disease compared with small bowel adenocarcinoma de novo. Inflamm Bowel Dis 2005;11(9):828–32.

[89] Kronberger IE, Graziadei IW, Vogel W. Small bowel adenocarcinoma in Crohn's disease: a case report and review of literature. World J Gastroenterol 2006;12(8):1317–20.

[90] Michelassi F, Testa G, Pomidor WJ, et al. Adenocarcinoma complicating Crohn's disease. Dis Colon Rectum 1993;36(7):654–61.

[91] Partridge SK, Hodin RA. Small bowel adenocarcinoma at a strictureplasty site in a patient with Crohn's disease: report of a case. Dis Colon Rectum 2004;47(5):778–81.

[92] Petras RE, Mir-Madjlessi SH, Farmer RG. Crohn's disease and intestinal carcinoma. A report of 11 cases with emphasis on associated epithelial dysplasia. Gastroenterology 1987;93(6):1307–14.

[93] Sigel JE, Petras RE, Lashner BA, et al. Intestinal adenocarcinoma in Crohn's disease: a report of 30 cases with a focus on coexisting dysplasia. Am J Surg Pathol 1999;23(6): 651–5.

[94] Tumbapura A, Kuwada S, DiSario JA. Adenocarcimoma of the small intestine. Curr Opin Gastroenterol 2000;2:51–8.

[95] Roy P, Kumar D. Intervention-free interval following strictureplasty for Crohn's disease. World J Surg 2006;30:1020–6.

[96] Horton KM, Fishman EK. Multidetector-row computed tomography and 3-dimensional computed tomography imaging of small bowel neoplasms: current concept in diagnosis. J Comput Assist Tomogr 2004;28(1):106–16.

[97] Schreyer AG, Geissler A, Albrich H, et al. Abdominal MRI after enteroclysis or with oral contrast in patients with suspected or proven Crohn's disease. Clin Gastroenterol Hepatol 2004;2(6):491–7.

[98] Gay G, Delvaux M, Fassler I. Outcome of capsule endoscopy in determining indication and route for push-and-pull enteroscopy. Endoscopy 2006;38(1):49–58.

[99] Kornbluth A, Legnani P, Lewis BS. Video capsule endoscopy in inflammatory bowel disease: past, present, and future. Inflamm Bowel Dis 2004;10(3):278–85.

[100] Triester SL, Leighton JA, Leontiadis GI, et al. A meta-analysis of the yield of capsule endoscopy compared to other diagnostic modalities in patients with non-stricturing small bowel Crohn's disease. Am J Gastroenterol 2006;101(5):954–64.

[101] Eliakim AR. Video capsule endoscopy of the small bowel (PillCam SB). Curr Opin Gastroenterol 2006;22(2):124–7.

[102] Urbain D, De Looze D, Demedts I, et al. video capsule endoscopy in small bowel malignancy: a multicenter Belgian study. Endoscopy 2006;38(4):408–11.

[103] Mata A, Llach J, Castells A, et al. A prospective trial comparing wireless capsule endoscopy and barium contrast series for small-bowel surveillance in hereditary GI polyposis syndromes. Gastrointest Endosc 2005;61(6):721–5.

[104] Abrahams NA, Halverson A, Fazio VW, et al. Adenocarcinoma of the small bowel: a study of 37 cases with emphasis on histologic prognostic factors. Dis Colon Rectum 2002;45(11):1496–502.

[105] Dabaja BS, Suki D, Pro B, et al. Adenocarcinoma of the small bowel: presentation, prognostic factors, and outcome of 217 patients. Cancer 2004;101(3):518–26.

[106] Andersson P, Olaison G, Hallbook O, et al. Segmental resection or subtotal colectomy in Crohn's colitis? Dis Colon Rectum 2002;45(1):47–53.

[107] Tekkis PP, Purkayastha S, Lanitis S, et al. A comparison of segmental vs subtotal/total colectomy for colonic Crohn's disease: a meta-analysis. Colorectal Dis 2006;8(2): 82–90.

[108] Aylett SO. Ileorectal anastomosis: review 1952–1968. Proc R Soc Med 1971;64(9): 967–71.

[109] Stocchi L, Nelson H. Minimally invasive surgery for colorectal carcinoma. Ann Surg Oncol 2005;12(12):960–70.

[110] Chang GJ, Nelson H. Laparoscopic colectomy. Curr Gastroenterol Rep 2005;7(5): 396–403.

[111] Clinical Outcomes of Surgical Therapy. A comparison of laparoscopically assisted and open colectomy for colon cancer. N Engl J Med 2004;350(20):2050–9.

[112] Peters WR. Laparoscopic total proctocolectomy with creation of ileostomy for ulcerative colitis: report of two cases. J Laparoendosc Surg 1992;2(3):175–8.

[113] Larson DW, Dozois EJ, Piotrowicz K, et al. Laparoscopic-assisted vs. open ileal pouch-anal anastomosis: functional outcome in a case-matched series. Dis Colon Rectum 2005;48(10):1845–50.

[114] Ouaissi M, Alves A, Bouhnik Y, et al. Three-step ileal pouch-anal anastomosis under total laparoscopic approach for acute or severe colitis complicating inflammatory bowel disease. J Am Coll Surg 2006;202(4):637–42.

[115] Kienle P, Z'Graggen K, Schmidt J, et al. Laparoscopic restorative proctocolectomy. Br J Surg 2005;92(1):88–93.

[116] Larson DW, Cima RR, Dozois EJ, et al. Safety, feasibility, and short-term outcomes of laparoscopic ileal-pouch-anal anastomosis: a single institutional case-matched experience. Ann Surg 2006;243(5):667–72.

[117] Aziz O, Constantinides V, Tekkis PP, et al. Laparoscopic versus open surgery for rectal cancer: a meta-analysis. Ann Surg Oncol 2006;13(3):413–24.

[118] Lowney JK, Dietz DW, Birnbaum EH, et al. Is there any difference in recurrence rates in laparoscopic ileocolic resection for Crohn's disease compared with conventional surgery? A long-term, follow-up study. Dis Colon Rectum 2006;49(1):58–63.

[119] Hassan I, Cima RC, Sloan JA. Assessment of quality of life outcomes in the treatment of advanced colorectal malignancies. Gastroenterol Clin North Am 2006;35(1):53–64.

[120] Simmonds PC. Palliative chemotherapy for advanced colorectal cancer: systematic review and meta-analysis. Colorectal Cancer Collaborative Group. BMJ 2000;321(7260): 531–5.

[121] Choti MA. Surgical management of hepatocellular carcinoma: resection and ablation. J Vasc Interv Radiol 2002;13(9 Pt 2):S197–203.

[122] Goldberg RM. Advances in the treatment of metastatic colorectal cancer. Oncologist 2005;10(Suppl 3):40–8.

[123] Meyerhardt JA, Mayer RJ. Systemic therapy for colorectal cancer. N Engl J Med 2005;352(5):476–87.

[124] Czito BG, Bendell J, Willett CG. Radiation therapy for resectable colon cancer. Is there a role in the modern chemotherapy era? Oncology 2006;20(2):179–87.

[125] Choti MA. Advances in treatment of liver metastases from colorectal cancer. Medscape Hematology-Oncology 2006;9(1):1–10.

[126] Hotta T, Takifuji K, Arii K, et al. Clinical impact of adjuvant chemotherapy on patients with stage III colorectal cancer: I-LV/5FU chemotherapy as a modified RPMI regimen is an independent prognostic factor for survival. Anticancer Res 2006;26(2B):1425–32.

[127] Shah SA, Haddad R, Al-Sukhni W, et al. Surgical resection of hepatic and pulmonary metastases from colorectal carcinoma. J Am Coll Surg 2006;202(3):468–75.

[128] Pfister DG, Benson AB III, Somerfield MR. Clinical practice. Surveillance strategies after curative treatment of colorectal cancer. N Engl J Med 2004;350(23):2375–82.

[129] Schwartz RW, McKenzie S. Update on postoperative colorectal cancer surveillance. Curr Surg 2005;62(5):491–4.

[130] Anthony T. Colorectal cancer follow-up in 2005. Surg Oncol Clin N Am 2006;15(1): 175–93. [viii].

[131] Ohlsson B, Palsson B. Follow-up after colorectal cancer surgery. Acta Oncol 2003;42(8): 816–26.

[132] Meyerhardt JA, Mayer RJ. Follow-up strategies after curative resection of colorectal cancer. Semin Oncol 2003;30(3):349–60.

[133] Anthony T, Simmang C, Hyman N, et al. Practice parameters for the surveillance and follow-up of patients with colon and rectal cancer. Dis Colon Rectum 2004;47(6):807–17.

[134] Desch CE, Benson AB III, Somerfield MR, et al. Colorectal cancer surveillance: 2005 update of an American Society of Clinical Oncology practice guideline. J Clin Oncol 2005;23(33):8512–9.

[135] Rodriguez-Moranta F, Salo J, Arcusa A, et al. Postoperative surveillance in patients with colorectal cancer who have undergone curative resection: a prospective, multicenter, randomized, controlled trial. J Clin Oncol 2006;24(3):386–93.

[136] Titu LV, Breen DJ, Nicholson AA, et al. Is routine magnetic resonance imaging justified for the early detection of resectable liver metastases from colorectal cancer? Dis Colon Rectum 2006;49(6):810–5.

[137] Juweid ME, Cheson BD. Positron-emission tomography and assessment of cancer therapy. N Engl J Med 2006;354(5):496–507.

[138] Kornbluth A, Sachar DB. Ulcerative colitis practice guidelines in adults (update): American College of Gastroenterology, Practice Parameters Committee. Am J Gastroenterol 2004;99(7):1371–85.

[139] Solomon MJ, Schnitzler M. Cancer and inflammatory bowel disease: bias, epidemiology, surveillance, and treatment. World J Surg 1998;22(4):352–8.

[140] Louhimo J, Carpelan-Holmstrom M, Alfthan H, et al. Serum HCG beta, CA 72–4 and CEA are independent prognostic factors in colorectal cancer. Int J Cancer 2002;101(6): 545–8.

[141] Duffy MJ. Carcinoembryonic antigen as a marker for colorectal cancer: is it clinically useful? Clin Chem 2001;47(4):624–30.

[142] Carpelan-Holmstrom M, Louhimo J, Stenman UH, et al. CEA, CA 242, CA 19-9, CA 72-4 and hCGbeta in the diagnosis of recurrent colorectal cancer. Tumour Biol 2004;25(5–6): 228–34.

[143] Duffy MJ, van Dalen A, Haglund C, et al. Clinical utility of biochemical markers in colorectal cancer: European Group on Tumour Markers (EGTM) guidelines. Eur J Cancer 2003;39(6):718–27.

[144] Lyall MS, Dundas SR, Curran S, et al. Profiling markers of prognosis in colorectal cancer. Clin Cancer Res 2006;12(4):1184–91.

Gastroenterol Clin N Am 35 (2006) 675–712

GASTROENTEROLOGY CLINICS
OF NORTH AMERICA

Chemoprevention: Risk Reduction with Medical Therapy of Inflammatory Bowel Disease

Erick P. Chan, MD[a], Gary R. Lichtenstein, MD[a,b],*

[a]Division of Gastroenterology, Department of Medicine, University of Pennsylvania School of Medicine, 3400 Spruce Street, Third Floor, Ravdin Building, Philadelphia, PA 19104-4283, USA
[b]Center for Inflammatory Bowel Disease, Division of Gastroenterology, University of Pennsylvania School of Medicine, Philadelphia, PA, USA

Patients with long-standing inflammatory bowel disease (IBD) are at increased risk for the development of colorectal cancer. Chemoprevention, which aims to mitigate this risk through the administration of medications, is a promising strategy that has been gaining prominence over the past decade. A number of studies have examined the anti-neoplastic potential of several medications, including: 5-aminosalicylates (5-ASA), nonsteroidal anti-inflammatory drugs (NSAIDs), corticosteroids, immunomodulators, ursodeoxycholic acid (UDCA), folate, calcium, and statins. The majority of evidence supports the chronic administration of aminosalicylates for the purpose of chemoprevention in patients with IBD. Although the data are not conclusive, folate also appears to have a role in cancer prevention. In patients with ulcerative colitis (UC) complicated by primary sclerosis cholangitis, UDCA has been demonstrated to have a beneficial effect. NSAIDs, corticosteroids, immune modulators, calcium supplementation, and statins cannot be recommended for chemoprevention. While systemic corticosteroids have shown a protective effect, their potential benefits are outweighed by known toxicities associated with chronic use. Azathioprine and 6-mercaptopurine do not appear to confer any reduction in cancer risk, while inadequate data exist on the efficacy of NSAIDs, calcium, and statins. Additional studies of these and other

Dr. Lichtenstein has disclosed the following commercial relations: research: Abbott Corporation, Berlex, Centocor, Human Genome Sciences, Inkine, Intesco Corporation, ISIS Corporation, Millenium Pharmaceuticals, Otsuka Corporation, Protein Design Labs, Protomed Scientific, and Salix Pharmaceuticals; consultant: Abbott Corporation, Astra-Zeneca, Axcan Corporation, Bristol-Myers Squibb, Centocor, Elan, Gilead, Human Genome Sciences, GlaxoSmithKline, Proctor and Gamble, Prometheus Laboratories, Protein Design Labs, Protomed Scientific, Salix Pharmaceuticals, Schering-Plough Corporation, Serono, Shire Pharmaceuticals, Solvay Pharmaceuticals, Synta Pharmaceuticals, UCB, and Wyeth; speakers bureau: Astra-Zeneca, Axcan Corporation, Centocor, Proctor and Gamble, Salix Pharmaceuticals, Schering-Plough Corporation, Shire Pharmaceuticals, and Solvay Pharmaceuticals; honorarium: Falk Pharm.

*Corresponding author. E-mail address: grl@uphs.upenn.edu (G.R. Lichtenstein).

0889-8553/06/$ – see front matter
doi:10.1016/j.gtc.2006.07.003
© 2006 Elsevier Inc. All rights reserved.
gastro.theclinics.com

medications are needed to determine how chemoprevention can best be applied in the management of patients with IBD.

The association between colorectal cancer (CRC) and IBD has been recognized since Crohn and Rosenberg first described a patient with chronic UC who developed rectal adenocarcinoma [1]. A large meta-analysis published in 2001 determined the cumulative risk of CRC to be 2% after 10 years, 8% after 20 years, and 18% after 30 years of UC [2]. Crohn's colitis, like UC, also confers an increased risk of CRC [3,4]. Because the development of cancer is one of the most serious and feared complications of long-standing IBD, intense efforts have focused on mitigating this risk. Prophylactic proctocolectomy is available as a therapy to eliminate the development of CRC completely. Understandably, patients and physicians have not favored such a radical solution and have looked for more moderate yet effective options. Despite the widespread use of endoscopic surveillance programs in patients with IBD, there have been no prospective studies that demonstrate a reduction in mortality from IBD-associated CRC as a result of surveillance. Additionally, many limitations to surveillance colonoscopy have been well documented [5]: significant sampling error as a consequence of an inadequate number of biopsies [6–8], interobserver variability among pathologists [9–11], and patient noncompliance [9]. Despite its imperfections, endoscopic surveillance does allow for earlier detection of dysplasia and carcinoma [12,13] and has been incorporated into most clinical guidelines for the management of patients with IBD [14–17].

Although surveillance colonoscopy aims to identify premalignant conditions and early neoplastic lesions (ie, dysplasia) as a means of secondary prevention of CRC, increasing attention has been directed to chemoprevention, the strategy of primary prevention of CRC though the regular administration of medications. Wattenberg [18] was the first to describe this concept in a 1966 review of specific compounds that could inhibit carcinogenesis in animal models. Ten years later, Sporn and colleagues [19] coined the term *chemoprevention*, which they defined as "an attempt...to arrest or reverse premalignant cells during their progression to invasive malignancy, using physiological mechanisms that are not cytotoxic." A more concise definition of chemoprevention is the use of pharmacologic or natural agents for the "prevention of initiation, promotion, and progression of carcinogenesis to cancer [20]." In recent years, many successful examples of chemoprevention have been incorporated into the standard of care for certain high-risk patients. These include the use of tamoxifen and finasteride for the prevention and delay of breast and prostate cancers, respectively [21,22]. A landmark study on aspirin use and colon cancer by Thun and colleagues [23] in 1991 provided the first prospective evidence to support chemoprevention of a gastrointestinal malignancy. They studied a cohort of 662,424 men and women from the Cancer Prevention Study II and found that regular use of aspirin (defined as at least 16 doses per month for 1 year) conferred a relative risk (RR) of death from colon cancer of 0.60 and 0.58 in men and women, respectively, when compared with individuals who took no aspirin [23]. Since then, many additional studies of aspirin and other

NSAIDs have confirmed a protective effect on adenomas and CRC. A recent Cochrane review concluded that aspirin significantly reduces the recurrence of sporadic adenomatous polyps (RR = 0.77, 95% confidence interval [CI], 0.61–0.96) and that NSAIDs (sulindac or celecoxib) were associated with regression of adenomas in patients with familial adenomatous polyposis (FAP) [24].

By the mid-1990s, in the context of a growing body of literature supporting the use of aspirin and NSAIDs in the prevention of sporadic CRC and FAP-related CRC, investigators began to study potential chemoprevention of CRC in patients with long-standing IBD. In this review, we examine the use of mesalamine and other 5-ASA compounds, NSAIDs, corticosteroids, immune modulators, UDCA, folate, calcium, and statins in the chemoprevention of IBD-related CRC. We discuss putative mechanisms of action, summarize the available literature, and offer our recommendations on the use of these medications in chemoprevention.

COLORECTAL CARCINOGENESIS IN INFLAMMATORY BOWEL DISEASE

A familiarity with the carcinogenesis of CRC is requisite for an understanding of the strategies to prevent these cancers. Most sporadic CRCs arise as the result of the "adenoma-carcinoma" sequence, whereby sequential mutations result in the loss of tumor suppressor proteins (APC, p53) and activation of oncogenes (k-ras) [25]. In particular, loss of APC is characteristically an early event in the molecular pathogenesis of sporadic CRC. Loss of p53 is typically a late event that results in the formation of carcinoma from advanced adenomas. Although many of the same genes and mechanisms are similar to those of sporadic CRC, the molecular pathogenesis of colitis-related CRC has several important distinctions. Whereas the premalignant lesion in sporadic CRC is the adenoma, in IBD-related CRC, inflammation and dysplasia are the precursors to carcinoma. In this "inflammation-dysplasia-carcinoma" sequence (Fig. 1), loss of p53 occurs by mutation or loss of hetcrozygosity (LOH) and

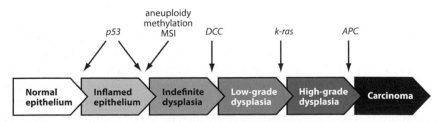

Fig. 1. Inflammation-dysplasia-carcinoma sequence of colitis-associated CRC. Sequential mutations in tumor suppressor proteins (APC, DCC, and p53) and proto-oncogenes (k-ras) result in progression of carcinogenesis. Mutation of p53 or loss of heterozygosity is characteristically early, whereas APC mutations are infrequent and represent later events in the pathway to carcinoma. MSI, microsatellite instability.

is an instrumental early step in carcinogenesis [26,27]. Conversely, *APC* mutations are infrequently found and likely represent later events in the pathway to carcinoma in patients with long-standing IBD [28].

Several observations support the important role of inflammation in the development of colitis-related CRC. First, the duration of colitis has consistently been the most important risk factor for the development of carcinoma, with CRC rarely found in patients with colitis for less than 7 years [2]. Second, the extent of colitis is another important risk factor. CRC risk rises dramatically with an increasing amount of mucosa involved with colitis. In a Swedish cohort of 3117 patients with UC, patients with pancolitis had a 14.8-fold higher incidence of CRC than expected in the general population (standardized incidence ratio) [29]. Those with left-sided colitis or ulcerative proctitis had standardized incidence ratios for the development of CRC of only 2.8 and 1.7, respectively [29]. Other studies have confirmed that patients with left-sided colitis have a lower risk of CRC than those with extensive colitis [30]. Third, the severity of colitis—specifically, the degree of inflammation—has been shown to be an additional risk factor for CRC. In a review of colectomy specimens performed on patients with UC and CRC, malignancies were identified in regions of the colon that were grossly free of disease [31]. These regions uniformly had histologic evidence of colitis, however, suggesting that microscopic rather than gross inflammation may better correlate with CRC risk [31]. Two recent case-control studies specifically found that the degree of histologic inflammation was directly associated with cancer risk in UC [32,33]. Finally, anti-inflammatory medications, particularly 5-ASAs, have been associated with decreased CRC risk in patients with IBD [34]. The data supporting a chemoprotective effect of 5-ASAs in the prevention of CRC are now reviewed in detail.

5-AMINOSALICYLATES

Aminosalicylate medications have been the mainstay of therapy for IBD, particularly for the management of mild to moderately active disease as well as for the maintenance of remission for UC [35]. Sulfasalazine, the original 5-ASA–containing medication, is split into two active molecules in the intestine: sulfapyridine, which has bacteriostatic activity, and 5-ASA (or mesalamine), which has potent anti-inflammatory activity. Because the 5-ASA moiety is believed to be the active agent in the treatment of colitis, many different formulations of mesalamine have been developed for use in IBD; these formulations result in differential delivery of mesalamine to the small bowel and colon. Because 5-ASA and aspirin (acetylsalicylic acid) are both derivatives of salicylic acid, they share structural similarities: aspirin has an acetyl group at position 2, whereas 5-ASA has an amino group at position 5 of the benzene ring (Fig. 2).

Initial inquiries into potential protective effects of 5-ASAs in colitis were largely based on its similarity to aspirin and aspirin's proven record in the chemoprevention of sporadic CRC and adenomas. Furthermore, the widespread use of mesalamine and its established safety profile make 5-ASA an ideal candidate for chemoprevention.

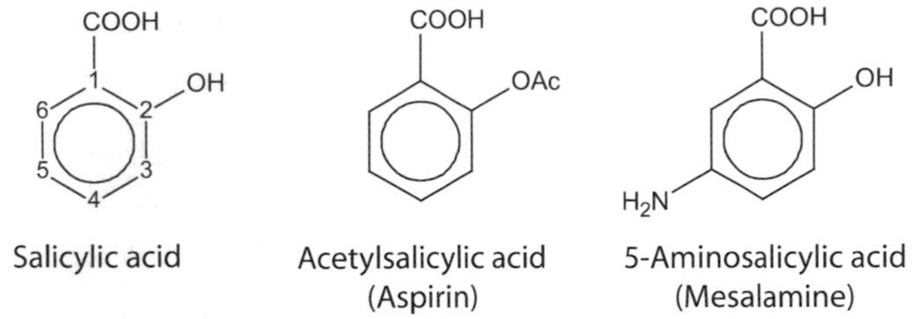

Fig. 2. Chemical structures of salicylic acid, acetylsalicylic acid (aspirin), and 5-ASA (mesalamine). Aspirin and mesalamine are derivatives of salicylic acid, with aspirin having an acetyl group at position 2 and mesalamine having an amino group at position 5.

Putative Mechanisms of 5-Aminosalicylates

Although the precise mechanisms by which NSAIDs and aspirin interfere with CRC carcinogenesis remain unknown, NSAIDs are thought to exert an antineoplastic effect through cyclooxygenase (COX)-2–dependent and COX-2–independent mechanisms. COX is the critical enzyme involved in the metabolism of arachidonic acid into prostaglandins, which are important signaling mediators. Two distinct COX isoforms have been identified: COX-1 and COX-2. Whereas COX-1 is generally constitutively expressed, COX-2 is inducible and upregulated in specific tissues during inflammation, wound healing, and neoplasia. In particular, increased expression of COX-2 has been identified in colorectal adenomas and carcinomas and is implicated as an early step in adenomatous polyp formation [36]. A number of in vitro experiments have shown that NSAIDs result in the stimulation of apoptosis, suppression of proliferation, and inhibition of angiogenesis [37]. These may be the result of changes not only in COX-2 activity but of many other mediators, including peroxisome proliferator–activated receptor-γ (PPARγ), *c-myc*, nuclear factor-κB (NF-κB), and *p38*/mitogen-activated protein (MAP) kinase [38].

5-ASAs are also believed to exert antitumor effects through a multitude of other mechanisms [39,40]. In addition to nonselective COX inhibitory activity, 5-ASAs have been shown to result in enhanced apoptosis through inhibition of NF-κB and MAP kinases [41–43]. The induction of apoptosis by 5-ASAs in vitro has been supported by in vivo findings. In a cohort of patients with sporadic carcinoma of the sigmoid or rectum, a 14-day treatment with topical mesalamine resulted in selectively increased apoptosis in malignant tissue when compared with adjacent normal mucosa [44]. A recent set of experiments suggests 5-ASAs may exert their antitumor effect through an alternate mechanism: improvement in the fidelity of DNA replication. Mesalamine treatment of HCT116 colon cancer cell lines (with and without intact mismatch repair genes) resulted in a lowered mutation rate (in mismatch repair–deficient cells) and improved replication fidelity (in mismatch repair–proficient cells) as assayed by flow cytometry [45]. Other potential mechanisms of anticancer action include the inhibition of reactive oxygen species [46–48], downregulation of oncogenes (eg, *c-myc*) and transcription factors [49], and reduction in aberrant stem cell activation [50].

Epidemiologic Studies of 5-Aminosalicylates

Because 5-ASAs remain a mainstay in the medical treatment of IBD, sulfasalazine and mesalamine have been the subjects of multiple studies on chemoprevention (Tables 1 and 2). In 1989, Lashner and colleagues [51] provided the earliest indirect evidence that 5-ASAs may have a protective effect against colitis-related CRC. The authors conducted a case-control study of 99 patients with long-standing colitis to determine associations between various exposures and the development of dysplasia or CRC. They made a striking finding that patients with sulfa allergy, and thus unable to take sulfasalazine, had a markedly increased likelihood of developing CRC (odds ratio [OR] = 11.71, 95% CI, 1.65–83.10) [51]. Paradoxically, sulfasalazine use was associated with a mildly elevated but nonstatistically significant increase in CRC risk (OR = 1.50, 95% CI, 0.43–5.19) [51].

Additional studies designed to examine the role of UDCA in the prevention of CRC in patients with UC and primary sclerosing cholangitis (PSC) have also addressed possible effects of 5-ASAs and have had mixed results. Tung and coworkers [52] performed a cross-sectional study of patients with UC with concomitant PSC. Although a history of sulfasalazine therapy was associated with an increased chance of dysplasia on surveillance (OR = 3.3, 95% CI, 0.8–14), mesalamine therapy had a mild protective effect (OR = 0.88, 95% CI, 0.25–3.2), although neither finding achieved statistical significance. This may be explained, in part, by the relatively small sample size (59 patients). In 2003, Pardi and colleagues [53] at the Mayo clinic analyzed data from a previously published, prospective, randomized controlled trial (RCT) of UDCA in patients with UC and PSC [54]. They found no significant association between the use of 5-ASAs and the development of dysplasia or cancer. None of these studies included duration or dosing of sulfasalazine or mesalamine treatment in their analyses. Furthermore, in the UDCA studies, it may be difficult to extrapolate these findings to the general population with long-standing colitis in the absence of PSC, because patients with UC with PSC carry a higher risk of developing CRC [55,56]. In a recent small study of patients with IBD and PSC, however, investigators found that the use of mesalamine with UDCA may decrease the risk of colorectal dysplasia when compared with UDCA alone [57]. The authors studied 24 patients, all of whom were taking UDCA for confirmed PSC in the setting of IBD (80% of patients had UC). Of the 5 patients not taking mesalamine, 1 (20%) developed dysplasia. Of the 19 patients taking mesalamine, only 1 (5%) developed dysplasia, thus conferring a protective effect of mesalamine in this population (RR = 0.26, 95% CI, 0.02–3.51). Although these numbers are small and not statistically significant, they do suggest that although 5-ASAs alone may not offer a protective effect in the high-risk group of patients with IBD and PSC, they may add incremental benefit when used in conjunction with UDCA.

Table 1
Summary of cohort studies of the use of aminosalicylates in the chemoprevention of inflammatory bowel disease (IBD)–related cancer or dysplasia

Author (year)	Subjects (case/controls)	IBD population	Study medication	Medication duration	Medication dose	Study period	Study location (setting)	End point	RR	Significant protection?
Moody, et al (1996)	10/158	UC	SSZ	"long term"	NR	1972–1992	UK (population)	Cancer	0.11	Yes
Lashner, et al (1997)	29/69	UC	SSZ Mes	≥6 mo	NR	1986–1992	US (university hospital)	Cancer or dysplasia	0.95 (SSZ) 0.88 (Mes)	No (SSZ) No (Mes)
Lindberg, et al (2001)	53/90	UC	SSZ	≥6 mo	NR	1973–1993	Sweden university hospital)	Cancer or dysplasia	0.76	No
Pardi, et al (2003)[a]	11/52	UC + PSC	5-ASA	NR	NR	1989–1995	US (multicenter, university hospitals)	Cancer or dysplasia	—[b]	No
Smith and Swaroop (2006)[c]	2/22	CD/UC + PSC (on UDCA)	Mes	NR	NR	1995–2005	US (university hospital)	Dysplasia	0.26	No

Abbreviations: 5-ASA, 5-aminosalicylates; Mes, mesalamine; mo, months; NR, not recorded; PSC, primary sclerosing cholangitis; RR, relative risk; SSZ, sulfasalazine; UC, ulcerative colitis; UDCA, ursodeoxycholic acid.
[a]Cohort of patients from a previously performed randomized controlled trial.
[b]RR cannot be calculated.
[c]Abstract publication.

Table 2
Summary of case-control and cross-sectional studies of the use of aminosalicylates in the chemoprevention of inflammatory bowel disease (IBD)–related cancer or dysplasia

Author (year)	Subjects (case/controls)	IBD population	Study medication	5-ASA duration	5-ASA dose	Study period	Study location (setting)	End point	OR	Significant protection?
Lashner, et al (1989)	35/64	UC	SSZ	NR	NR	NR	US (university hospital)	Cancer or dysplasia	1.50	No
Pinczowski, et al (1994)	102/196	UC	SSZ	≥3 mo	NR	1965–1983	Sweden (population)	Cancer	0.38	Yes
Eaden, et al (2000)	102/102	UC	SSZ Mes	5–10 y	S ≥2 g/d M ≥1.2 g/d	Late 1980s	UK (community)	Cancer	0.25 (any) 0.85 (SSZ) 0.19 (Mes)	Yes (any) No (SSZ) Yes (Mes)
Tung, et al (2001)[a]	26/33	UC + PSC	SSZ Mes	NR	NR	NR	US (university hospital)	Dysplasia	3.3 (SSZ) 0.88 (Mes)	No (SSZ) No (Mes)
Rubin, et al (2003)[b]	26/96	UC	SSZ Mes	NR	M ≥1.2 g/d	NR	US (university hospital)	Cancer or dysplasia	0.28	Yes
Bernstein, et al (2003)	25/348	CD or UC	SSZ	≥2 mo	NR	1997–2000	Canada (population)	Cancer	1.46	No

Study	Cases/controls	Disease	Agent	Exposure		Years	Setting	Outcome	OR	PSC
Rutter, et al (2004)	68/136	UC	SSZ Mes	>10 y	NR	1988–2002	UK (university hospital)	Cancer or dysplasia	1.58 (SSZ) 0.65 (Mes)	No (SSZ) No (Mes)
van Staa, et al (2005)	100/600	CD or UC	5-ASA	"regular"	NR	NR	UK (population)	Cancer	0.60	Yes
Terdiman, et al (2005)[b]	197/NR	CD or UC	5-ASA	≥3			prescriptions	NR	2000–2003	US
Siegel, et al (2006)[b]	27/27	CD	5-ASA	"regular"	NR	Since 1990	(population) US (university hospital)	Cancer Cancer	0.47 0.30	Yes No
Velayos, et al (2006)	188/188	UC	5-ASA	Cumulative use 1–5 y	NR	1976–2002	US (university hospital)	Cancer	0.4	Yes

Abbreviations: 5-ASA, 5-aminosalicylates; CD, Crohn's disease; mo, months; NR, not recorded; OR, odds ratio; PSC, primary sclerosing cholangitis; Mes, mesalamine; SSZ, sulfasalazine; UC, ulcerative colitis; yr, years.

[a]Cross-sectional study (all others are case-control studies).

[b]Abstract publication.

Although these studies provide inconsistent evidence for a protective role of 5-ASAs, additional trials designed to assess whether 5-ASAs can modulate the risk of developing CRC generally seem to support a chemoprotective effect of these medications. Twelve trials (3 cohort and 9 case-control studies) and a recent meta-analysis addressing this question have been published since 1994.

In 1994, Pinczowski and colleagues [58] provided the first compelling evidence that 5-ASA use was associated with a decreased risk of CRC in patients with IBD. In this case-control study drawn from a cohort of 3112 Swedish patients with UC, the authors compared 102 cases of patients with CRC with 196 cancer-free matched controls. They found that any pharmacotherapy (including sulfasalazine and corticosteroids) for a duration of at least 3 months was associated with a protective effect against the development of CRC (RR = 0.45, 95% CI, 0.25–0.81) when compared with no therapy or therapy for less than 3 months; specific treatment with at least 3 months of sulfasalazine was associated with a more pronounced protective effect (RR = 0.34, 95% CI, 0.19–0.62). Because this effect was maintained even after adjusting for disease activity using multivariate analysis (sulfasalazine: RR = 0.38, 95% CI, 0.20–0.69), the authors concluded that sulfasalazine had an independent protective effect.

Two years later, Moody and coworkers [59] in the United Kingdom published similar findings. They followed a cohort of 168 patients with long-standing UC for 10 years; during this time, 10 patients developed CRC. Using compliance with medical therapy as a surrogate for sulfasalazine use, the authors found a 3% risk of CRC in compliant patients compared with a 31% risk of CRC in noncompliant patients ($P<.001$). Thus, in this cohort, patients compliant with sulfasalazine therapy had a significantly lower risk of developing CRC.

Together with his colleagues, Lashner [60], now at the Cleveland Clinic, analyzed a historical cohort of 98 patients with pancolitis of at least 8 years' duration. These patients were followed for development of dysplasia or cancer. Patients who took sulfasalazine and mesalamine therapy for at least 6 months' duration had minimal and nonsignificant reductions in the risk of dysplasia or CRC (RR = 0.95, 95% CI, 0.34–2.70; RR = 0.88, 95% CI, 0.21–3.73, respectively). No information about 5-ASA dosing was reported.

A rigorous case-control study of patients drawn from gastroenterology practices across the United Kingdom was published by Eaden and coworkers [61] in 2000. Results of multivariate analysis of the 102 cases of UC complicated by CRC and 102 matched controls showed a 75% reduction (OR = 0.25, 95% CI, 0.13–0.48) in cancer risk in patients who took regular 5-ASA (defined as treatment for 5–10 years). Unlike previous studies, these authors then analyzed cancer risk associated with specific medications and doses. Mesalamine at a dose of 1.2 g/d or greater reduced CRC risk by 81% (OR = 0.19, 95% CI, 0.06–0.61), whereas sulfasalazine at a dose of 2 g/d or greater had less of an effect (OR = 0.85, 95% CI, 0.32–2.26). Two criticisms of this study concern the control population. Although cases were drawn from throughout the United Kingdom and from teaching and community hospitals, the control population was drawn exclusively from the IBD database at Leicestershire General Hospital, a large referral center. Additionally, the case and control populations differed significantly in their ethnic composition, with Asian patients being overrepresented in controls (43%) compared with cases (6%). Nevertheless, according to these authors, unpublished analyses have determined that neither factor affected the final results [61,62].

The next two studies to be published found no beneficial effect of 5-ASA use. Lindberg and colleagues [63] followed a cohort of 143 Swedish patients with pancolitis of more than 10 years' duration. Over the course of 20 years of follow-up in a surveillance colonoscopy program, 51 patients developed dysplasia or cancer. Their primary finding confirmed PSC to be an independent risk factor for the development of CRC (63% compared with 30% in patients with UC without PSC). The authors then examined the effect of sulfasalazine or 5-ASA treatment. They defined the "treatment group" as those who received either medication for at least 6 months; the remaining patients had no treatment or were treated for less than 6 months. Treated patients did have a slightly lower risk of dysplasia and CRC (34%) compared with nontreated patients (44%), but this difference did not reach statistical significance. A post-hoc analysis demonstrated that this study was underpowered, however, suggesting that a larger sample size could have yielded significant results [63].

In 2003, a Canadian group led by Bernstein [64] studied 25 cases of IBD with CRC compared with 348 matched control patients who did not develop cancer. All patients were culled from the Manitoba Inflammatory Bowel Disease Epidemiology Database, and their medication use was linked to the province-wide prescription drug database. Unexpectedly, the investigators found that continuous use of 5-ASAs for at least 2 months was associated with an increased risk of CRC (OR = 1.46, 95% CI, 0.58–3.73), although this was not statistically significant. Slight differences in the mean duration of treatment (400.9 days for patients with CRC compared with 420.2 days for controls) and the average prescribed daily dose of 5-ASA (2295 mg in patients with CRC compared with 1811 mg for controls) were also not significant. Notably, the study by Bernstein and coworkers [64] was the first chemoprevention study to include patients with Crohn's disease (CD) as well as UC. Although control patients with UC and CD had similar use of 5-ASAs (25% and 26%, respectively), CRC cases differed slightly: 45% of patients with UC with CRC had regular use of 5-ASAs compared with only 14% of patients with CD.

Also in 2003, Rubin and colleagues [65] at the University of Chicago published in abstract form an analysis of 26 cases of UC complicated by dysplasia (18 patients) or CRC (8 patients) compared with 96 matched control patients without neoplasia. They recorded all 5-ASA products used during the duration of disease and converted doses to average daily mesalamine equivalents. Using conditional logistic regression analysis adjusting for disease duration, age at diagnosis, and family history of CRC, the authors found that an average daily dose of mesalamine of 1.2 g or greater was associated with a significant reduction in the risk of CRC or dysplasia (OR = 0.28, 95% CI, 0.09–0.85). Furthermore, they found a dose-dependent response: increasing doses of mesalamine resulted in incremental decreased risk.

These findings were not reproduced by Rutter and coworkers [32] in the United Kingdom, who published the results of their own case-control study in 2004. From a population of 525 patients with UC enrolled in a colonoscopic surveillance program, the authors identified 68 with CRC who were matched with 136 control patients. Importantly, they produced the first controlled evidence that severity of inflammation (graded colonoscopically and histologically) was associated with an increased rate of CRC in long-standing UC. Unexpectedly, univariate analysis showed a nonsignificant trend toward increased CRC risk with increasing 5-ASA duration of use. When compared with patients who never used 5-ASA (or used it for less than 3 cumulative months), patients who used 5-ASA for up to 10 years had an increased risk of CRC (OR = 1.74, 95% CI, 0.45–6.70); those with cumulative use of 5-ASA of greater than 10 years had an even higher risk for CRC (OR = 2.38, 95% CI, 0.67–8.54). The authors then analyzed CRC risk by specific 5-ASA compound: sulfasalazine or nonsulfasalazine. Sulfasalazine use showed no statistically significant effect (up to 10 years: OR = 0.97, 95% CI, 0.41–2.26; greater than 10 years: OR = 1.58, 95% CI, 0.71–3.51). Nevertheless, there was a trend toward a dose-dependent protective effect of nonsulfasalazine 5-ASA medications (up to 10 years: OR = 0.79, 95% CI, 0.40–1.55; greater than 10 years: OR = 0.65, 95% CI, 0.26–1.62), although neither effect was statistically significant.

In one of the largest population-based studies of its kind, van Staa and coworkers [66] used the United Kingdom's General Practice Research Database (GPRD) to study 18,969 patients with IBD and active prescriptions for 5-ASA medications. In a nested case-control analysis, each incident case of CRC with 5-ASA use in the 6 months before cancer diagnosis was matched to 6 control patients. They identified 100 cases of CRC (76 patients had UC, 15 had CD, and 9 had unspecified CRC). When patients were stratified by "regularity" of 5-ASA use, as measured by the number of 5-ASA prescriptions filled in the previous 12 months, the authors found that when compared with nonregular users of 5-ASA, regular users (6 or more 5-ASA prescriptions) had a significant reduction in CRC risk (OR = 0.60, 95% CI, 0.38–0.96). The authors found no decreased risk of CRC with mesalamine or sulfasalazine users with 6 to 12 prescriptions (OR = 1.13, 95% CI, 0.49–2.59; OR = 0.95, 95% CI, 0.22–4.11, respectively). In those patients who filled more 5-ASA prescriptions, however, mesalamine use seemed to have more profound reductions in CRC risk when compared with sulfasalazine. In mesalamine users with 13 to 30 prescriptions or greater than 30 prescriptions, there was a statistically significant protective effect (OR = 0.30, 95% CI, 0.11–0.83; OR = 0.31, 95% CI, 0.11–0.84, respectively). In sulfasalazine users, there was a trend toward protection that was not statistically significant (OR = 0.41, 95% CI, 0.14–1.20; OR = 0.77, 95% CI, 0.37–1.60, respectively).

Terdiman and colleagues [67] presented preliminary results from a large case-control trial in the form of an abstract in 2005. Using a large health claims database, the authors identified 197 cases of CRC in patient with IBD. Their findings confirmed an increased risk of CRC in patients with IBD (OR = 1.89, 95% CI, 1.52–2.35). Patients with at least three 5-ASA prescriptions during the 2 years before CRC diagnosis were significantly less likely to develop cancer when compared with patients with only one or two prescriptions (OR = 0.47, 95% CI, 0.24–0.90), supporting a chemoprotective effect of these medications.

Siegel and colleagues [68] in Boston conducted the only case-control study of CRC in patients with CD and presented these results in the form of an abstract in 2006. They studied patients from the Massachusetts General Hospital patient database with Crohn's colitis involving at least one third of the colon, comparing 27 cases of CRC with 27 matched controls. Among their other findings, they reported that regular use of 5-ASA was associated with a trend toward a protective effect (OR = 0.30, 95% CI, 0.05–1.17).

The most recent study on this topic was performed by Velayos and co-workers [69], who published a large and rigorous case-control study of patients with UC followed at the Mayo Clinic. The authors studied risk factors associated with 188 patients with colitis-related CRC compared with 188 matched controls. Use of 5-ASA for 1 to 5 years was associated with a marked reduction in CRC risk (OR = 0.4, 95% CI, 0.2–0.9) when compared with that of those who used 5-ASA for less than 1 year. When 5-ASAs were used for greater than 6 years, their protective effect was somewhat diminished and no longer statistically significant (6–10 years: OR = 0.6, 95% CI, 0.3–1.4; >10 years: OR = 0.6, 95% CI, 0.3–1.3).

Although most of these studies support a reduction in CRC and dysplasia risk with regular 5-ASA use, there remains substantial heterogeneity among these trials. A prospective, double-blind, placebo-based RCT of 5-ASA in the prevention of colitis-associated CRC would be the ideal means to reach a definitive finding. Many factors make this impossible, however. Because 5-ASAs are currently a safe and widely used therapy for IBD (especially UC), significant ethical concerns exist about withholding these medications from trial participants receiving placebo [66,70]. Additionally, because CRC-complicating colitis is still a relatively rare event with a long latency period, such a trial would require decades to enroll an adequate number of patients to detect a significant protective effect [66,70,71].

Given that an RCT is unlikely to be performed, systematic review and meta-analysis provide the best interpretation of the available data. In 2005, Velayos and colleagues [34] published the results of their comprehensive meta-analysis of nine of the previously cited studies (three cohort and six case-control studies). They included only studies that had a defined exposure to 5-ASA medications (dosage or duration) and reported an RR or OR. The authors calculated pooled ORs for the development of dysplasia, CRC, and a combined end point of CRC or dysplasia. They found no protective effect of 5-ASAs against the development of dysplasia (OR = 1.18, 95% CI, 0.41–3.43), although only two studies addressed this end point. Nevertheless, there was a significant risk reduction associated with 5-ASA use and the development of CRC (OR = 0.51, 95% CI, 0.37–0.69) and CRC/dysplasia (OR = 0.51, 95% CI, 0.38–0.69).

5-Aminosalicylates and Dysplasia Progression

Although these studies have generally examined the utility of 5-ASAs in primary prevention of dysplasia or CRC, investigators have more recently studied whether 5-ASAs may have a benefit in secondary prevention by retarding the progression of dysplasia to carcinoma. Two recent abstracts from 2006 have addressed this possibility. Akram and coworkers [72] studied factors that may influence the progression of dysplasia in patients with UC. They identified 32 patients with indefinite dysplasia (IND) or low-grade dysplasia (LGD) and followed them for progression or regression of neoplasia. They found that patients with regression had an average daily dose of 5-ASA that was significantly higher than that of the group with progression or persistence of dysplasia (2.3 g and 1.5 g, respectively; $P = .01$). These findings imply that chronic higher dose use of 5-ASAs may have continued utility even after the development of dysplasia.

Velayos and colleagues [73] presented an abstract that included the first data suggesting a CRC-mortality benefit of 5-ASA use. They studied 76 patients with long-standing colitis complicated by CRC. Increasing 5-ASA use in the 2 years before CRC diagnosis was associated with decreasing CRC-related 5-year mortality ("infrequent" use = 63%, "intermittent" use = 35%, and "regular" use = 10%). When adjusting for other variables, regular and intermittent use of 5-ASA had significantly lower cancer mortality when compared with that of infrequent users (hazard ratio [HR] = 0.1, 95% CI, 0.01–0.4; HR = 0.3, 95% CI, 0.1–0.8, respectively).

In 2003, Ullman and colleagues [74] analyzed the progression of flat low-grade dysplasia (fLGD) to advanced neoplasia in 46 patients with UC and found a protective, although nonsignificant, effect of mesalamine use (defined as 6 months or greater or more than one course of treatment; OR = 0.40, 95% CI, 0.09–1.87). This same group has recently completed an analysis of a large cohort of patients with UC with no dysplasia, IND, or fLGD, and found that 5-ASA use was associated with a chemoprotective (but not statistically significant) effect only in patients with no dysplasia or IND (T.A. Ullman, MD, personal communication, 2006). No protective effect was identified in patients with fLGD, leading the authors to suggest that the beneficial action of 5-ASAs may be more important in the prevention of dysplasia formation rather than in the progression of dysplasia to carcinoma (T.A. Ullman, MD, personal communication, 2006).

These studies are potentially important because they suggest that the benefits of 5-ASAs may not be limited to the primary chemoprevention of CRC. Rather, chronic use of 5-ASAs may favorably alter the natural course of dysplasia or CRC in patients with IBD. Additional trials are needed to clarify the role of 5-ASAs in neoplastic progression.

NONSTEROIDAL ANTI-INFLAMMATORY DRUGS

Although the data support a protective effect of NSAIDs and aspirin in the prevention of sporadic CRC and adenomas [24], few studies have been conducted to look for a similar effect in colitis-related CRC. This may be explained, in part, by the hesitancy of physicians to prescribe NSAIDs for patients with IBD, given the conventionally held belief that NSAID use is associated with clinical exacerbations of IBD [75–77]. Several recent studies suggest that short courses of low-dose NSAIDs, particularly selective COX-2 inhibitors, may be safe for use in patients with IBD, however [78–80].

Two studies have suggested NSAIDs have a beneficial effect in the prevention of colitis-related CRC. In a 1996 case-control study of 11,446 patients with IBD from a Veterans Affairs (VA) database of hospital discharges, Bansal and Sonnenberg [81] provided encouraging evidence that the protective effect of NSAIDs might also extend to colitis-related CRC. They found that patients with IBD with concomitant diseases that are typically treated with chronic NSAIDs had a lower risk of CRC and CRC-related death (OR = 0.84, 95% CI, 0.65–1.09; OR = 0.68, 95% CI, 0.65–0.72, respectively). A recent case-control study of patients with UC by Velayos and colleagues [69] found a protective effect of aspirin (OR = 0.3, 95% CI, 0.1–0.8) and NSAID use (OR = 0.1, 95% CI, 0.03–0.5). Of note, no patients in this study took selective COX-2 inhibitors. Although these results are intriguing, the role of NSAIDs in chemoprevention remains unclear until additional studies can confirm the safety of long-term NSAIDs in patients with IBD.

CORTICOSTEROIDS

Because one of the principal putative mechanisms whereby mesalamine exerts an anticancer effect is through suppression of inflammation, many have reasoned that other medications that reduce colonic inflammation in IBD may also decrease neoplastic risk. Although their precise modes of action are unknown, corticosteroids are among the most potent anti-inflammatory medications and are one of the most commonly used therapies in the treatment of acute flares of UC or CD. Because of the high risk of multiple side effects (including but not limited to cataracts, osteoporosis, fractures, infections, and glucose intolerance), corticosteroids are not used long term for maintenance of remission in patients with IBD. As such, systemic steroids have limited appeal as chemopreventative agents, although topical agents or steroids (eg, budesonide) with high first-pass metabolism, low systemic absorption, and improved side-effect profiles may hold more promise. Several studies have queried whether steroids exert a protective effect, and their results have been mixed (Tables 3 and 4).

One of the primary findings in the study by Pinczowski and colleagues [58] suggested that corticosteroids might contribute to a beneficial effect. When taken for at least 3 months, pharmacologic therapy (including sulfasalazine and systemic or local corticosteroids) was associated with a significant

Table 3
Summary of cohort studies of the use of corticosteroids in the chemoprevention of inflammatory bowel disease (IBD)–related cancer or dysplasia

Author (year)	Subjects (cases/ controls)	IBD population	Study medication	Medication duration	Medication dose	Study period	Study location (setting)	End point	RR	Significant protection?
Lashner, et al (1997)	29/69	UC	Prednisone	≥6 mo	NR	1986–1992	US (university hospital)	Cancer or dysplasia	1.52	No

Abbreviations: mo, months; NR, not recorded; RR, relative risk; UC, ulcerative colitis.

Table 4
Summary of case-control studies of the use of corticosteroids in the chemoprevention of inflammatory bowel disease (IBD)–related cancer or dysplasia

Author (year)	Subjects (cases/controls)	IBD population	Study medication	Medication duration	Medication dose	Study period	Study location (setting)	End point	OR	Significant protection?
Lashner, et al (1989)	35/64	UC	Prednisone	NR	NR	NR	US (university hospital)	Cancer or dysplasia	0.43	No
Eaden, et al (2000)	102/102	UC	Systemic and local	5–10 y	NR	Late 1980s	UK (community)	Cancer	0.26 (systemic) 0.44 (local)	Yes (systemic) No (local)
Tung, et al (2001)[a]	26/33	UC + PSC	Prednisone	NR	NR	NR	US (university hospital)	Dysplasia	0.50	No
van Staa, et al (2005)	100/600	CD or UC	Oral glucocorticoid	Use within prior 6 mo	NR	NR	UK (population)	Cancer	1.83	No
Velayos, et al (2006)	188/188	UC	Unspecified	Use ≥1 y	NR	1976–2002	US (university hospital)	Cancer	0.4	Yes

Abbreviations: CD, Crohn's disease; mo, months; NR, not recorded; OR, odds ratio; PSC, primary sclerosing cholangitis; UC, ulcerative colitis; yr, years.
[a] Cross-sectional study (all others are case-control studies).

decreased risk of CRC (OR = 0.45, 95% CI, 0.25–0.81). Multivariate analysis of sulfasalazine use itself demonstrated that the bulk of this protective effect was likely from sulfasalazine (OR = 0.38, 95% CI, 0.20–0.69) rather than from other medications, such as corticosteroids, however. In their 2005 case-control analysis of CRC risk in patients with IBD, van Staa and coworkers [66] found that use of oral glucocorticoids in the prior 6 months resulted in an increased risk of CRC (OR = 1.83, 95% CI, 1.17–2.88).

Most other studies have found corticosteroids to confer some degree of protection. In the earlier case-control study of Lashner and colleagues [51], they found prednisone use to have a nonsignificant protective effect (OR = 0.43, 95% CI, 0.11–1.68) against the development of dysplasia or CRC. Interpretation of these findings regarding steroid use is limited, because no information on dose or duration of prednisone was included. Lashner and coworkers [60] did include this information in a subsequent study but did not arrive at the same conclusion. In this cohort study, prednisone use for greater than 6 months was associated with a nonsignificant increased risk for neoplasia (RR = 1.52, 95% CI, 0.55–4.16).

In the study of patients with UC with PSC by Tung and coworkers [52], the authors included corticosteroid use in their analysis. Dysplasia was found in 19 (50%) of 38 patients without prednisone use and in only 7 (33.3%) of 21 patients with prednisone use (OR = 0.50, 95% CI, 0.16–1.5), although this difference did not achieve statistical significance. No dose or duration information was recorded, and the authors did not clearly state which criteria they used to categorize patients as having used or not used prednisone.

Two additional studies have also supported a chemoprotective effect of corticosteroid use. In the case-control study by Eaden and coworkers [61], regular use of topical steroids in the 5 to 10 years before CRC diagnosis was associated with a protective, although not significant, effect (OR = 0.44, 95% CI, 0.19–1.02). The beneficial effect of systemic steroids was even more pronounced and did achieve significance (OR = 0.26, 95% CI, 0.01–0.70). No dose-response effect was demonstrated for either formulation of corticosteroids. In the case-control study of patients with UC by Velayos and colleagues [69], cumulative use of systemic steroids for at least 1 year was associated with a 60% reduction in CRC risk (OR = 0.4, 95% CI, 0.2–0.8).

IMMUNOMODULATORS

Immune-modulating medications, such as the purine analogues (6-mercaptopurine [6MP] and azathioprine [AZA]), cyclosporine (CsA), and methotrexate (MTX), are commonly prescribed for the treatment of IBD. Although their mechanisms of efficacy are also unknown, they are effective in reducing colonic inflammation and are widely used for the treatment of active and steroid-refractory IBD as well as for the maintenance of quiescent disease [82,83]. Initial concerns about these immunosuppressive medications focused attention not on whether they would decrease risk of CRC but on whether they were associated with an increased risk of malignancies, including CRC. Indeed, experience with AZA in organ transplantation and for the treatment of rheumatoid arthritis has demonstrated an increased risk of malignancy in particular skin cancers and non-Hodgkin's lymphoma [84–86]. A recent meta-analysis supports an increased risk of lymphoma in patients with CD treated with AZA or 6MP (RR = 4.18, 95% CI, 2.07–7.51) [87]. The authors point out that the effects of 6MP or AZA use and disease severity could not be separated, however. Several studies of immune-modulating therapy in IBD have found no increased rates of CRC [88,89].

Connell and colleagues [88] analyzed CRC rates of patients with long-standing pancolitis as part of their study to determine whether AZA therapy was associated with an elevated risk for malignancy. They compared 86 such patients who had received standard treatment with AZA at a dose of 2 mg/kg with 180 matched controls who did not receive AZA. The mean duration of AZA therapy was 12.5 months (range: 2 days to 15 years). Eight patients developed CRC in the AZA group, whereas 15 patients developed CRC in the control group. This difference in CRC rates between the treated and untreated groups was not significant. A similar study by Fraser and coworkers [89] arrived at the same conclusion. There was no difference in the combined rate of CRC and high-grade dysplasia (HGD) in patients with UC treated (2.2%) and not treated (2.8%) with AZA. Importantly, because significantly more patients with pancolitis were in the AZA-treated group (38% compared with 30%), any protective effect of AZA may have been underestimated in their analysis. The authors did not specify AZA doses, although mean exposure was 27.1 months (range: 1–222 months).

Several studies have included immune modulators as variables in chemoprevention studies (Tables 5 and 6). In the 1997 cohort study of Lashner and colleagues [60], use of at least 6 months of AZA or 6MP showed no benefit (RR = 1.12, 95% CI, 0.26–4.77), although dosages were unspecified. In their study of dysplasia in patients with PSC who had UC, Tung and coworkers [52] found no significant protection associated with AZA (OR = 0.68, 95% CI, 0.17–2.6), CsA (OR = 0.57, 95% CI, 0.15–2.2), or MTX (OR = 2.7, 95% CI, 0.23–31). In the study of neoplasia in patients with UC by Rutter and colleagues [32], there was a trend toward lower cancer risk in patients with total AZA use of 1 to 5 years and greater than 5 years' duration (OR = 0.34, 95% CI, 0.09–1.25; OR = 0.73, 95% CI, 0.30–1.78, respectively), although they could not exclude the null hypothesis. van Staa and coworkers [66] also reported no protective effect of immune modulators (AZA, 6MP, or CsA use in the prior 6 months) on CRC risk (OR = 0.85, 95% CI, 0.25–2.94). Most recently, Velayos and colleagues [69] found that immunosuppressive use for greater than 1 year was associated with an increased risk of CRC (OR = 3.0, 95% CI, 0.7–13.6). None of these studies provided information on dosing of these agents.

The most recent and rigorous study of the immune modulators was published in 2005 by Matula and colleagues [90] at Mount Sinai Hospital. The

Table 5
Summary of cohort studies of the use of immune modulators in the chemoprevention of inflammatory bowel disease (IBD)–related cancer or dysplasia

Author (year)	Subjects (cases/controls)	IBD population	Study medication	Medication duration	Medication dose	Study period	Study location (setting)	End point	RR	Significant protection?
Connell, et al (1994)	23/243	CD or UC	AZA	Mean 12.5 mo	2 mg/kg	1962–1991	UK (university hospital)	Cancer	1.11	No
Fraser, et al (2002)	36/1313	CD or UC	AZA	Mean 27 mo	NR	NR	UK (university hospital)	Cancer or dysplasia	0.8	No
Lashner, et al (1997)	29/69	UC	AZA or 6MP	≥6 mo	NR	1986–1992	US (university hospital)	Cancer or dysplasia	1.12	No
Matula, et al (2005)	54/261	UC	AZA or 6MP	≥3 mo	Mean 60.6 mg 6MP	1996–1997	US (university hospital)	Cancer or dysplasia	1.06[a]	No
van Staa, et al (2005)	100/600	CD or UC	AZA or 6MP or CsA	Use within prior 6 mo	NR	NR	UK (population)	Cancer	0.85	No

Abbreviations: AZA, azathioprine; CD, Crohn's disease; CsA, cyclosporine A; mo, months; 6MP, 6-mercaptopurine; NR, not recorded; RR, relative risk; UC, ulcerative colitis.
[a] Hazard ratio.

Table 6
Summary of case-control and cross-sectional studies of the use of immune-modulators in the chemoprevention of inflammatory bowel disease (IBD)–related cancer or dysplasia

Author (year)	Subjects (case/ controls)	IBD population	Study medication	Medication duration	Dose	Study period	Study location (setting)	End point	OR	Significant protection?
Tung, et al (2001)[a]	26/33	UC + PSC	AZA CsA MTX	NR	NR	NR	US (university hospital)	Dysplasia	0.68 (AZA) 0.57 (CsA) 2.7 (MTX)	No (AZA) No (CsA) No (MTX)
Rutter, et al (2004)	68/136	UC	AZA	1–5 y	NR	1988–2002	UK (university hospital)	Cancer or dysplasia	0.34	No
Velayos, et al (2006)	188/188	UC	Unspecified	Use ≥1 y	NR	1976–2002	US (university hospital)	Cancer	3.0	No

Abbreviations: AZA, azathioprine; CsA, cyclosporine A; MTX, methotrexate; NR, not recorded; OR, odds ratio; PSC, primary sclerosing cholangitis; UC, ulcerative colitis; yr, years.
[a]Cross-sectional study.

authors conducted a retrospective cohort study of 315 patients with long-standing colitis (defined as greater than 7 years) with an initial surveillance colonoscopy that was negative for dysplasia. Ninety-six of these patients had continuous use of 6MP or AZA and were classified as "exposed." The average use of these medications was 6MP equivalents at a dose of 60.6 ± 29.5 mg/d for 7.4 years. At 8 years of follow-up, rates of progression to neoplasia were similar in the exposed (16%) and unexposed (18%) groups. Proportional hazards analysis confirmed no significant beneficial effect of the 6MP/AZA group on the progression to any neoplasia (HR = 1.06, 95% CI, 0.59–1.93) or to advanced neoplasia (HR = 1.30, 95% CI, 0.45–3.75). The major criticism of this study is unavoidable in a retrospective cohort analysis like this: there are likely to be inherent and important differences between these groups of patients, because immune modulators are typically reserved for patients with more clinically severe disease and often for steroid-refractory IBD [91]. Indeed, the fact that colectomy rates (for indications unrelated to findings of HGD or CRC) were substantially higher in the 6MP/AZA group (11.5% compared with 5.5%) would suggest that patients receiving these medications had greater disease severity [90]. Nevertheless, this was a well-conducted study with few other limitations, and it provides the best evidence to date that the purine analogues seem to have no beneficial effect in the prevention of CRC.

Although the data are mixed, the current literature suggests that immune modulators do not protect against the development of colitis-related CRC. Future studies to address this issue might study immune modulators in conjunction with other potential chemoprotective agents or focus on the subset of patients with documented mucosal healing.

URSODEOXYCHOLIC ACID

Patients with UC and concomitant PSC are at even greater risk for the development of CRC [55,56]. In a Swedish study of patients with PSC with long-standing pancolitis, cumulative rates of CRC and dysplasia were 9%, 31%, and 50% at 10, 20, and 25 years of disease duration, respectively [92]. These rates were markedly higher than those of matched control patients with pancolitis but without PSC (2%, 5%, and 10%, respectively). Conventional doses of UDCA, a synthetic bile acid used in the treatment of PSC, improve biochemical indices of liver function but do not delay the clinical progression of cholestatic liver disease [53], although higher doses of UDCA have been shown to improve the 4-year expected survival of patients with PSC [93]. Additionally, emerging evidence has accumulated to support anticancer effects of UDCA. As the 7-β-epimer of chenodeoxycholic acid, UDCA reduces the colonic concentration of deoxycholic acid, a cytotoxic secondary bile acid that has been implicated in colorectal carcinogenesis [94,95]. Other potential mechanisms of UDCA in the prevention of CRC may include direct antiproliferative activity [96] and antioxidant effects [97].

Four human studies have examined the effect of UDCA on rates of CRC in patients with PSC and long-standing UC, and their conclusions have been mixed (Tables 7 and 8). Tung and his colleagues [52] performed a cross-sectional study of 59 patients with UC and PSC enrolled in the surveillance program at their institution. Use of UDCA was associated with a decreased prevalence of dysplasia. Dysplasia was found in 13 (32%) of 41 patients taking UDCA compared with 13 (72%) of 18 patients not taking UDCA (OR = 0.18, 95% CI, 0.05–0.61). No significant difference in cumulative UDCA exposure was found between the UDCA-treated patients who did and did not develop dysplasia. Several limitations to this study have been cited [98]. First, the number of patients followed was relatively small. Second, the reported prevalence of dysplasia in untreated patients (72%) was substantially higher than reported elsewhere in the literature (up to 50% after 25 years of disease duration) [92], raising doubts about the generalizability of these findings to patients at other institutions. Last, patients in the untreated group had a significantly younger age at diagnosis and longer disease duration than the UDCA-treated group (21.0 years compared with 14.3 years, respectively); both differences are likely to bias results in favor of UDCA.

In 2003, a Mayo Clinic group led by Pardi [53] studied a cohort of 52 patients with concomitant UC drawn from an earlier placebo-based RCT of UDCA in PSC. Most of these patients had pancolitis. Twenty-nine patients were treated with UDCA at a dose of 13 to 15 mg/kg for a median of 42 months and were followed an average of 6.5 years. CRC or dysplasia developed in 8 patients (35%) in the placebo group and in only 3 patients (10%) treated with UDCA (RR = 0.26, 95% CI, 0.06–0.92). Even after some placebo-treated patients were converted to open-label UDCA, the magnitude of protection remained significant and unchanged (RR = 0.26, 95% CI, 0.07–0.99). These results must be interpreted with some caution, however, given the relatively low number of colonic biopsies obtained at each surveillance examination. Prior studies have shown that a minimum of 33 and 56 biopsies are needed to exclude dysplasia with 90% and 95% confidence, respectively [7]. Because Pardi and colleagues [53] performed an average of only 22 biopsies in the patients given UDCA and 20 biopsies in the patients given placebo, existing dysplasia is likely to have been missed. Nevertheless, as a prospective RCT, this study offers substantial support to a beneficial effect of UDCA.

Sjöqvist and coworkers [99] conducted a prospective RCT of UDCA treatment in the prevention of neoplastic progression of patients with IBD with existing LGD. Their study population included patients with CD and UC and was not limited to those with concomitant PSC. Nineteen patients (13 with UC and 6 with CD) with prior findings of LGD were randomized to receive UDCA at a dose of 500 mg twice daily (n = 10) or placebo (n = 9) and were followed for 2 years. Because neoplastic progression of LGD is associated with characteristic histologic and chromosomal changes (ie, aneuploidy), the authors developed a scoring system ("neoplastic score") incorporating both determinants. Surveillance colonoscopy and DNA flow

Table 7

Summary of cohort studies of the use of ursodeoxycholic acid in the chemoprevention of inflammatory bowel disease (IBD)–related cancer or dysplasia

Author (year)	Subjects (cases/ controls)	IBD population	Medication	Duration	Dose	Study period	Study location (setting)	End point	RR	Significant protection?
Pardi, et al (2003)	11/52	UC + PSC	UDCA	NR	13–15 mg/kg	1989–1995	US (multi-center, university hospitals)	Cancer or dysplasia	0.26	Yes
Wolf, et al (2005)	35/120	UC + PSC	UDCA	≥ 6 mo	NR	1976–1994	US (university hospital)	Cancer or dysplasia	0.59	No

Abbreviations: mo, months; NR, not recorded; PSC, primary sclerosing cholangitis; RR, relative risk; UC, ulcerative colitis; UDCA, ursodeoxycholic acid.

Table 8
Summary of cross-sectional studies of the use of ursodeoxycholic acid in the chemoprevention of inflammatory bowel disease (IBD)–related cancer or dysplasia

Author (year)	Subjects (case/controls)	IBD population	Medication	Duration	Dose	Study period	Study location (setting)	End point	OR	Significant protection?
Tung, et al (2001)	26/33	UC + PSC	UDCA	NR	NR	NR	US (university hospital)	Dysplasia	0.18	Yes

Abbreviations: NR, not recorded; OR, odds ratio; PSC, primary sclerosing cholangitis; UC, ulcerative colitis; UDCA, ursodeoxycholic acid.

cytometry were performed at baseline and every 6 months. The authors found no significant differences in the neoplastic scores between the UDCA- and placebo-treated groups. Two patients in the placebo group had progression of LGD (1to HGD and 1 to a dysplasia-associated lesion or mass), whereas no patients in the UDCA group had neoplastic progression. The principal drawback of this study was the short follow-up time of 2 years, which was probably inadequate to detect any significant benefit of UDCA therapy. Furthermore, the scoring system, although making empiric sense, had not been previously validated for this study population.

Most recently, Wolf and coworkers [100] at the Cleveland Clinic performed a historical cohort study of 120 patients with PSC and UC. Twenty-eight patients received UDCA daily for at least 6 months (mean duration of 3.4 years), whereas the remaining 92 did not. They found no significant differences in the rate of neoplasia: 5 (17.9%) patients in the UDCA group developed dysplasia and 3 (10.7%) developed CRC, compared with 12 (13.0%) and 15 (16.3%), respectively, in the untreated group (RR = 0.59, 95% CI, 0.26–1.36). Furthermore, no dose-response effect was identified. There were significantly fewer deaths (from all causes) among the UDCA-treated patients (RR = 0.44, 95% CI, 0.22–0.90), however. Although both groups were generally similar, the UDCA-treated group had a higher rate of 5-ASA use (96% compared with 79%), which may have magnified any beneficial effect of UDCA.

FOLATE

Folate is an important cofactor in multiple cellular processes, including methylation and nucleotide synthesis. Experimental and epidemiologic studies have implicated low folate levels as a risk factor for the development of sporadic CRC. Folate deficiency can result in DNA strand breaks in the *p53* tumor suppressor gene [101] as well as in DNA hypomethylation [102], which are two mechanisms implicated in colorectal carcinogenesis. The Nurses Health Study showed that women with high daily folate intake (greater than 0.4 mg) had a lower prevalence of CRC compared with those taking 0.2 mg or less (RR = 0.69, 95% CI, 0.52–0.93) [103]. A similar study of men and women demonstrated that populations with low folate diets had higher incidences of colorectal adenomas [104]. Patients with IBD are at increased risk for folate deficiency as a result of multiple mechanisms. Active disease may result in poor nutritional intake with lower folate consumption as well as in enhanced intestinal losses through inflamed mucosa [105,106]. Sulfasalazine, long a common therapy for IBD, can also decrease folate absorption by greater than 30% through competitive inhibition of folate transport enzymes and direct inhibition of folate metabolism [107,108].

A number of studies have examined the role of folate supplementation in the development of colitis-related CRC (Tables 9 and 10). The first study was conducted by Lashner and colleagues [51] at the University of Chicago. They studied 99 patients with pancolitis (of greater than 7 years' duration) enrolled in

Table 9
Summary of cohort studies of the use of folate in the chemoprevention of inflammatory bowel disease inflammatory bowel disease (IBD)–related cancer or dysplasia

Author (year)	Subjects (cases/ controls)	IBD population	Medication	Duration	Dose	Study period	Study location (setting)	End point	RR	Significant protection?
Lashner, et al (1997)	29/69	UC	Folate	≥6 mo	1.0 mg	1986–1992	US (university hospital)	Cancer or dysplasia	0.54	No
Pardi, et al (2003)[a]	11/52	UC + PSC	Folate	NR	NR	1989–1995	US (multi-center, university hospitals)	Cancer or dysplasia	0.68	No
Smith and Swaroop (2006)[b]	2/22	CD/UC + PSC (on UDCA)	Folate	NR	NR	1995–2005	US (university hospital)	Dysplasia	—[c]	No

Abbreviations: mo, months; NR, not recorded; PSC, primary sclerosing cholangitis; RR, relative risk; UC, ulcerative colitis.
[a] Cohort of patients from a previously performed randomized controlled trial.
[b] Abstract publication.
[c] RR cannot be calculated.

Table 10
Summary of case-control studies of the use of folate in the chemoprevention of inflammatory bowel disease (IBD)–related cancer or dysplasia

Author (year)	Subjects (case/controls)	IBD population	Medication	Duration	Dose	Study period	Study location (setting)	End point	OR	Significant protection?
Lashner, et al (1989)	35/64	UC	Folate	NR	0.4 or 1.0 mg	NR	US (university hospital)	Cancer or dysplasia	0.38	No
Lashner, et al (1993)	6/61	UC	Folate	NR	NR	NR	US (university hospital)	Cancer or dysplasia	0.82[a]	Yes
Rutter, et al (2004)	68/136	UC	Folate	NR	NR	1988–2002	UK (university hospital)	Cancer or dysplasia	0.40	No

Abbreviations: mo, months; NR, not recorded; OR, odds ratios; RR, relative risk; UC, ulcerative colitis.
[a] OR = 0.82 for every 10-ng/mL increase in red blood cell folate levels.

a surveillance program. Thirty-five patients with dysplasia or cancer were compared with 64 matched controls. Folate supplementation of at least 0.4 mg/d was associated with a 62% lower incidence of neoplasia compared with no supplementation (OR = 0.38, 95% CI, 0.12–1.20). This result did not achieve statistical significance, partially as a result of a relatively small sample size. Although duration of treatment was not reported, the authors found no apparent differences in neoplasia rates with different folate doses (0.4 mg compared with 1 mg).

In 1993, Lashner [109] conducted a follow-up case-control study of 67 patients with chronic pancolitis, of whom 6 had dysplasia (n = 4) or cancer (n = 2). He found an inverse relation between folate levels and risk of colorectal neoplasia. Using red blood cell (RBC) folate levels as a measure of intermediate-term folate stores, he reported markedly lower levels of RBC folate in patients compared with controls. For every 10-ng/mL incremental increase in RBC folate, the risk of dysplasia or CRC decreased by 18% (OR = 0.82, 95% CI, 0.68–0.99). Serum folate, which reflects short-term folate stores, was not different between the two groups.

The third study by Lashner and colleagues [60], now at the Cleveland Clinic, followed a cohort of 98 patients with long-standing pancolitis. Thirty-nine patients used folate (as a 0.4-mg multivitamin supplement or a 1.0-mg sole supplement) for at least 6 months' duration. Folate use was associated with a protective, although not significant, effect (RR = 0.72, 95% CI, 0.28–1.83). Unlike the earlier study, the authors did find a dose-response effect of higher folate supplementation (for 0.4 mg: RR = 0.76, 95% CI, 0.36–1.61; for 1.0 mg: RR = 0.54, 95% CI, 0.20–1.48). Furthermore, folate use seemed to offer additional protection against advanced neoplasia, such that the risk reduction was highest in the prevention of cancer (RR = 0.45, 95% CI, 0.05–3.80), intermediate for HGD (RR = 0.52, 95% CI, 0.16–1.77), and lowest for LGD (RR = 0.75, 95% CI, 0.28–2.02). An important caveat in interpreting the studies by these investigators is their dependence on medical records to report folate supplementation and doses. It is plausible that folate use would be underestimated and that patients in the untreated groups may have actually been receiving folate supplementation, thereby biasing the results in favor of folate efficacy.

Biasco and coworkers [110] conducted a small pilot RCT of folate (folinic acid) versus placebo in 12 patients with chronic UC in remission. The authors had previously correlated neoplastic risk in UC with specific cell proliferation abnormalities detected by immunohistochemistry [111]. In the current trial, they found that treatment with folate for 3 months resulted in reduction of cell proliferation. This coincided with significant increases in serum and RBC folate levels, supporting a causal relation between folate use and the prevention of colonic dysplasia [110].

In the case-control study by Rutter and colleagues [32] of risk factors for the development of dysplasia in long-standing UC, the authors reported findings consistent with those of prior folate studies. Any exposure to folate supplementation had a nonsignificant protective effect (OR = 0.40, 95% CI, 0.05–3.42). Folate doses and duration of treatment were not recorded. Because the overall number of patients treated with folate was extremely low (one patient in the dysplasia group and five patients in the control group), extrapolation of these findings must be made with caution.

In their prospective trial of UDCA in patients with UC and concomitant PSC, Pardi and colleagues [53] performed univariate analysis and Cox proportional hazards regression and did not find a significant association between the use of folic acid and the development of dysplasia or CRC (univariate, $P = .50$; Cox proportional hazards, $P = .22$). Because this population of patients with PSC represents a unique subset of patients with colitis with an even higher risk for CRC, it is unclear if their findings can be generalized to the general IBD population.

Finally, in another study involving this patient population, Smith and Swaroop [57] presented results from a small cohort of 24 patients with PSC and IBD, all of whom also received UDCA. They compared rates of folate use in patients with and without dysplasia. Of the 19 patients without folate use, 2 (11%) developed dysplasia. Of the 5 patients who did use folate, none developed dysplasia. Although these findings did not achieve statistical significance, they do join a growing body of literature generally supporting a chemoprotective role for folate.

CALCIUM

Calcium is among several dietary factors that have been studied as chemoprotective agents against sporadic CRC. Calcium binds to potentially cytotoxic bile acids in the intestinal lumen. This results in saponification of the bile acids, thereby neutralizing their carcinogenic effects on the colonic mucosa [112,113]. Although the data are conflicting, a recent systematic review of two RCTs by the Cochrane group found only a modest protective effect in the prevention of recurrent adenomatous polyps (OR = 0.74, 95% CI, 0.58–0.95) [114]. More recently, the largest RCT to date was performed as part of the Women's Health Initiative and found no beneficial effect of calcium and vitamin D supplementation [115]. In this trial, 36,282 postmenopausal women were randomized to receive daily elemental calcium (1000 mg) and vitamin D (400 IU) or matched placebo. Incidence of CRC was the designated secondary end point. After an average of 7 years of follow-up, the authors found no statistically significant difference between these groups (HR = 1.08, 95% CI, 0.86–1.34).

Bostick and colleagues [116] performed the only study of calcium supplementation in UC. They randomized 31 patients with UC to treatment with daily elemental calcium or matching placebo for 2 months at a dose of 2 g. Rectal biopsies were obtained at baseline and at the end of treatment, and proliferation was determined by immunohistochemistry. They found no significant effect of calcium supplementation on the proliferation of colonic epithelial cells. Principal limitations of this study are its small sample size and extremely short follow-up, although it was designed to be a pilot study.

STATINS

3-Hydroxy-3-methylglutaryl coenzyme A (HMG-CoA) reductase inhibitors (commonly referred to as statins), through inhibition of the rate-limiting step of sterol synthesis, are potent cholesterol-lowering medications commonly used in the treatment and prevention of cardiovascular disease. Recently, potential anticancer effects have emerged and may be mediated through anti-inflammatory, immunomodulatory, antiangiogenic, proapoptotic, and antiproliferative mechanisms [117]. Recently, Khurana and colleagues [118,119] conducted two large case-control studies using a large VA database and found that statin use was associated with a significant protective effect against pancreatic cancer (OR = 0.41, 95% CI, 0.33–0.51) [118] and esophageal cancer (OR = 0.44, 95% CI, 0.36–0.53) [119].

Data supporting a beneficial effect of statins in the prevention of CRC followed shortly. Poynter and coworkers [120] conducted a large, population-based, case-control study in Israel and found that statin use for at least 5 years was associated with a significant reduction in overall CRC risk (OR = 0.53, 95% CI, 0.38–0.74). Intriguingly, an even more profound protective effect was identified when the analysis was limited to the subgroup of 55 patients with concomitant IBD. They found that patients with IBD who used statins, when compared with nonusers, had a marked reduction in risk of colitis-related CRC (OR = 0.06, 95% CI, 0.006–0.55). Although the data supporting a chemoprotective benefit of statins in colitis-related CRC are suggestive, enthusiasm must be tempered by this study's relatively small sample size. Furthermore, because the study was conducted in Israel, there was a disproportionate representation of Jewish patients of Ashkenazi descent, a population known to be at significantly higher risk for CRC [121]. Further studies are needed to clarify the potential role of statins in the reduction of CRC risk.

POTENTIAL CHEMOPREVENTATIVE AGENTS

Although most chemoprevention studies have focused on medications that are currently part of the armamentarium of conventional IBD therapies, additional novel agents are likely to be studied in the near future. Anti-tumor necrosis factor (TNF)-α agents, such as infliximab, have rapidly become part of the standard treatment regimen for otherwise refractory IBD. Their effect on dysplasia and CRC has not been studied, although their high cost may be prohibitive for widespread use in chemoprevention. Potential areas of future study include COX-2 inhibitors, short-chain fatty acids, antioxidants, and thiazolidinediones. Preliminary data from in vitro experiments and animal models have yielded encouraging results [122–127], and additional studies are needed.

SUMMARY AND RECOMMENDATIONS

The ideal chemopreventative agent, in addition to being efficacious in the prevention of cancer, must be easily administered, affordable, safe, and well tolerated, with minimal side effects. In the past decade, a growing body of literature has emerged on the prevention of CRC in patients with long-standing CD and

UC. The data are not definitive and consist almost exclusively of retrospective case-control and cohort studies rather than the more rigorous prospective RCTs. 5-ASA compounds have been most thoroughly studied, and most of the existing data support the use of 5-ASA in the prevention of CRC. Although the precise dose and duration are unclear, studies suggest that chronic systemic administration of 5-ASA at a dose of at least 1.2 g/d is most likely to be effective [61,65]. A beneficial effect of folate, albeit not statistically significant, has been consistently shown in every study performed for this purpose. Folate supplementation, which is safe and affordable, should also be recommended for all patients with IBD, especially those taking sulfasalazine. UDCA has been shown to exert a protective effect in most studies on patients with UC and concomitant PSC. Because this patient population is at particularly high risk for CRC, it is advisable to consider UDCA in all patients with colitis complicated by PSC. For patients without PSC, sufficient data do not exist to recommend it for the purpose of cancer prevention.

Five of the six corticosteroid studies have found a beneficial effect of systemic steroids, although most did not reach statistical significance. Regardless, given the frequent and serious adverse effects associated with chronic steroid use, systemic corticosteroids should not be prescribed for this indication. Budesonide, an oral corticosteroid with minimal systemic absorption, is a potential alternative, although it has not yet been studied as a chemopreventative agent. Similarly, until the long-term safety of chronic NSAID use can be demonstrated in patients with IBD, the role of NSAIDs in chemoprevention remains undefined. Although the data are conflicting, immune-modulating medications, such as AZA, do not seem to confer any reduction in the risk of dysplasia or CRC. The data on calcium supplementation and statin use are still too limited to endorse their use for the prevention of colitis-related CRC.

Chemoprevention is an area that holds great promise in the reduction of morbidity and mortality associated with IBD. Further studies, including prospective trials when possible and cost-effectiveness analyses, need to be performed to develop an optimal strategy for the reduction of cancer risk in patients with IBD.

References
[1] Crohn BB, Rosenberg H. The sigmoidoscopic picture of chronic ulcerative colitis. Am J Med Sci 1925;170:220–8.
[2] Eaden JA, Abrams KR, Mayberry JF. The risk of colorectal cancer in ulcerative colitis: a meta-analysis. Gut 2001;48(4):526–35.
[3] Gillen CD, Walmsley RS, Prior P, et al. Ulcerative colitis and Crohn's disease: a comparison of the colorectal cancer risk in extensive colitis. Gut 1994;35(11):1590–2.
[4] Bernstein CN, Blanchard JF, Kliewer E, et al. Cancer risk in patients with inflammatory bowel disease: a population-based study. Cancer 2001;91(4):854–62.
[5] Chan EP, Lichtenstein GR. Endoscopic evaluation for cancer and dysplasia in patients with inflammatory bowel disease. Techniques in Gastrointestinal Endoscopy 2004;6(4):169–74.
[6] Woolrich AJ, DaSilva MD, Korelitz BI. Surveillance in the routine management of ulcerative colitis: the predictive value of low-grade dysplasia. Gastroenterology 1992;103(2):431–8.

[7] Rubin CE, Haggitt RC, Burmer GC, et al. DNA aneuploidy in colonic biopsies predicts future development of dysplasia in ulcerative colitis. Gastroenterology 1992;103(5): 1611–20.

[8] Eaden JA, Ward BA, Mayberry JF. How gastroenterologists screen for colonic cancer in ulcerative colitis: an analysis of performance. Gastrointest Endosc 2000;51(2):123–8.

[9] Connell WR, Lennard-Jones JE, Williams CB, et al. Factors affecting the outcome of endoscopic surveillance for cancer in ulcerative colitis. Gastroenterology 1994;107(4): 934–44.

[10] Lim CH, Dixon MF, Vail A, et al. Ten year follow-up of ulcerative colitis patients with and without low grade dysplasia. Gut 2003;52(8):1127–32.

[11] Eaden J, Abrams K, McKay H, et al. Inter-observer variation between general and specialist gastrointestinal pathologists when grading dysplasia in ulcerative colitis. J Pathol 2001;194(2):152–7.

[12] Mpofu C, Watson AJ, Rhodes JM. Strategies for detecting colon cancer and/or dysplasia in patients with inflammatory bowel disease. Cochrane Database Syst Rev 2004;2: CD000279.

[13] Rutter MD, Saunders BP, Wilkinson KH, et al. Thirty-year analysis of a colonoscopic surveillance program for neoplasia in ulcerative colitis. Gastroenterology 2006;130(4):1030–8.

[14] Eaden JA, Mayberry JF. Guidelines for screening and surveillance of asymptomatic colorectal cancer in patients with inflammatory bowel disease. Gut 2002;51(Suppl 5):V10–2.

[15] Winawer S, Fletcher SR, Rex D, et al. Colorectal cancer screening and surveillance: clinical guidelines and rationale—update based on new evidence. Gastroenterology 2003;124(2):544–60.

[16] Kornbluth A, Sachar DB. Ulcerative colitis practice guidelines in adults (update): American College of Gastroenterology, Practice Parameters Committee. Am J Gastroenterol 2004;99(7):1371–85.

[17] Itzkowitz SH, Present DH. Consensus conference: colorectal cancer screening and surveillance in inflammatory bowel disease. Inflamm Bowel Dis 2005;11(3):314–21.

[18] Wattenberg LW. Chemoprophylaxis of carcinogenesis: a review. Cancer Res 1966;26(7): 1520–6.

[19] Sporn MB, Dunlop NM, Newton DL, et al. Prevention of chemical carcinogenesis by vitamin A and its synthetic analogs (retinoids). Fed Proc 1976;35(6):1332–8.

[20] Theisen C. Chemoprevention: what's in a name? J Natl Cancer Inst 2001;93(10):743.

[21] Fisher B, Costantino JP, Wickerham DL, et al. Tamoxifen for prevention of breast cancer: report of the National Surgical Adjuvant Breast and Bowel Project P-1 Study. J Natl Cancer Inst 1998;90(18):1371–88.

[22] Thompson IM, Goodman PG, Tangen CM, et al. The influence of finasteride on the development of prostate cancer. N Engl J Med 2003;349(3):215–24.

[23] Thun MJ, Namboodiri MM, Heath CW Jr. Aspirin use and reduced risk of fatal colon cancer. N Engl J Med 1991;325(23):1593–6.

[24] Asano TK, McLeod RS. Non steroidal anti-inflammatory drugs (NSAID) and aspirin for preventing colorectal adenomas and carcinomas. Cochrane Database Syst Rev 2004;2: CD004079.

[25] Vogelstein B, Fearon ER, Hamilton SR, et al. Genetic alterations during colorectal-tumor development. N Engl J Med 1988;319(9):525–32.

[26] Itzkowitz SH, Yio X. Inflammation and cancer. IV. Colorectal cancer in inflammatory bowel disease: the role of inflammation. Am J Physiol Gastrointest Liver Physiol 2004;287(1): G7–17.

[27] Brentnall TA, Crispin DA, Rabinovitch PS, et al. Mutations in the p53 gene: an early marker of neoplastic progression in ulcerative colitis. Gastroenterology 1994;107(2):369–78.

[28] Tarmin L, Yin J, Harpaz N, et al. Adenomatous polyposis coli gene mutations in ulcerative colitis-associated dysplasias and cancers versus sporadic colon neoplasms. Cancer Res 1995;55(10):2035–8.

[29] Ekbom A, Helmick C, Zack M, et al. Ulcerative colitis and colorectal cancer. A population-based study. N Engl J Med 1990;323(18):1228–33.

[30] Gyde SN, Prior P, Allan RN, et al. Colorectal cancer in ulcerative colitis: a cohort study of primary referrals from three centres. Gut 1988;29(2):206–17.

[31] Mathy C, Schneider K, Chen YY, et al. Gross versus microscopic pancolitis and the occurrence of neoplasia in ulcerative colitis. Inflamm Bowel Dis 2003;9(6):351–5.

[32] Rutter M, Saunders B, Wilkinson K, et al. Severity of inflammation is a risk factor for colorectal neoplasia in ulcerative colitis. Gastroenterology 2004;126(2):451–9.

[33] Rubin DT, Huo D, Rothe JA, et al. Increased inflammatory activity is an independent risk factor for dysplasia and colorectal cancer in ulcerative colitis: a case-control analysis with blinded prospective pathology review. Gastroenterology 2006;130(4 Suppl. 2):A-2.

[34] Velayos FS, Terdiman JP, Walsh JM. Effect of 5-aminosalicylate use on colorectal cancer and dysplasia risk: a systematic review and metaanalysis of observational studies. Am J Gastroenterol 2005;100(6):1345–53.

[35] Bergman R, Parkes M. Systematic review: the use of mesalazine in inflammatory bowel disease. Aliment Pharmacol Ther 2006;23(7):841–55.

[36] Eberhart CE, Coffey RJ, Radhika A, et al. Up-regulation of cyclooxygenase 2 gene expression in human colorectal adenomas and adenocarcinomas. Gastroenterology 1994;107(4):1183–8.

[37] Rao CV, Reddy BS. NSAIDs and chemoprevention. Curr Cancer Drug Targets 2004;4(1):29–42.

[38] Janne PA, Mayer RJ. Chemoprevention of colorectal cancer. N Engl J Med 2000;342(26):1960–8.

[39] Allgayer H, Kruis W. Aminosalicylates: potential antineoplastic actions in colon cancer prevention. Scand J Gastroenterol 2002;37(2):125–31.

[40] Allgayer H. Review article: mechanisms of action of mesalazine in preventing colorectal carcinoma in inflammatory bowel disease. Aliment Pharmacol Ther 2003;18(Suppl 2):10–4.

[41] Egan LJ, Mays DC, Huntoon CJ, et al. Inhibition of interleukin-1-stimulated NF-kappaB RelA/p65 phosphorylation by mesalamine is accompanied by decreased transcriptional activity. J Biol Chem 1999;274(37):26448–53.

[42] Kaiser GC, Yan F, Polk DB. Mesalamine blocks tumor necrosis factor growth inhibition and nuclear factor kappaB activation in mouse colonocytes. Gastroenterology 1999;116(3):602–9.

[43] Weber CK, Liptay S, Wirth T, et al. Suppression of NF-kappaB activity by sulfasalazine is mediated by direct inhibition of IkappaB kinases alpha and beta. Gastroenterology 2000;119(5):1209–18.

[44] Bus PJ, Nagtegaal ID, Verspaget HW, et al. Mesalazine-induced apoptosis of colorectal cancer: on the verge of a new chemopreventive era? Aliment Pharmacol Ther 1999;13(11):1397–402.

[45] Gasche C, Goel A, Natarajan L, et al. Mesalazine improves replication fidelity in cultured colorectal cells. Cancer Res 2005;65(10):3993–7.

[46] Allgayer H, Hofer P, Schmidt M, et al. Superoxide, hydroxyl and fatty acid radical scavenging by aminosalicylates. Direct evaluation with electron spin resonance spectroscopy. Biochem Pharmacol 1992;43(2):259–62.

[47] Allgayer H, Rang S, Klotz U, et al. Superoxide inhibition following different stimuli of respiratory burst and metabolism of aminosalicylates in neutrophils. Dig Dis Sci 1994;39(1):145–51.

[48] McKenzie SM, Doe WF, Buffinton GD. 5-Aminosalicylic acid prevents oxidant mediated damage of glyceraldehyde-3-phosphate dehydrogenase in colon epithelial cells. Gut 1999;44(2):180–5.

[49] Chu E, Chai J, Tarnawski AS. Mesalamine downregulates oncogene c-myc and genes encoding transcription factors and signaling transduction molecules involved in cell survival

and proliferation in colon cancer cells: molecular basis for chemopreventative action. Gastroenterology 2006;130(4 Suppl 2):A-184.

[50] Grimm G, Lee G, Dirisina R, et al. Dose-dependent inhibition of stem cell activation by 5-ASA: a possible explanation for the chemo preventative effect of %-ASA therapy in colitis-induced cancer. Gastroenterology 2006;130(4 Suppl 2):A-693.

[51] Lashner BA, Heidenreich PA, Su GL, et al. Effect of folate supplementation on the incidence of dysplasia and cancer in chronic ulcerative colitis. A case-control study. Gastroenterology 1989;97(2):255–9.

[52] Tung BY, Emond MJ, Haggitt RC, et al. Ursodiol use is associated with lower prevalence of colonic neoplasia in patients with ulcerative colitis and primary sclerosing cholangitis. Ann Intern Med 2001;134(2):89–95.

[53] Lindor KD. Ursodiol for primary sclerosing cholangitis. Mayo Primary Sclerosing Cholangitis-Ursodeoxycholic Acid Study Group. N Engl J Med 1997;336(10):691–5.

[54] Pardi DS, Loftus EV Jr, Kremers WK, et al. Ursodeoxycholic acid as a chemopreventive agent in patients with ulcerative colitis and primary sclerosing cholangitis. Gastroenterology 2003;124(4):889–93.

[55] Shetty K, Rybicki L, Brzezinski A, et al. The risk for cancer or dysplasia in ulcerative colitis patients with primary sclerosing cholangitis. Am J Gastroenterol 1999;94(6):1643–9.

[56] Brentnall TA, Haggitt RC, Rabinovitch PS, et al. Risk and natural history of colonic neoplasia in patients with primary sclerosing cholangitis and ulcerative colitis. Gastroenterology 1996;110(2):331–8.

[57] Smith T, Swaroop P. Mesalamine reduces the rate of colorectal dysplasia in patients with inflammatory bowel disease and primary sclerosing cholangitis who are on ursodeoxycholic acid. Gastroenterology 2006;130(4 Suppl 2):A-653.

[58] Pinczowski D, Ekbom A, Baron J, et al. Risk factors for colorectal cancer in patients with ulcerative colitis: a case-control study. Gastroenterology 1994;107(1):117–20.

[59] Moody GA, Jayanthi V, Probert CS, et al. Long-term therapy with sulphasalazine protects against colorectal cancer in ulcerative colitis: a retrospective study of colorectal cancer risk and compliance with treatment in Leicestershire. Eur J Gastroenterol Hepatol 1996;8(12):1179–83.

[60] Lashner BA, Provencher KS, Seidner DL, et al. The effect of folic acid supplementation on the risk for cancer or dysplasia in ulcerative colitis. Gastroenterology 1997;112(1):29–32.

[61] Eaden J, Abrams K, Ekbom A, et al. Colorectal cancer prevention in ulcerative colitis: a case-control study. Aliment Pharmacol Ther 2000;14(2):145–53.

[62] Eaden J. Review article: the data supporting a role for aminosalicylates in the chemoprevention of colorectal cancer in patients with inflammatory bowel disease. Aliment Pharmacol Ther 2003;18(Suppl 2):15–21.

[63] Lindberg BU, Broome U, Persson B. Proximal colorectal dysplasia or cancer in ulcerative colitis. The impact of primary sclerosing cholangitis and sulfasalazine: results from a 20-year surveillance study. Dis Colon Rectum 2001;44(1):77–85.

[64] Bernstein CN, Blanchard JF, Metge C, et al. Does the use of 5-aminosalicylates in inflammatory bowel disease prevent the development of colorectal cancer? Am J Gastroenterol 2003;98(12):2784–8.

[65] Rubin DT, Djordjevic A, Dezheng H, et al. Use of 5-ASA is associated with decreased risk of dysplasia and colon cancer (CRC) in ulcerative colitis (UC). Gastroenterology 2003;124(4 Suppl 1):A-36.

[66] van Staa TP, Card T, Logan RF, et al. 5-Aminosalicylate use and colorectal cancer risk in inflammatory bowel disease: a large epidemiological study. Gut 2005;54(11):1573–8.

[67] Terdiman JP, Ullman T, Blumentals WA, et al. A case-control of 5-aminosalicylic acid therapy in the prevention of colitis-related colorectal cancer. Gastroenterology 2005;128(4 Suppl 2):A-299.

[68] Siegel CA, Kamin I, Sands BE. Risk factors for colorectal cancer in Crohn's colitis: a case-control study. Gastroenterology 2006;130(4 Suppl 2):A-2.

[69] Velayos FS, Loftus EV Jr, Jess T, et al. Predictive and protective factors associated with colorectal cancer in ulcerative colitis: a case-control study. Gastroenterology 2006;130(7):1941–9.

[70] Giannini EG, Kane SV, Testa R, et al. 5-ASA and colorectal cancer chemoprevention in inflammatory bowel disease: can we afford to wait for 'best evidence'? Dig Liver Dis 2005;37(10):723–31.

[71] Rubin DT, Lashner BA. Will a 5-ASA a day keep the cancer (and dysplasia) away? Am J Gastroenterol 2005;100(6):1354–6.

[72] Akram S, Loftus EV, Tremaine WJ, et al. Determinants of progression of indefinite or low-grade dysplasia to advance dysplasia in ulcerative colitis. Gastroenterology 2006;130(4 Suppl 2):A-647.

[73] Velayos F, Loftus EV, Jess T, et al. Colorectal cancer survival in ulcerative colitis is associated with prior use of 5-aminosalicylic acid but not surveillance colonoscopy. Gastroenterology 2006;130(4 Suppl 2):A-2.

[74] Ullman T, Croog V, Harpaz N, et al. Progression of flat low-grade dysplasia to advanced neoplasia in patients with ulcerative colitis. Gastroenterology 2003;125(5):1311–9.

[75] Kaufmann HJ, Taubin HL. Nonsteroidal anti-inflammatory drugs activate quiescent inflammatory bowel disease. Ann Intern Med 1987;107(4):513–6.

[76] Felder JB, Korelitz BI, Rajapakse R, et al. Effects of nonsteroidal antiinflammatory drugs on inflammatory bowel disease: a case-control study. Am J Gastroenterol 2000;95(8): 1949–54.

[77] Evans JM, McMahon AD, Murray FE, et al. Non-steroidal anti-inflammatory drugs are associated with emergency admission to hospital for colitis due to inflammatory bowel disease. Gut 1997;40(5):619–22.

[78] Bonner GF, Fakhri A, Vennamaneni SR. A long-term cohort study of nonsteroidal anti-inflammatory drug use and disease activity in outpatients with inflammatory bowel disease. Inflamm Bowel Dis 2004;10(6):751–7.

[79] Takeuchi K, Smale S, Premchand P, et al. Prevalence and mechanism of nonsteroidal anti-inflammatory drug-induced clinical relapse in patients with inflammatory bowel disease. Clin Gastroenterol Hepatol 2006;4(2):196–202.

[80] Sandborn WJ, Stenson WF, Brynskov J, et al. Safety of celecoxib in patients with ulcerative colitis in remission: a randomized, placebo-controlled, pilot study. Clin Gastroenterol Hepatol 2006;4(2):203–11.

[81] Bansal P, Sonnenberg A. Risk factors of colorectal cancer in inflammatory bowel disease. Am J Gastroenterol 1996;91(1):44–8.

[82] Present DH, Korelitz BI, Wisch N, et al. Treatment of Crohn's disease with 6-mercaptopurine. A long-term, randomized, double-blind study. N Engl J Med 1980;302(18): 981–7.

[83] Bouhnik Y, Lemann M, Mary JY, et al. Long-term follow-up of patients with Crohn's disease treated with azathioprine or 6-mercaptopurine. Lancet 1996;347(8996):215–9.

[84] Jones M, Symmons D, Finn J, et al. Does exposure to immunosuppressive therapy increase the 10 year malignancy and mortality risks in rheumatoid arthritis? A matched cohort study. Br J Rheumatol 1996;35(8):738–45.

[85] Asten P, Barrett J, Symmons D. Risk of developing certain malignancies is related to duration of immunosuppressive drug exposure in patients with rheumatic diseases. J Rheumatol 1999;26(8):1705–14.

[86] Agraharkar ML, Cinclair RD, Kuo YF, et al. Risk of malignancy with long-term immunosuppression in renal transplant recipients. Kidney Int 2004;66(1):383–9.

[87] Kandiel A, Fraser AG, Korelitz BI, et al. Increased risk of lymphoma among inflammatory bowel disease patients treated with azathioprine and 6-mercaptopurine. Gut 2005;54(8): 1121–5.

[88] Connell WR, Kamm MA, Dickson M, et al. Long-term neoplasia risk after azathioprine treatment in inflammatory bowel disease. Lancet 1994;343(8908):1249–52.

[89] Fraser AG, Orchard TR, Robinson EM, et al. Long-term risk of malignancy after treatment of inflammatory bowel disease with azathioprine. Aliment Pharmacol Ther 2002;16(7): 1225–32.

[90] Matula S, Croog V, Itzkowitz S, et al. Chemoprevention of colorectal neoplasia in ulcerative colitis: the effect of 6-mercaptopurine. Clin Gastroenterol Hepatol 2005;3(10): 1015–21.

[91] Su C, Lichtenstein GR. Treatment of inflammatory bowel disease with azathioprine and 6-mercaptopurine. Gastroenterol Clin North Am 2004;33(2):209–34.

[92] Broome U, Lofberg R, Veress B, et al. Primary sclerosing cholangitis and ulcerative colitis: evidence for increased neoplastic potential. Hepatology 1995;22(5):1404–8.

[93] Harnois DM, Angulo P, Jorgensen RA, et al. High-dose ursodeoxycholic acid as a therapy for patients with primary sclerosing cholangitis. Am J Gastroenterol 2001;96(5): 1558–62.

[94] Hill MJ, Melville DM, Lennard-Jones JE, et al. Faecal bile acids, dysplasia, and carcinoma in ulcerative colitis. Lancet 1987;2(8552):185–6.

[95] Nagengast FM, Grubben MJ, van Munster IP. Role of bile acids in colorectal carcinogenesis. Eur J Cancer 1995;31A(7–8):1067–70.

[96] Martinez JD, Stratagoules ED, LaRue JM, et al. Different bile acids exhibit distinct biological effects: the tumor promoter deoxycholic acid induces apoptosis and the chemopreventive agent ursodeoxycholic acid inhibits cell proliferation. Nutr Cancer 1998;31(2):111–8.

[97] Mitsuyoshi H, Nakashima T, Sumida Y, et al. Ursodeoxycholic acid protects hepatocytes against oxidative injury via induction of antioxidants. Biochem Biophys Res Commun 1999;263(2):537–42.

[98] Hawk ET, Viner JL. Chemoprevention in ulcerative colitis: narrowing the gap between clinical practice and research. Ann Intern Med 2001;134(2):158–60.

[99] Sjoqvist U, Tribukait B, Ost A, et al. Ursodeoxycholic acid treatment in IBD-patients with colorectal dysplasia and/or DNA-aneuploidy: a prospective, double-blind, randomized controlled pilot study. Anticancer Res 2004;24(5B):3121–7.

[100] Wolf JM, Rybicki LA, Lashner BA. The impact of ursodeoxycholic acid on cancer, dysplasia and mortality in ulcerative colitis patients with primary sclerosing cholangitis. Aliment Pharmacol Ther 2005;22(9):783–8.

[101] Kim YI, Pogribny IP, Basnakian AG, et al. Folate deficiency in rats induces DNA strand breaks and hypomethylation within the p53 tumor suppressor gene. Am J Clin Nutr 1997;65(1):46–52.

[102] Goelz SE, Vogelstein B, Hamilton SR, et al. Hypomethylation of DNA from benign and malignant human colon neoplasms. Science 1985;228(4696):187–90.

[103] Giovannucci E, Stampfer MJ, Colditz GA, et al. Multivitamin use, folate, and colon cancer in women in the Nurses' Health Study. Ann Intern Med 1998;129(7):517–24.

[104] Giovannucci E, Stampfer MJ, Colditz GA, et al. Folate, methionine, and alcohol intake and risk of colorectal adenoma. J Natl Cancer Inst 1993;85(11):875–84.

[105] Elsborg L, Larsen L. Folate deficiency in chronic inflammatory bowel diseases. Scand J Gastroenterol 1979;14(8):1019–24.

[106] Swinson CM, Perry J, Lumb M, et al. Role of sulphasalazine in the aetiology of folate deficiency in ulcerative colitis. Gut 1981;22(6):456–61.

[107] Franklin JL, Rosenberg HH. Impaired folic acid absorption in inflammatory bowel disease: effects of salicylazosulfapyridine (Azulfidine). Gastroenterology 1973;64(4):517–25.

[108] Selhub J, Dhar GJ, Rosenberg IH. Inhibition of folate enzymes by sulfasalazine. J Clin Invest 1978;61(1):221–4.

[109] Lashner BA. Red blood cell folate is associated with the development of dysplasia and cancer in ulcerative colitis. J Cancer Res Clin Oncol 1993;119(9):549–54.

[110] Biasco G, Zannoni U, Paganelli GM, et al. Folic acid supplementation and cell kinetics of rectal mucosa in patients with ulcerative colitis. Cancer Epidemiol Biomarkers Prev 1997;6(6):469–71.

[111] Biasco G, Paganelli GM, Miglioli M, et al. Rectal cell proliferation and colon cancer risk in ulcerative colitis. Cancer Res 1990;50(4):1156–9.

[112] Newmark HL, Wargovich MJ, Bruce WR. Colon cancer and dietary fat, phosphate, and calcium: a hypothesis. J Natl Cancer Inst 1984;72(6):1323–5.

[113] Van der Meer R, Lapre JA, Govers MJ, et al. Mechanisms of the intestinal effects of dietary fats and milk products on colon carcinogenesis. Cancer Lett 1997;114(1–2):75–83.

[114] Weingarten MA, Zalmanovici A, Yaphe J. Dietary calcium supplementation for preventing colorectal cancer and adenomatous polyps. Cochrane Database Syst Rev 2005;3: CD003548.

[115] Wactawski-Wende J, Kotchen JM, Anderson GL, et al. Calcium plus vitamin D supplementation and the risk of colorectal cancer. N Engl J Med 2006;354(7):684–96.

[116] Bostick RM, Boldt M, Darif M, et al. Calcium and colorectal epithelial cell proliferation in ulcerative colitis. Cancer Epidemiol Biomarkers Prev 1997;6(12):1021–7.

[117] Demierre MF, Higgins PD, Gruber SB, et al. Statins and cancer prevention. Nat Rev Cancer 2005;5(12):930–42.

[118] Khurana V, Barkin JS, Caldito G, et al. Statins reduce the risk of pancreatic cancer in humans: half a million US veterans' case control study. Gastroenterology 2005; 128(4 Suppl 2):A-62.

[119] Khurana V, Chalasani R, Caldito G, et al. Statins reduce the incidence of esophageal cancer: a study of half a million US veterans. Gastroenterology 2005;128(4 Suppl 2):A-93.

[120] Poynter JN, Gruber SB, Higgins PD, et al. Statins and the risk of colorectal cancer. N Engl J Med 2005;352(21):2184–92.

[121] Bat L, Pines A, Ron E, et al. Colorectal adenomatous polyps and carcinoma in Ashkenazi and non-Ashkenazi Jews in Israel. Cancer 1986;58(5):1167–71.

[122] Kohno H, Suzuki R, Sugie S, et al. Suppression of colitis-related mouse colon carcinogenesis by a COX-2 inhibitor and PPAR ligands. BMC Cancer 2005;5(1):46.

[123] D'Argenio G, Cosenza V, Delle Cave M, et al. Butyrate enemas in experimental colitis and protection against large bowel cancer in a rat model. Gastroenterology 1996;110(6): 1727–34.

[124] Kohno H, Yoshitani S, Takashima S, et al. Troglitazone, a ligand for peroxisome proliferator-activated receptor gamma, inhibits chemically-induced aberrant crypt foci in rats. Jpn J Cancer Res 2001;92(4):396–403.

[125] Tanaka T, Kohno H, Yoshitani S, et al. Ligands for peroxisome proliferator-activated receptors alpha and gamma inhibit chemically induced colitis and formation of aberrant crypt foci in rats. Cancer Res 2001;61(6):2424–8.

[126] Takeda J, Kitajima K, Fujii S, et al. Inhibitory effects of etodolac, a selective COX-2 inhibitor, on the occurrence of tumors in colitis-induced tumorigenesis model in rats. Oncol Rep 2004;11(5):981–5.

[127] Seril DN, Liao J, Ho KL, et al. Inhibition of chronic ulcerative colitis-associated colorectal adenocarcinoma development in a murine model by N-acetylcysteine. Carcinogenesis 2002;23(6):993–1001.

Gastroenterol Clin N Am 35 (2006) 713–727

GASTROENTEROLOGY CLINICS
OF NORTH AMERICA

ELSEVIER
SAUNDERS

Systemic Treatment of Patients Who Have Colorectal Cancer and Inflammatory Bowel Disease

Wolfram Goessling, MD, PhD[a-d], Robert J. Mayer, MD[a,b],*

[a]Department of Medical Oncology, Dana-Farber Cancer Institute, 44 Binney Street,
Boston, MA 02115, USA
[b]Department of Medicine, Brigham and Women's Hospital, Harvard Medical School,
75 Francis Street, Boston, MA 02115, USA
[c]Gastrointestinal Unit, Department of Medicine, Massachusetts General Hospital,
55 Fruit Street, Boston, MA 02114, USA
[d]Stem Cell Program and Division of Hematology/Oncology, Children's Hospital,
300 Longwood Avenue, Boston, MA 02115, USA

Inflammatory bowel disease (IBD) is an acknowledged predisposing factor for the development of intestinal and extraintestinal cancers [1,2]. In general, an increased risk for colorectal cancer exists for patients who have both ulcerative colitis (UC) and Crohn's disease (CD). Small bowel tumors are extremely rare in the general population, but their incidence is enhanced 40-fold in patients who have CD, and include adenocarcinoma, leiomyosarcoma, lymphoma, and neuroendocrine tumors [2–7]. Chronic perineal inflammation in CD may be responsible for the increased incidence of squamous cell carcinomas of the anus [8] and vulva [9]. UC confers a marginally increased risk for myeloid leukemia, whereas patients who have CD may have a trend toward a higher incidence of lymphoma, possibly related to the disease itself or to the use of immunosuppressive therapy [10–16]. Although epidemiologic and molecular aspects of carcinogenesis and screening strategies for patients who have IBD are covered elsewhere in this issue, this article reviews the therapeutic options for the most common malignant complication, colorectal carcinoma, as well as specific recommendations regarding the impact of the underlying disease upon the tolerance and efficacy of chemotherapy. Detailed aspects of the treatment of these tumors in the setting of IBD have not been dealt with in the past. This article focuses on the role of the oncologist in the treatment of colorectal cancer in the setting of IBD.

*Corresponding author. Department of Medical Oncology, Dana-Farber Cancer Institute, 44 Binney Street, Boston, MA 02115. E-mail address: robert_mayer@dfci.harvard.edu (R.J. Mayer).

0889-8553/06/$ – see front matter
doi:10.1016/j.gtc.2006.07.006
© 2006 Elsevier Inc. All rights reserved.
gastro.theclinics.com

COLORECTAL CANCER

Colorectal cancer is the third most common malignancy and the second most frequent cause of cancer-related death in the United States [17]. It is anticipated that almost 150,000 new cases will be diagnosed in 2006, resulting in more than 55,000 deaths. Patients with long-standing extensive UC and CD have an increased risk for developing colorectal cancer as well as extraintestinal cancers when compared with the general population; this association has been reported for UC and CD in population-based and referral center studies, as well as meta-analyses [6,18]. The risk progresses with longer duration of the IBD, extent of colonic involvement, and severity of inflammation [5,7,19,20]. The tumors appear earlier in life than do sporadic colorectal cancers and a higher percentage are proximal to the splenic flexure, which reflects the differences in biology and carcinogenic mechanism [21]. These observations have led to the emergence of endoscopic surveillance programs [22]; several reports have suggested a lower 5-year mortality from colorectal cancer for patients who undergo such surveillance [23–25]; however, a recent statistical analysis of the available literature argues that convincing outcome results are lacking to support such a surveillance practice [26]. Only one retrospective study is available that compared the overall outcome for patients who had colon cancer and IBD with patients who had colorectal cancer alone. No difference in 5-year survival was found between 290 patients who had colorectal cancer and IBD at the Mayo Clinic when compared with age- and sex-matched patients who had colorectal cancer but not IBD [21]. Furthermore, no data are available to assess the specific treatment options in patients who have IBD who develop colorectal cancer. Therefore, this article highlights the difficulties that oncologists face when caring for patients who have IBD and colorectal cancer. It focuses on the available information regarding tolerability of different treatment regimens in the general patient population, combined with personal experience in the care of these patients. It emphasizes the need for prospective interdisciplinary studies to provide the best possible care for these patients as the treatment options for colorectal cancer continue to evolve.

DIAGNOSTIC CHALLENGES

Although screening programs in the general population seem to be detecting more colorectal cancers at an earlier stage, many patients still are diagnosed because of such symptoms as bloating, abdominal pain, intermittent diarrhea, and bloody stools, in addition to systemic symptoms, such as weight loss, anorexia, and fatigue. All of these symptoms also are associated with IBD in the absence of malignancy, which makes it extremely difficult to distinguish subtle clinical changes that may herald the appearance of cancer [27]. It is this overlap in symptoms between the underlying disease and the secondary malignancy that makes regular endoscopic surveillance so theoretically appealing. Even with endoscopic surveillance, however, making a diagnosis of cancer remains difficult because as many as two thirds of the tumors that arise in patients who have IBD do not arise from polyps and even may be missed on serial biopsies [28,29]. Furthermore, malignancies may arise in strictures; the symptoms of benign strictures are identical to those of malignant ones, and endoscopic (ie, superficial) biopsies of such strictures may reveal only inflammation where a carcinoma—subsequently identified through surgical resection—is actually present [30]. More sensitive endoscopic techniques, such as chromoendoscopy and endoscopic optical coherence tomography, are being developed and will allow in vivo molecular and functional imaging to enhance the rate of cancer detection [31]. See article by Kiesslich and Neurath elsewhere in this issue for a discussion of these new imaging modalities.

CHEMOTHERAPY

The pathologic stage at presentation is the most important prognostic factor for patients who have colorectal cancer, and it dictates the treatment options. Depth of tumor invasion through the bowel wall and regional lymph node involvement, as used in the TNM staging system, are the main predictors of outcome (Table 1). Chemotherapy reduces mortality in the adjuvant setting and prolongs survival for patients who have metastatic disease. For decades, treatment with

Table 1
TNM staging system for colorectal cancer

Primary tumor (T)

T_x	Primary tumor cannot be assessed
T_{is}	Carcinoma in situ
T_1	Tumor invades submucosa
T_2	Tumor invades muscularis propia
T_3	Tumor invades through the muscularis propia into the subserosa
T_4	Tumor directly invades other organs or structures, or perforates visceral peritoneum

Regional lymph nodes (N)

N_x	Regional lymph nodes cannot be assessed
N_0	No regional lymph node metastases
N_1	Metastases in one to three regional lymph nodes
N_2	Metastases in four or more regional lymph nodes

Distant metastases (M)

M_x	Presence or absence of distant metastases cannot be determined
M_0	No distant metastases detected
M_1	Distant metastases detected

Stage grouping and 5-yr survival

Stage	TNM classification	5-yr survival
I	T_{1-2}, N_0, M_0	>90%
IIA	T_3, N_0, M_0	60–85%
IIB	T_4, N_0, M_0	
IIIA	T_{1-2}, N_1, M_0	55–60%
IIIB	T_{3-4}, N_1, M_0	35–42%
IIIC	T_{1-4}, N_2, M_0	25–27%
IV	T_{1-4}, N_{0-2}, M_1	5–7%

Adapted from Meyerhardt JA, Mayer RJ. Systemic therapy for colorectal cancer. N Engl J Med 2005;352(5):478; with permission. © 2005 Massachusetts Medical Society.

fluoropyrimidines has been the backbone of therapy; however, recently, additional chemotherapeutic agents and targeted drugs have proven useful as well.

FLUOROPYRIMIDINES

Fluorouracil (5-FU), a fluorinated pyrimidine, is believed to act primarily by inhibiting thymidylate synthase, and, thereby, impairs nucleotide synthesis and DNA replication. Almost 50 years after its development, 5-FU remains the central drug of colon cancer therapy and typically is given with leucovorin (also known as folinic acid), which enhances the binding of the drug to its target, thymidylate synthase. The combination of 5-FU and leucovorin results in an objective response rate of 20% (ie, shrinkage of tumor size by >50%) and prolongs the median survival in patients who have metastatic disease from approximately 6 months to 11 months [32]. Data regarding specific therapeutic considerations for patients who have advanced colorectal cancer and also have clinically active IBD are virtually nonexistent. In one small retrospective study, 19 such patients who were treated with 5-FU–based chemotherapy at Memorial Sloan-Kettering Cancer Center over a 10-year period from 1985 to 1995 were reviewed; 9 patients had UC, whereas 10 patients had CD [33]. Most of these patients (14 of 19) had colon cancer, 1 patient had anal cancer, and 2 patients each had esophageal and gastric cancer. The treatment dose schedules varied among this heterogeneous group of patients, some of whom were given adjuvant therapy after surgery, whereas others were treated palliatively for metastatic disease. All received some form of 5-FU, and most received the combination of 5-FU and leucovorin. Five patients received concurrent or subsequent radiation therapy. Of the 19 patients, 53% (10 patients) experienced dose-limiting diarrhea compared with the 5% to 15% figure that typically is associated with this treatment in randomized trials [34–36]. The diarrhea led to discontinuation of therapy in 5 patients and dose reduction in another 5 patients. Patient age, type of IBD, and dosing schedule of 5-FU did not seem to influence the frequency of severe diarrhea. The degree of disease activity of IBD before treatment had no effect or predictive value for the development of diarrhea. In particular, the absence of active inflammation did not confer a lower incidence of diarrhea, which implies that the presence of the underlying disease leaves the mucosa more vulnerable to the effects of chemotherapy. None of the patients in this study experienced a catastrophic event, such as treatment-related deaths or bowel perforation while undergoing chemotherapy. The study does not report on the response rates to chemotherapy or on the overall outcome (eg, 5-year survival or time to progression). These observations led the investigators to recommend that patients who have IBD and gastrointestinal malignancies should be administered full treatment doses, but should be monitored carefully for increased toxicity and prophylactic dose reductions.

Several 5-FU dosing regimens have been established to treat colorectal cancer. Although these regimens are equivalent therapeutically, they have distinguishing toxicity profiles. Diarrhea occurs more frequently when 5-FU is given in a bolus manner (Table 2) [37–43]. In the so-called "Roswell Park

Table 2
Drugs used in the treatment of colon cancer and their use in patients who have inflammatory bowel disease

Drug	Administration regimen	Dosing	Schedule	Major toxicity	Recommended treatment with IBD
5-FU/ leucovorin	Mayo (bolus)	5-FU 425 mg/m² bolus on days 1–5 LV 20 mg/m² bolus on days 1–5	Every 4–5 wk	Diarrhea, neutropenia	No
	Roswell Park (bolus)	5-FU 500 mg/m² bolus LV 500 mg/m² over 2 h	Weekly for 6 out of 8 wk	Diarrhea	No
	Continuous infusion	5-FU 400 mg/m² bolus on days 1,2 + 600 mg/m² IVCI over 22 h on days 1,2 LV 200 mg/m² over 2 h on days 1,2	Every 2 wk	Hand-foot syndrome	Yes
Capecitabine		1250 mg/m² orally twice per day on days 1–14	Every 3 wk	Hand-foot syndrome	Needs further study
Irinotecan	IFL	5-FU 500 mg/m² bolus LV 20 mg/m² bolus Irinotecan 125 mg/m²	Weekly for 4 out of 6 wk	Diarrhea, neutropenia, sepsis	No
	FOLFIRI	5-FU 400 mg/m² bolus on day 1 + 2400–3000 mg/m² IVCI over 46 h on days 1,2 LV 400 mg/m² over 2 h on day 1 Irinotecan 180 mg/m² on day 1	Every 2 wk	Diarrhea, neutropenia, sepsis	No
Oxaliplatin	FOLFOX	5-FU 400 mg/m² bolus + 600 mg/m² IVCI over 22 h on days 1,2 LV 200 mg/m² over 2 h on days 1,2 Oxaliplatin 85 mg/m² on day 1	Every 2 wk	Neuropathy, myelosuppression	Yes
Cetuximab		Cetuximab 250 mg/m² on days 1,8 (first dose only: 400 mg/m²) Irinotecan 180 mg/m² on day 1	Every 2 wk	Rash	Yes, needs further study
Bevacizumab		Bevacizumab 5 mg/kg on day 1 with fluorouracil-based chemotherapy	Every 2 wk	Intestinal perforation	No, needs further study

Abbreviations: LV, leucovorin; IVCI, intravenous continuous infusion.
Modified from Wolpin BM, Meyerhardt JA, Mamon HJ, et al. Adjuvant therapy in colorectal cancer. CA Cancer J Clin 2006; in press; with permission.

regimen," bolus fluorouracil and leucovorin are administered weekly for 6 out of 8 weeks; significant diarrhea is observed frequently with the diarrhea occasionally being bloody and extremely watery, which may lead to severe dehydration [44]. The so-called "Mayo Clinic regimen" consists of bolus fluorouracil and leucovorin administered daily for 5 days every 4 to 5 weeks; neutropenia, stomatitis, and diarrhea (less than that associated with the Roswell Park regimen) are the most common side effects. The disruption of mucosal integrity as the result of mucositis in the neutropenic patient may facilitate bacterial entry into the bloodstream and resultant sepsis. Continuous infusional 5-FU, given for several weeks through a pump on an ambulatory basis, is more expensive and inconvenient for the patient than are the other regimens; however, it has the lowest incidence of diarrhea and hematologic toxicities [42] and it has been tolerated well anecdotally in patients who had IBD. Its major side effect is the hand-foot syndrome, a reversible erythematous, painful rash that involves the palms and soles. An oral formulation, capecitabine, undergoes a three-step enzymatic conversion to the active compound fluorouracil and has a similar side effect profile and median survival to that of continuous infusion 5-FU. The incidence of diarrhea seems to be higher for capecitabine than for infusional 5-FU, but it is still lower than when 5-FU is given in a bolus manner [45–47].

IRINOTECAN

Irinotecan is a semisynthetic topoisomerase I inhibitor that causes the persistence of DNA strand breaks during replication. It is a prodrug that is hydrolyzed in the liver into the active compound, SN-38. The most common dose-limiting toxicity of the drug is delayed-onset diarrhea, which occurs in up to 33% of treated patients (see Table 2). Typically, the diarrhea begins during the second or third week of treatment on a weekly infusion schedule. The degree of diarrhea can be improved by intensive and early therapy with oral loperamide [48]. The drug is glucuronidated by hepatic uridine diphosphate glucuronosyltransferase 1A1, and polymorphisms of this enzyme have been linked to differences in drug metabolism that influence and predict for the incidence and severity of toxicity [49–52]. For the treatment of advanced colorectal cancer, irinotecan is used in combination with weekly bolus 5-FU/leucovorin ("IFL") or with infusional 5-FU/leucovorin every 2 weeks [53,54]. The gastrointestinal and hematologic toxicities of irinotecan and 5-FU are additive, especially when bolus 5-FU is a component as in the IFL regimen; the diarrhea that is experienced by patients who are treated in this manner can be far more severe than in patients who are treated with 5-FU alone. Furthermore, the combination of neutropenia and injury to the intestinal mucosal that is due to irinotecan enhances the risk for sepsis greatly [55–58]. No reports are available for the use of irinotecan in patients who have IBD, but one would expect a high rate of dose-limiting diarrhea and possible sepsis given the experience with 5-FU alone [33]. This drug probably should be avoided in patients who have IBD.

OXALIPLATIN

Oxaliplatin is a platinum compound that induces DNA damage by forming DNA adducts or cross-links and inducing apoptosis. Its administration leads to a cumulative, but usually reversible, sensory neuropathy, predominantly in the hands and feet [59]. It acts synergistically with 5-FU, in regards to therapeutic efficacy and also in relation to myelosuppression and diarrhea (see Table 2). Oxaliplatin has little activity in colon cancer as a single agent, but it has been combined successfully with infusional 5-FU and leucovorin (FOLFOX) to treat metastatic disease [60,61] or as adjuvant therapy [62]. It also has been combined effectively with bolus 5-FU and leucovorin as adjuvant therapy [63]. The incidence of severe diarrhea in regimens that contain oxaliplatin and 5-FU seems to be less than in those using irinotecan with 5-FU. Therefore, FOLFOX seems to be a more appropriate treatment choice for patients who have IBD-associated colorectal cancer in the adjuvant and palliative setting. This may be of particular importance for patients who have active intestinal inflammation.

TARGETED THERAPIES
Monoclonal Antibodies Against the Epidermal Growth Factor Receptor: Cetuximab and Panitumumab

The epidermal growth factor receptor (EGFR) is a 170,000-kd transmembrane protein that belongs to the c-ErbB group of growth factor receptors that also includes Her2/neu. Its activation affects several signaling pathways that result in cellular growth, differentiation, and proliferation [64]. Cetuximab is a recombinant, chimeric, monoclonal antibody that binds specifically to EGFR on normal and tumor cells, and competitively inhibits the binding of epidermal growth factor (EGF) and other ligands, such as transforming growth factor-α. Binding of the antibody inhibits receptor activation and subsequent autophosphorylation and signal transduction [65]. The predominant side effect that is associated with cetuximab is an acneiform rash that correlates with an increased likelihood of response [66–68]. Cetuximab is effective as a second-line agent, either alone or in combination with irinotecan, in patients who have advanced colorectal cancer whose disease had progressed previously following treatment with an irinotecan-containing regimen [66,69,70]. The likelihood of such benefit seems to be unrelated to the extent of EGFR expression on the surface of tumor cells. Panitumumab is a fully humanized monoclonal antibody to EGFR that seems to have similar activity as cetuximab in single-agent trials in patients who have metastatic colorectal cancer. Several studies using panitumumab, either in combination with chemotherapy or alone, are ongoing.

In general, growth factor–dependent signaling pathways are not only important in carcinogenesis but also in early embryonal development. The observed paucity of severe gastrointestinal side effects in patients who are treated with cetuximab might be due to the selectivity of the drug for a target and the relative quiescence of the targeted pathway in homeostatic adult tissue. During acute or chronic inflammation or injury, these pathways may be activated to induce processes of tissue regeneration, repair, and growth. It has been postulated that the up-regulation of pathways, such as EGF, may be a promoting factor in carcinogenesis in patients who have IBD [71]. Activation of the EGF pathway also could be instrumental to repair processes in colitis [72]. Mice that are deficient for the EGF receptor protein (waved-2) are more susceptible to chemically (dextran) induced diarrhea [73], whereas inhibition of EGFR tyrosine kinase results in growth inhibition of cultured gut explants [74]. In various mouse models of colitis, the addition of EGF reduced intestinal apoptosis [75], improved erosions [76], and restored colonic ion transport [77]. Furthermore, when used in combination, EGF and another growth factor, trefoil factor, reduced the histologic colitis score in dextran-induced diarrhea by more than 40% [78], and were beneficial in indomethacin-induced gastric damage in the rat [79]. For these reasons, EGF therapy has been suggested as a possible treatment of neonatal necrotizing enterocolitis [80]. These data suggest that the EGF pathway plays an important role in repair of the inflamed colon. Although EGFR inhibition does not seem to affect patients who do not have mucosal abnormalities, theoretically, it could exacerbate the severity of the underlying disease in patients who have IBD. There have been no significant gastrointestinal side effects reported with cetuximab, however. Hence, despite these theoretic concerns, its use seems reasonable in patients who have IBD. More studies are needed in this patient population to define the impact of EGFR inhibition on the underlying disease better.

Bevacizumab

Bevacizumab is a humanized, monoclonal antibody that targets the vascular endothelial growth factor, which is responsible for the stimulation of blood vessel growth in tumors. Its most common side effects are hypertension and proteinuria; however, hemoptysis, intestinal perforation, and delayed wound healing have been reported [81,82]. Bevacizumab improved response rates and overall survival in patients who had metastatic colon cancer when given in combination with IFL [83–85] and FOLFOX chemotherapy [86]; it also improved response rates and time to tumor progression when given with 5-FU/leucovorin alone [87]. Bevacizumab is approved by the US Food and Drug Administration for first-line treatment of advanced colorectal cancer in combination with any 5-FU–containing regimen. Because of the possibility of intestinal perforation, one needs to be more cautious about its use in patients who have IBD. Any special considerations or interactions with these drugs with regard to inflammatory bowel disease are hypothetic and have been inferred largely from preclinical studies.

MUCOSA-PROTECTIVE AGENTS

In addition to the possible enteric side effects of chemotherapy, it may prove beneficial to administer drugs that have a protective effect on the intestinal mucosal by inhibiting inflammatory cytokines. One such drug is RDP58, a novel decapeptide, which inhibits the production of tumor necrosis factor (TNF)-α, interferon-γ, and interleukin 12. In rodent models it reduced irinotecan- and 5-FU–induced diarrhea [88] and chemical colitis [89]. Based on these studies, it has been used successfully in an early clinical trial in patients who had UC [90].

TREATMENT COMPLICATIONS

The onset of diarrhea during chemotherapy for colon cancer may be due to the treatment regimen, but it also may be caused by a flare of the underlying IBD [90]. In patients who have CD who have undergone a partial bowel resection, increasing diarrhea could indicate further IBD activity. Furthermore, frequent bowel movements are common in patients who have UC after total colectomy and ileal pouch anal anastomosis. There is no symptom-based method of distinguishing chemotherapy-induced diarrhea from IBD-associated diarrhea. In patients who have IBD, and undergo chemotherapy for colorectal cancer who develop diarrhea, it seems prudent to assume a disease flare and treat with aminosalicylates. Immunosuppressive drugs, such as corticosteroids, 6-mercaptopurine, or TNF-α antagonists, generally should be avoided during chemotherapy because they may lead to a higher incidence of hematologic toxicitics. Endoscopic studies and biopsies may be needed in patients who have persistent diarrhea during or after chemotherapy.

OUTLOOK

In recent years, the treatment of IBD and colorectal cancer has benefited greatly from newly designed pharmacologic approaches, namely TNF-α antagonists in IBD and novel chemotherapy and targeted therapy in colorectal cancer. For patients who have IBD and develop intestinal malignancies, no data are available to select the optimal treatment rationally. Given the prevalence of colorectal cancer in patients who have IBD and the potentially detrimental effects of chemotherapy in these patients, prospective, interdisciplinary studies that bridge the fields of gastroenterology and oncology are needed to provide a basis for the optimal care of this patient population (Box 1). These studies need to address the overall treatment outcomes for patients who have colorectal cancer and IBD compared on a stage-for-stage basis with those reported in patients who have colorectal cancer but do not have IBD; the optimal chemotherapy regimen for these patients; and the potentially preventative effects of IBD-specific therapy on tumor incidence. In addition, it will be important to assess any impact of targeted therapies, such as EGFR antagonists or bevacizumab, on IBD. It is conceivable that these drugs will impact signaling pathways that are important for tissue repair or regeneration and cause significant worsening of the disease during the treatment for cancer.

SUMMARY

Colorectal cancer is the most common malignant complication in patients who have IBD. The disease is difficult to diagnose because there is an overlap in

Box 1: Areas of study for possible clinical studies in patients who have inflammatory bowel disease and colorectal cancer

Prevention

Role of disease-modifying agents on cancer incidence: possible protective effects of aminosalicylates, folic acid, ursodiol, and the immunomodulators

Disease Outcome

Stage-for-stage comparison of mortality and survival data between patients who have colorectal cancer and who do or do not have IBD; delineation of differences in outcome between CD and UC

Chemotherapy Regimen

Study of several treatment regimens for colorectal cancer to evaluate which ones are tolerated best and have the fewest severe side effects, and the ability of patients to complete these regimens compared with patients who do not have IBD

Targeted Therapies

Characterization of the effects of targeted therapies, such as anti-EGFR and antiangiogenic treatment, on the inflammatory activity and long-term outcome of the underlying IBD and the colorectal cancer

symptoms in patients who have colon cancer and those who have IBD. Much has been learned about the incidence of colorectal cancer in patients who have IBD and its correlation with disease activity, duration, and anatomic location; however, almost no data are available regarding specific therapeutic considerations during adjuvant or palliative chemotherapy for these patients with respect to their underlying disease. Patients who have IBD who develop colorectal cancer are at higher risk for developing severe diarrhea during chemotherapy that may be due to the toxic effects of cytotoxic drugs or a flare of the IBD. Continuous infusional 5-FU alone, in combination with leucovorin, or in combination with oxaliplatin (FOLFOX) seems to be tolerated best. Bolus infusions of 5-FU (Roswell Park or Mayo regimens) and combination therapy of irinotecan with 5-FU should be avoided because of severe diarrhea and the possibility of sepsis. When diarrhea develops or worsens, empiric aminosalicylates may be given. Although it is theoretically possible that anti-EGFR therapies could affect IBD activity adversely, clinical experience with cetuximab in patients who have colorectal cancer has not shown any significant gastrointestinal side effects. Therefore, it seems reasonable to use it in patients who have colorectal cancer and IBD. The administration of bevacizumab has been associated with rare episodes of intestinal perforation; it should be used with great care in patients who have IBD. More studies and an integrative, multidisciplinary approach from oncologists and gastroenterologists are needed to provide optimal care for patients who have IBD during chemotherapy for colorectal cancer.

References

[1] Bernstein CN, Blanchard JF, Kliewer E, et al. Cancer risk in patients with inflammatory bowel disease: a population-based study. Cancer 2001;91(4):854–62.

[2] Jess T, Loftus EV Jr, Velayos FS, et al. Risk of intestinal cancer in inflammatory bowel disease: a population-based study from Olmsted County, Minnesota. Gastroenterology 2006;130(4):1039–46.

[3] Jess T, Winther KV, Munkholm P, et al. Intestinal and extra-intestinal cancer in Crohn's disease: follow-up of a population-based cohort in Copenhagen County, Denmark. Aliment Pharmacol Ther 2004;19(3):287–93.

[4] Persson PG, Karlen P, Bernell O, et al. Crohn's disease and cancer: a population-based cohort study. Gastroenterology 1994;107(6):1675–9.

[5] Gillen CD, Walmsley RS, Prior P, et al. Ulcerative colitis and Crohn's disease: a comparison of the colorectal cancer risk in extensive colitis. Gut 1994;35(11):1590–2.

[6] Canavan C, Abrams KR, Mayberry J. Meta-analysis: colorectal and small bowel cancer risk in patients with Crohn's disease. Aliment Pharmacol Ther 2006;23(8):1097–104.

[7] Greenstein AJ, Sachar DB, Smith H, et al. A comparison of cancer risk in Crohn's disease and ulcerative colitis. Cancer 1981;48(12):2742–5.

[8] Connell WR, Sheffield JP, Kamm MA, et al. Lower gastrointestinal malignancy in Crohn's disease. Gut 1994;35(3):347–52.

[9] Prezyna AP, Kalyanaraman U. Bowen's carcinoma in vulvovaginal Crohn's disease (regional enterocolitis): report of first case. Am J Obstet Gynecol 1977;128(8):914–6.

[10] Askling J, Brandt L, Lapidus A, et al. Risk of haematopoietic cancer in patients with inflammatory bowel disease. Gut 2005;54(5):617–22.

[11] Caspi O, Polliack A, Klar R, et al. The association of inflammatory bowel disease and leukemia—coincidence or not? Leuk Lymphoma 1995;17(3–4):255–62.

[12] Farrell RJ, Ang Y, Kileen P, et al. Increased incidence of non-Hodgkin's lymphoma in inflammatory bowel disease patients on immunosuppressive therapy but overall risk is low. Gut 2000;47(4):514–9.

[13] Kwon JH, Farrell RJ. The risk of lymphoma in the treatment of inflammatory bowel disease with immunosuppressive agents. Crit Rev Oncol Hematol 2005;56(1):169–78.

[14] Kandiel A, Fraser AG, Korelitz BI, et al. Increased risk of lymphoma among inflammatory bowel disease patients treated with azathioprine and 6-mercaptopurine. Gut 2005;54(8):1121–5.

[15] Greenstein AJ, Gennuso R, Sachar DB, et al. Extraintestinal cancers in inflammatory bowel disease. Cancer 1985;56(12):2914–21.

[16] Raderer M, Puspok A, Birkner T, et al. Primary gastric mantle cell lymphoma in a patient with long standing history of Crohn's disease. Leuk Lymphoma 2004;45(7):1459–62.

[17] Jemal A, Siegel R, Ward E, et al. Cancer statistics, 2006. CA Cancer J Clin 2006;56(2): 106–30.

[18] Jess T, Gamborg M, Matzen P, et al. Increased risk of intestinal cancer in Crohn's disease: a meta-analysis of population-based cohort studies. Am J Gastroenterol 2005;100(12): 2724–9.

[19] Rutter M, Saunders B, Wilkinson K, et al. Severity of inflammation is a risk factor for colorectal neoplasia in ulcerative colitis. Gastroenterology 2004;126(2):451–9.

[20] Jess T, Loftus EV Jr, Harmsen WS, et al. Survival and cause-specific mortality in patients with inflammatory bowel disease: a long-term outcome study in Olmsted County, Minnesota, 1940–2004. Gut 2006, in press.

[21] Delaunoit T, Limburg PJ, Goldberg RM, et al. Colorectal cancer prognosis among patients with inflammatory bowel disease. Clin Gastroenterol Hepatol 2006;4(3):335–42.

[22] Itzkowitz SH, Present DH. Consensus conference: colorectal cancer screening and surveillance in inflammatory bowel disease. Inflamm Bowel Dis 2005;11(3):314–21.

[23] Choi PM, Nugent FW, Schoetz DJ Jr, et al. Colonoscopic surveillance reduces mortality from colorectal cancer in ulcerative colitis. Gastroenterology 1993;105(2):418–24.

[24] Karlen P, Kornfeld D, Brostrom O, et al. Is colonoscopic surveillance reducing colorectal cancer mortality in ulcerative colitis? A population-based case control study. Gut 1998;42(5): 711–4.

[25] Lindberg J, Stenling R, Palmqvist R, et al. Efficiency of colorectal cancer surveillance in patients with ulcerative colitis: 26 years' experience in a patient cohort from a defined population area. Scand J Gastroenterol 2005;40(9):1076–80.

[26] Collins P, Mpofu C, Watson A, et al. Strategies for detecting colon cancer and/or dysplasia in patients with inflammatory bowel disease. Cochrane Database Syst Rev 2006;(2): CD000279.

[27] Greenstein AJ. Cancer in inflammatory bowel disease. Mt Sinai J Med 2000;67(3): 227–40.

[28] Chawla A, Judge TA, Lichtenstein GR. Evaluation of polypoid lesions in inflammatory bowel disease. Gastrointest Endosc Clin N Am 2002;12(3):525–34.

[29] Itzkowitz SH, Harpaz N. Diagnosis and management of dysplasia in patients with inflammatory bowel diseases. Gastroenterology 2004;126(6):1634–48.

[30] Yamazaki Y, Ribeiro MB, Sachar DB, et al. Malignant colorectal strictures in Crohn's disease. Am J Gastroenterol 1991;86(7):882–5.

[31] Kiesslich R, Hoffman A, Neurath MF. Colonoscopy, tumors, and inflammatory bowel disease - new diagnostic methods. Endoscopy 2006;38(1):5–10.

[32] Meyerhardt JA, Mayer RJ. Systemic therapy for colorectal cancer. N Engl J Med 2005;352(5):476–87.

[33] Tiersten A, Saltz LB. Influence of inflammatory bowel disease on the ability of patients to tolerate systemic fluorouracil-based chemotherapy. J Clin Oncol 1996;14(7):2043–6.

[34] Chau I, Norman AR, Cunningham D, et al. A randomised comparison between 6 months of bolus fluorouracil/leucovorin and 12 weeks of protracted venous infusion fluorouracil as adjuvant treatment in colorectal cancer. Ann Oncol 2005;16(4):549–57.

[35] Andre T, Colin P, Louvet C, et al. Semimonthly versus monthly regimen of fluorouracil and leucovorin administered for 24 or 36 weeks as adjuvant therapy in stage II and III colon cancer: results of a randomized trial. J Clin Oncol 2003;21(15):2896–903.

[36] Haller DG, Catalano PJ, Macdonald JS, et al. Phase III study of fluorouracil, leucovorin, and levamisole in high-risk stage II and III colon cancer: final report of Intergroup 0089. J Clin Oncol 2005;23(34):8671–8.

[37] Erlichman C, Fine S, Wong A, et al. A randomized trial of fluorouracil and folinic acid in patients with metastatic colorectal carcinoma. J Clin Oncol 1988;6(3):469–75.

[38] Poon MA, O'Connell MJ, Moertel CG, et al. Biochemical modulation of fluorouracil: evidence of significant improvement of survival and quality of life in patients with advanced colorectal carcinoma. J Clin Oncol 1989;7(10):1407–18.

[39] Cocconi G, Cunningham D, Van Cutsem E, et al. Open, randomized, multicenter trial of raltitrexed versus fluorouracil plus high-dose leucovorin in patients with advanced colorectal cancer. Tomudex Colorectal Cancer Study Group. J Clin Oncol 1998;16(9):2943–52.

[40] Petrelli N, Douglass HO Jr, Herrera L, et al. The modulation of fluorouracil with leucovorin in metastatic colorectal carcinoma: a prospective randomized phase III trial. Gastrointestinal Tumor Study Group. J Clin Oncol 1989;7(10):1419–26.

[41] Buroker TR, O'Connell MJ, Wieand HS, et al. Randomized comparison of two schedules of fluorouracil and leucovorin in the treatment of advanced colorectal cancer. J Clin Oncol 1994;12(1):14–20.

[42] Toxicity of fluorouracil in patients with advanced colorectal cancer: effect of administration schedule and prognostic factors. Meta-Analysis Group In Cancer. J Clin Oncol 1998;16(11):3537–41.

[43] Wolpin BM, Meyerhardt JA, Mamon HJ, et al. Adjuvant therapy in colorectal cancer. CA Cancer J Clin 2006, in press.

[44] Fata F, Ron IG, Kemeny N, et al. 5-Fluorouracil-induced small bowel toxicity in patients with colorectal carcinoma. Cancer 1999;86(7):1129–34.

[45] Van Cutsem E, Twelves C, Cassidy J, et al. Oral capecitabine compared with intravenous fluorouracil plus leucovorin in patients with metastatic colorectal cancer: results of a large phase III study. J Clin Oncol 2001;19(21):4097–106.
[46] Hoff PM, Ansari R, Batist G, et al. Comparison of oral capecitabine versus intravenous fluorouracil plus leucovorin as first-line treatment in 605 patients with metastatic colorectal cancer: results of a randomized phase III study. J Clin Oncol 2001;19(8):2282–92.
[47] Twelves C, Wong A, Nowacki MP, et al. Capecitabine as adjuvant treatment for stage III colon cancer. N Engl J Med 2005;352(26):2696–704.
[48] Abigerges D, Armand JP, Chabot GG, et al. Irinotecan (CPT-11) high-dose escalation using intensive high-dose loperamide to control diarrhea. J Natl Cancer Inst 1994;86(6):446–9.
[49] Ando M, Hasegawa Y, Ando Y. Pharmacogenetics of irinotecan: a promoter polymorphism of UGT1A1 gene and severe adverse reactions to irinotecan. Invest New Drugs 2005;23(6):539–45.
[50] Mehra R, Murren J, Chung G, et al. Severe irinotecan-induced toxicities in a patient with uridine diphosphate glucuronosyltransferase 1A1 polymorphism. Clin Colorectal Cancer 2005;5(1):61–4.
[51] Innocenti F, Undevia SD, Iyer L, et al. Genetic variants in the UDP-glucuronosyltransferase 1A1 gene predict the risk of severe neutropenia of irinotecan. J Clin Oncol 2004;22(8):1382–8.
[52] Massacesi C, Terrazzino S, Marcucci F, et al. Uridine diphosphate glucuronosyl transferase 1A1 promoter polymorphism predicts the risk of gastrointestinal toxicity and fatigue induced by irinotecan-based chemotherapy. Cancer 2006;106(5):1007–16.
[53] Saltz LB, Cox JV, Blanke C, et al. Irinotecan plus fluorouracil and leucovorin for metastatic colorectal cancer. Irinotecan Study Group. N Engl J Med 2000;343(13):905–14.
[54] Douillard JY, Cunningham D, Roth AD, et al. Irinotecan combined with fluorouracil compared with fluorouracil alone as first-line treatment for metastatic colorectal cancer: a multicentre randomised trial. Lancet 2000;355(9209):1041–7.
[55] Kuehr T, Ruff P, Rapoport BL, et al. Phase I/II study of first-line irinotecan combined with 5-fluorouracil and folinic acid Mayo Clinic schedule in patients with advanced colorectal cancer. BMC Cancer 2004;4:36.
[56] Blanke CD, Haller DG, Benson AB, et al. A phase II study of irinotecan with 5-fluorouracil and leucovorin in patients with previously untreated gastric adenocarcinoma. Ann Oncol 2001;12(11):1575–80.
[57] Rougier P, Bugat R, Douillard JY, et al. Phase II study of irinotecan in the treatment of advanced colorectal cancer in chemotherapy-naive patients and patients pretreated with fluorouracil-based chemotherapy. J Clin Oncol 1997;15(1):251–60.
[58] Sargent DJ, Niedzwiecki D, O'Connell MJ, et al. Recommendation for caution with irinotecan, fluorouracil, and leucovorin for colorectal cancer. N Engl J Med 2001;345(2):144–5.
[59] Lehky TJ, Leonard GD, Wilson RH, et al. Oxaliplatin-induced neurotoxicity: acute hyperexcitability and chronic neuropathy. Muscle Nerve 2004;29(3):387–92.
[60] de Gramont A, Figer A, Seymour M, et al. Leucovorin and fluorouracil with or without oxaliplatin as first-line treatment in advanced colorectal cancer. J Clin Oncol 2000;18(16):2938–47.
[61] Kemeny N, Garay CA, Gurtler J, et al. Randomized multicenter phase II trial of bolus plus infusional fluorouracil/leucovorin compared with fluorouracil/leucovorin plus oxaliplatin as third-line treatment of patients with advanced colorectal cancer. J Clin Oncol 2004;22(23):4753–61.
[62] Andre T, Boni C, Mounedji-Boudiaf L, et al. Oxaliplatin, fluorouracil, and leucovorin as adjuvant treatment for colon cancer. N Engl J Med 2004;350(23):2343–51.
[63] Wolmark N, Wieand HS, Keubler JP, et al. A phase III trial comparing FULV to FULV + oxaliplatin in stage II or III carcinoma of the colon: results of the NSABP protocol C-07 [abstract]. J Clin Oncol 2005;23(16S):246s.

[64] Baselga J, Arteaga CL. Critical update and emerging trends in epidermal growth factor receptor targeting in cancer. J Clin Oncol 2005;23(11):2445–59.

[65] Roskoski R Jr. The ErbB/HER receptor protein-tyrosine kinases and cancer. Biochem Biophys Res Commun 2004;319(1):1–11.

[66] Cunningham D, Humblet Y, Siena S, et al. Cetuximab monotherapy and cetuximab plus iri-notecan in irinotecan-refractory metastatic colorectal cancer. N Engl J Med 2004;351(4): 337–45.

[67] Laux I, Jain A, Singh S, et al. Epidermal growth factor receptor dimerization status deter-mines skin toxicity to HER-kinase targeted therapies. Br J Cancer 2006;94(1):85–92.

[68] Perez-Soler R, Saltz L. Cutaneous adverse effects with HER1/EGFR-targeted agents: is there a silver lining? J Clin Oncol 2005;23(22):5235–46.

[69] Saltz LB, Meropol NJ, Loehrer Sr PJ, et al. Phase II trial of cetuximab in patients with refrac-tory colorectal cancer that expresses the epidermal growth factor receptor. J Clin Oncol 2004;22(7):1201–8.

[70] Folprecht G, Lutz MP, Schoffski P, et al. Cetuximab and irinotecan/5-fluorouracil/folinic acid is a safe combination for the first-line treatment of patients with epidermal growth factor receptor expressing metastatic colorectal carcinoma. Ann Oncol 2006;17(3):450–6.

[71] Malecka-Panas E, Kordek R, Biernat W, et al. Differential activation of total and EGF recep-tor (EGF-R) tyrosine kinase (tyr-k) in the rectal mucosa in patients with adenomatous polyps, ulcerative colitis and colon cancer. Hepatogastroenterology 1997;44(14):435–40.

[72] Bernal NP, Stehr W, Coyle R, et al. Epidermal growth factor receptor signaling regulates Bax and Bcl-w expression and apoptotic responses during intestinal adaptation in mice. Gastro-enterology 2006;130(2):412–23.

[73] Egger B, Buchler MW, Lakshmanan J, et al. Mice harboring a defective epidermal growth factor receptor (waved-2) have an increased susceptibility to acute dextran sulfate-induced colitis. Scand J Gastroenterol 2000;35(11):1181–7.

[74] Abud HE, Watson N, Heath JK. Growth of intestinal epithelium in organ culture is dependent on EGF signalling. Exp Cell Res 2005;303(2):252–62.

[75] Clark JA, Lane RH, Maclennan NK, et al. Epidermal growth factor reduces intestinal apopto-sis in an experimental model of necrotizing enterocolitis. Am J Physiol Gastrointest Liver Physiol 2005;288(4):G755–62.

[76] Procaccino F, Reinshagen M, Hoffmann P, et al. Protective effect of epidermal growth factor in an experimental model of colitis in rats. Gastroenterology 1994;107(1):12–7.

[77] McCole DF, Rogler G, Varki N, et al. Epidermal growth factor partially restores colonic ion transport responses in mouse models of chronic colitis. Gastroenterology 2005;129(2): 591–608.

[78] FitzGerald AJ, Pu M, Marchbank T, et al. Synergistic effects of systemic trefoil factor family 1 (TFF1) peptide and epidermal growth factor in a rat model of colitis. Peptides 2004;25(5): 793–801.

[79] Chinery R, Playford RJ. Combined intestinal trefoil factor and epidermal growth factor is pro-phylactic against indomethacin-induced gastric damage in the rat. Clin Sci (Lond) 1995;88(4):401–3.

[80] Dvorak B. Epidermal growth factor and necrotizing enterocolitis. Clin Perinatol 2004;31(1):183–92.

[81] Lordick F, Geinitz H, Theisen J, et al. Increased risk of ischemic bowel complications during treatment with bevacizumab after pelvic irradiation: report of three cases. Int J Radiat Oncol Biol Phys 2006;64(5):1295–8.

[82] Scappaticci FA, Fehrenbacher L, Cartwright T, et al. Surgical wound healing complications in metastatic colorectal cancer patients treated with bevacizumab. J Surg Oncol 2005;91(3):173–80.

[83] Hurwitz HI, Fehrenbacher L, Hainsworth JD, et al. Bevacizumab in combination with fluoro-uracil and leucovorin: an active regimen for first-line metastatic colorectal cancer. J Clin Oncol 2005;23(15):3502–8.

[84] Kabbinavar FF, Hambleton J, Mass RD, et al. Combined analysis of efficacy: the addition of bevacizumab to fluorouracil/leucovorin improves survival for patients with metastatic colorectal cancer. J Clin Oncol 2005;23(16):3706–12.

[85] Hurwitz H, Fehrenbacher L, Novotny W, et al. Bevacizumab plus irinotecan, fluorouracil, and leucovorin for metastatic colorectal cancer. N Engl J Med 2004;350(23):2335–42.

[86] Giantonio BJ, Catalano PJ, Meropol NJ. High-dose bevacizumab improves survival when combined with FOLFOX4 in previously treated advanced colorectal cancer: Results from the Eastern Cooperative Oncology Group (ECOG) study E3200 [abstract]. J Clin Oncol 2005;23(16S):1s.

[87] Kabbinavar FF, Schulz J, McCleod M, et al. Addition of bevacizumab to bolus fluorouracil and leucovorin in first-line metastatic colorectal cancer: results of a randomized phase II trial. J Clin Oncol 2005;23(16):3697–705.

[88] Zhao J, Huang L, Belmar N, et al. Oral RDP58 allows CPT-11 dose intensification for enhanced tumor response by decreasing gastrointestinal toxicity. Clin Cancer Res 2004;10(8):2851–9.

[89] Bourreille A, Doubremelle M, de la Bletiere DR, et al. RDP58, a novel immunomodulatory peptide with anti-inflammatory effects. A pharmacological study in trinitrobenzene sulphonic acid colitis and Crohn disease. Scand J Gastroenterol 2003;38(5):526–32.

[90] Travis S, Yap LM, Hawkey C, et al. RDP58 is a novel and potentially effective oral therapy for ulcerative colitis. Inflamm Bowel Dis 2005;11(8):713–9.

GASTROENTEROLOGY CLINICS
OF NORTH AMERICA

**ELSEVIER
SAUNDERS**

INDEX

Note: Page numbers of article titles are in **boldface** type.

0889-8553/06/$ – see front matter
doi:10.1016/S0889-8553(06)00070-7

© 2006 Elsevier Inc. All rights reserved.
gastro.theclinics.com

—